# Pharmacology for Student and Pupil Nurses
and Students in Associated Professions

# Pharmacology
## for
# Student and Pupil Nurses
## and Students in Associated Professions

BERNARD R. JONES, F.P.S.

*formerly Group Pharmacist*
*South Warwickshire Hospital Group*

*Second Edition*

WILLIAM HEINEMANN MEDICAL BOOKS LIMITED
LONDON

First published 1971
Revised reprint 1973
Reprinted 1975
Second Edition 1978

ISBN 0 433 17542 7

PRINTED AND BOUND IN GREAT BRITAIN BY
R. J. ACFORD LTD., CHICHESTER, SUSSEX

# CONTENTS

# PREFACE TO THE SECOND EDITION

The two Revised Reprints of the First Edition made possible the inclusion of various changes and modifications in the drug scene, but, as is inevitable in this sphere, a distinct and thoroughly reassessed Edition is now called for. The format of the earlier Edition continues happily the same, and whilst certain deletions have become necessary, this has been more than counterbalanced by the incorporation of an abundance of new material—as is to be expected in view of the progress made in the realm of new therapy and the more complete exploration of drug trends already established.

The opportunity has been taken to introduce some forward-looking features, amongst them a section on Patient Counselling, an explanation of certain aspects of the International System of Units ("SI") as they concern the nursing sphere, and a discussion of the immune-response process as it affects certain specialised fields of treatment. However, the need to explain the subject matter in the clearest of terms has been ever in mind, and it is my hope that nursing personnel, and others concerned, will again be happy to turn the pages without it ever becoming tedious reading; this has been the gratifying comment hitherto, may it indeed continue.

B.R.J.

# INTRODUCTION

This book is the result of a desire to record, and at the same time bring up to date, the substance of lectures given during upwards of thirty years to nurses in training for the State Registration and State Enrolment Examinations, and also to Students in Dispensing. In the early years the subject was termed Materia Medica; it is now entitled Pharmacology.

Pharmacology is the science, or knowledge, of the action of drugs, and when applied to the treatment of disease it becomes Therapeutics. A knowledge of Pharmacology not only makes work on the ward more interesting and meaningful to the nurse, but may also assist to a more thorough understanding of the Medical and Surgical lectures, in which drugs are often referred to. Thus, the aim in these pages is to provide a readable, and, in its turn, understandable account of the drugs in general use today, and every effort has been made to include only those which are already established or appear certain or highly likely to become so. Chapter 15 includes an outline of the drugs used in certain of the more prominent tropical diseases; it is hoped this will be of interest, and of value, to student nurses who have come from abroad to do their training in this country.

References to the diseases concerned, and the therapeutic background, inevitably intrude into the narrative in the case of many of the drugs discussed; such references have been kept as simple as possible, and it should be borne in mind that they are necessarily of a generalised nature and are intended merely as a guide to the understanding of the main subject, which is the drugs themselves and their actions and uses.

The practical aspects of the Regulations governing the use of Poisons in the hospital ward are described, and also the ward routine as it applies to the handling of drugs generally and its liaison with the Pharmacy (this is the preferred name for the former "Dispensary"). Instruction is also included on how to perform calculations that may be required in the Qualifying Examinations or on the wards.

There has been no attempt to make this a book of reference by including the vast number of commercial preparations of each drug. The accent has been rather on mentioning a fair sample only of the branded preparations which are in common use, so avoiding a confused text.

It is hoped that the treatment of the subject will be neither too advanced for the S.E.N. Student to read with interest, nor too simplified for the S.R.N. Student to benefit from. A further aim has been to provide an easily assimilable background to Pharmacology for those members of the paramedical professions, e.g. Laboratory Technicians, Radiographers, Physiotherapists and Medical Secretaries, to whom a knowledge of the various aspects of drug therapy may be both relevant and useful; the Examination requirements of Student Pharmacy Technicians in both Hospital and General Practice are especially in mind.

## Terminology

It will be seen that, in general, drugs are described by their "approved" name together with the commercial ("brand" or "proprietary") name. The approved name is the one used to designate the drug in official books of reference, such as the B.P. (British Pharmacopoeia), B.P.C. (British Pharmaceutical Codex) and B.N.F. (British National Formulary), and is free from commercial association. Thus, chlorpromazine and ampicillin are the approved names for the drugs concerned, whereas the brand names, used by the firms who introduced them, are 'Largactil' and 'Penbritin' respectively. A drug is occasionally sold under more than one brand name, an example being oxytetracycline (approved name) which is available as 'Terramycin', 'Imperacin' and 'Clinimycin'. *Brand, or proprietary, names are in inverted commas throughout.*

The use of the approved name is now firmly established, as being more ethical and freeing the medical profession from commercial ties; however, this practice is not without its disadvantages. The problem is that approved names, in addition to being often long and complex, usually have a direct connection with the chemical nature of the drug, and as a number of different drugs may belong to the same family, i.e. be closely related, it may happen that the approved names are dangerously similar. Examples are the antihistamine, promethazine ('Phenergan'), and the tranquillizer, promazine ('Sparine'); the sedative, diazepam ('Valium'), and the hypnotic, nitrazepam ('Mogadon'); and the narcotic, levorphanol ('Dromoran'), and the stimulant, levallorphan ('Lorfan')—which incidentally, have generally opposing actions! Brand, or proprietary names, on the other hand, appear to be "vetted" carefully before drugs are marketed, so that no two are too much alike; this will be appreciated by a glance at the brand names above. There would appear to be a real need for a system of "approved" naming of drugs which will avoid as far as possible any chance of error in handling and administration; there is also much to be said for the writing of prescriptions in block lettering.

A further minor problem concerns the labelling of drugs *in manufacturers' containers,* for under the Medicines Act which comes into force during 1977 it is required that the *International* Non-proprietary Name (I.N.N.) must also appear on the label if it differs from the approved name employed in *this* country for the drug concerned. This can be confusing, and Nursing Staff should bear this in mind if they are ever by chance called upon to administer drugs from a manufacturer's original container.

The term "B.N.F." will be found attached to many preparations mentioned in the text and means that the preparation concerned is contained in the British National Formulary. This is an official publication containing information on prescribing, together with a wide range of carefully devised formulae for use by Doctors and Dispensary Staff; it is revised at regular intervals. The term "(see page )", or its abbreviation "(p. )", will also be met frequently in the text; this is not intended to indicate that the page referred to must be turned to each time. This could become a distraction, and it is stressed that the purpose of these references is merely to supplement the Index and offer a handier route to other aspects of the drugs concerned; they may also act as a useful reminder.

An additional point in this connection is that when a paragraph (or successive paragraphs) deals with several drugs of the same group, the brand names and doses are listed together at the end of the paragraph(s). This is done so that the flow of reading is not unduly interrupted by these details, and interest is thus maintained.

**"Hyper"** and **"Hypo"**—are two prefixes frequently met when discussing Pharmacology, e.g. *hyper*thyroidism and *hypo*thyroidism (p. 179). Hence the reminder that "hyper" indicates *raised* or *excessive,* and "hypo" *lowered* or *insufficient.*

## Dosage

The dose to be given of a drug is, of course, decided by the doctor prescribing, and the nurse duly administers accordingly. However, a knowledge of the normal dose of drugs in general use is helpful, as being an additional safeguard against error in administration. Hence this detail has been included where it is considered to be of relevant value.

It needs to be added that the range of dosage of a drug is often wide, and that the doses included here are, as stated, *average doses,* i.e. they may be considered "typical" or "medium". Likewise, it is stressed that, except where otherwise stated, *adult* doses are referred to.

It should also be noted that the doses are *single* doses, i.e. as given on each occasion; thus a stated dose may have to be given several times daily.

Factors which may have a bearing on drug dosage are discussed in the Appendix (p. 261).

The Metric System of Weights and Measures is now officially established in this country, hence all weights and measures are expressed in terms of the Metric System, an explanation of which will be found in Chapter 2.

### "Units"

It will be noted that the strength of certain preparations, e.g. insulin (p. 184), is expressed in terms of units. A unit is a measure of the activity of a drug in the same way that a term of actual weight is, e.g. milligram.

In some cases, a unit equals a definite weight of a drug, e.g. one unit of insulin $= 0.04167$ mg, and this may be a convenient and/or customary way of expressing its strength. More frequently, the drug may not be obtainable in the pure form and thus cannot be weighed to present a consistent and accurate dose; it then has to be tested for potency on living tissue and issued in terms of units. Each unit used is specific for the drug concerned.

A.C.T.H. (p. 193) is an interesting example. It is available both as the natural substance (obtained from pig pituitary) and in synthetic form (artificially prepared). The natural form is variable and never 100% pure, and thus the dosage is in units, each unit expressing a definite degree of potency determined by an official test of each batch. Synthetic A.C.T.H., however, is a 100% pure chemical, and the dose can be expressed by actual weight, i.e. milligrams.

**N.B.** *The following note on the International System of Units, or "SI", will assist in adapting the reader to those details of this new official system which are employed throughout the text.*

### "SI"—The International System of Units

This has been introduced in order to hasten the standardisation of the units in use for length, volume, weight and temperature, and its acceptance brings this country into line with those already employing it on the Continent. SI relates to the Metric System, and the reader will already be accustomed to many of the terms and abbreviations employed, e.g. gram (g) and millilitre (ml), etc.; of the terms which may not be familiar, three only would seem to concern the nurse-in-training in the present context.

Firstly, and in relation to temperature, the term Centigrade is now replaced by **Celsius**, but as the degree and the symbol (C) remain the same, this new term is easily accepted.

Secondly, the term **"millimole"** will now be seen on the labels of containers of intravenous infusion fluids, but this is explained more appropriately in Chapter 6, which deals with these fluids.

Then, the term calorie, which signifies the unit of heat/energy, is replaced by the term **joule**; but as reference to the heat/energy unit is used in the text merely to indicate physiological effect, e.g. in the case of dextrose (p. 45), opinions favour the retention of the familiar "calorie", and it appears as such (in Chapter 6).

Two further points may appear simple but deserve mention.

Firstly, the abbreviations for units in the Metric System (Chapter 2), e.g. mg for milligram, do not now carry an added "stop"—as has been customary. Thus—

      mg    g    kg    ml    l,
and not mg.  g.  kg.  ml.  1.

If at the end of a sentence, the normal full stop *is* used, of course.

Note also that capitals are not used, i.e. small g, not G; and kg, not Kg.

The second point refers to the way the figures in large numbers are set out. Hitherto, it has been common practice to insert a comma at the appropriate place in numbers indicating one thousand upwards, as, for example—

1,000     15,000     250,000     1,000,000

However, the convention now is to employ a *space* instead of the comma. Thus, the above examples become—

1 000     15 000     250 000     1 000 000

This is because on the Continent the comma is used as a decimal point, and this could lead to confusion.

Incidentally, SI states that the decimal point should be a stop on the line, but in this case the traditional raised point is preserved here in the text as an interim measure.

# ACKNOWLEDGEMENTS

## FIRST EDITION

My sincere thanks are due to the following:

Drs. Patricia Carpenter, Rosemary Davies, M. K. Alexander, R. N. Allan, P. A. Gordon, D. G. Larard, M. E. MacGregor, J. R. Moore, D. W. W. Newling, J. G. Powell, J. M. Wales, V. F. Weinstein and S. R. F. Whittaker, and Mr. J. A. Harpman, M.S., all of the South Warwickshire Hospital Group, have readily given of their time to read appropriate sections of the manuscript. In dealing with the less familiar subject matter of much of Chapter 15, I have had grateful recourse to "Clinical Tropical Diseases" (Adams and Maegraith), and have been further aided by suggestions from Professor H. V. Morgan of Birmingham University and by the reading of Dr. Dermot Grene of Warwick.

Miss Maureen Aston of the X-Ray Department of Warwick Hospital and Mr. Rodney Poulter of the Group Pathological Laboratory have been most helpful regarding technical aspects of their specialties; Professor Tom Whitehead of Birmingham University has also given valuable advice in this connection.

Mrs. Mary Gilbert, Clinical Teacher at Warwick Hospital, and Mr. Derek Pickard and other members of the Nursing Tutorial Staff have provided comment of great assistance in maintaining the desired level of approach to the subject.

Finally, Mr. John Baker and Mr. Robert Adamson, Group Chief Pharmacist and Senior Pharmacist, respectively, of Walsgrave Hospital, have placed their critical judgement freely at my disposal; Mr. Adamson's collaboration in the proof reading has been of additional support.

I take this opportunity to pay one further important tribute—it is to the Nursing Profession. No other body has to combine such a wide range of theoretical knowledge with so much practical application and selfless work for others; our debt to them is indeed profound.

## REVISED REPRINTS

It is my further duty and pleasure to pay tribute to the support given me by the following.

Dr. G. O. R. Holmgren, Medical Registrar at Warwick Hospital, and, again, Mr. John Baker and Mr. Robert Adamson, have all three given of their time to read the new material and have proffered valuable suggestions.

Likewise, I take this opportunity to repair an omission in the original Acknowledgements by recording my appreciation of the expert advice and cheerful comfort afforded me by Mr. Richard Emery of William Heinemann Medical Books Ltd.

## SECOND EDITION

It continues my pleasurable commitment to acknowledge the support afforded me so generously by the following.

Dr. T. E. Bucknall, Surgical Registrar at Warwick Hospital, has read and approved the new material which has been added, and has provided valuable suggestions; John Baker and Robert Adamson, now Area and Principal Pharmacists respectively at Walsgrave Hospital, have yet again given of their time to do likewise in the pharmaceutical context; and I am indebted once more to Professor H. V. Morgan for authoritative guidance in respect of the drugs discussed in Chapter 15.

As with the previous Editions, I have had the good fortune to be able to call on those many other friends in hospital practice, both medical and paramedical, for judgment regarding points relevant to their specialties; the personnel of the Pathological Laboratory at Warwick are particularly in mind. The availability of access to the Drug Information Section in my old Department at Warwick Hospital has been additionally useful when needing data re new drugs.

I have depended very much indeed on the audiotyping factor, entailing, as it has done, a vast amount of complex terminology, and I warmly record my deep appreciation of the dedication with which Barbara Ward has applied herself to this task.

Finally, I have continued to be greatly sustained by the advice and kind indulgence of Richard Emery and by the meticulous collaboration, on the production side, of Ninetta Martyn, also of William Heinemann Medical Books Ltd.

BERNARD JONES

# CHAPTER 1

# HOW DRUGS ARE ADMINISTERED
## — the main routes employed
## — the forms in which they are used

The route chosen for administering a drug will be influenced by several factors, such as convenience, speed of action, and the condition of the patient; also to be considered may be the drug itself—which may be active by one particular route only.

## THE ORAL ROUTE

—is the one most commonly employed. It is simple and normally acceptable, and absorption into the system from the gastro-intestinal tract is generally efficient (within the limits of the drug concerned). Certain drugs, e.g. the antacids, are taken orally for their effect within the stomach, and some are so prepared as to enable them to pass into the duodenum before their action commences (e.g. in the treatment of duodenal ulcer). Several of the drugs taken by mouth to treat bowel conditions are absorbed only to a very limited extent and are thus able to exert their action along the entire intestinal tract. An occasional disadvantage of oral medication is the gastro-intestinal disturbance that may be caused by certain drugs.

The liquid **mixture** (Latin "Mistura", abbreviation "Mist"), although rapidly giving way to tablets, etc., still continues in use. It has the advantage of flexibility of prescribing, reasonable accuracy in dosage (provided a measure is used), and, normally, ease of taking; the taste may sometimes be unpleasant and difficult to mask, however, even with a strong flavouring agent. Two points to be noted are that mixtures should be kept in a cool place, and they should always be shaken, even if clear and without sediment.

**Syrups** are thick and sugar based, **elixirs** are normally thinner; both are usually agreeably flavoured and commonly taken neat from the spoon. **Suspensions** are thickened mixtures containing a drug which is insoluble, and it is especially important that these are shaken well before use. **Linctuses** are again thick, viscous preparations, usually taken neat for their additional soothing effect on the throat.

**Emulsions** are permanent mixtures of oil, or fat, and water. A common example is liquid paraffin emulsion, in which liquid paraffin and water (which would normally separate when mixed and shaken) are made into a thick permanent cream with the aid of an emulsifying agent; an example in nature is milk, which is a stable mixture of fat and water. Emulsions have the advantage of being easily flavoured, and are thus usually far more palatable than the oils themselves.

**Tablets** are the most widely used form of oral medication; they are accurate in dosage and normally easy to swallow, and usually disintegrate quickly in the moisture of the stomach. They may be plain or "coated", the latter form masking the taste, which is an advantage if the drug is bitter. Occasionally tablets are required to pass through the stomach unchanged so that they disintegrate in the duodenum, or continue to do so gradually along the intestinal tract; in such cases they are specially coated to make them impervious to acid, and this ensures that they pass intact through the acid stomach into the alkaline duodenum before disintegrating. The employment of drugs in slow-release form, i.e. to achieve prolonged effect, is increasing significantly

Certain tablets are intended not to be swallowed when taking; these are the buccal and sublingual forms. The buccal tablet is usually lodged in the cavity between the cheek and gum, and the sublingual tablet is retained under the tongue; in both cases the tablet is allowed to dissolve (avoiding swallowing as far as possible) and the drug contained is absorbed into the circulation via the mucosa, thus bypassing the stomach and digestive processes. This routine is of value when the drug concerned is destroyed or partially inactivated in the stomach if swallowed in the usual way, and when a more rapid action is required; examples are the buccal tablet of 'Pitocin' (see page 109), and the sublingual tablets of methyltestoserone (p. 200) and trinitrin (p. 52).

**Powders** (Latin abbreviation "pulv.") are occasionally prescribed, each being usually wrapped in folded white paper; the method of taking is to pour the powder on to the tongue and swallow with a draught of liquid. Advantages are accuracy in dosage and the finely powdered form of the drug which may hasten absorption.

Two methods of facilitating the taking of drugs which are bitter or nauseous are the use of **cachets** and **capsules**. Cachets are made of rice paper and are dipped in water, placed in the mouth, and swallowed with a further draught of water; the rice paper softens when moistened, thus making swallowing easy, and finally disintegrates in the stomach to release the contents. The employment of drugs in cachet form has lessened greatly in recent years, but capsules, on the other hand, are an extremely popular form of drug presentation. These are made of hard gelatine, in two halves, one fitting over the other, and are used to contain drugs of bitter taste; the gelatine dissolves in the stomach moisture and the drug is then released. Such capsules can also be made acid-resistant, so enabling them to reach the duodenum before melting and releasing their contents. *Soft* gelatine capsules may be used to contain liquids of unpleasant taste, such as male-fern extract (p. 150). As with tablets, an advantage of these presentations is accuracy of dosage.

## THE INJECTION ROUTE

—is indicated in several circumstances. The drug concerned may be ineffective orally due to its being destroyed in, or not absorbed from, the gastro-intestinal tract; or the patient may be too ill for oral administration to be employed; or speed of action may be an urgent requirement; or an injection may be the only way for the drug to reach the required site, as in the case of local anaesthetics. The drug may be contained in—

(a) glass ampoules, the neck being filed and snapped off for extraction of the contents; some ampoules, usually with a coloured band on the neck, do not need filing before snapping. The drug is usually in solution, but if it is of a kind that deteriorates quickly it is issued as a powder ready for dissolving just before use. If in the form of an insoluble suspension, the ampoule should be shaken gently but thoroughly before opening.

(b) Multi-dose glass vials (e.g. from 1 ml to 20 ml or more) sealed with a rubber bung, through which the needle is inserted to withdraw the dose. Again the drug may be in powder form and need to be dissolved in water before use. Likewise, the vial will need to be shaken if it contains an insoluble suspension. A point to note is that when adding water to a vial of powder to produce a definite volume of solution or suspension, e.g. 5 ml, of which part only, say 1 ml, is to be injected, it is usually incorrect to add *5 ml,* for this *plus the powder* will make *more than 5 ml,* and the injection will be weaker than intended; in such cases, the volume to add to achieve the correct strength is usually stated on the leaflet or label.

Single-dose ampoules or vials are considered far preferable to multi-dose containers, which, although they provide for doses of varying volumes, carry the risk of contamination during repeated use.

(c) Half litre and one litre glass bottles or plastic containers, as used when giving intravenous "infusions".

In all injection routine, strict aseptic precautions must be observed, which means paying close attention to the disinfection of the patient's

skin at the site, and ensuring the sterility of both the injection
to be given and the equipment used (syringe, needle, rubber bung,
giving sets, etc.). The personal aspect (thoroughly cleansed hands,
etc.) is also an important factor in aseptic technique.

## Intradermal ("I /D") Injections

—are given between the dermis and epidermis, the inner and outer
layers of the skin; they are usually employed when testing the
patient's reaction to various substances; examples are the Mantoux
test, which is concerned with tuberculosis, and the prick tests in
allergic asthma, etc. (see page 165).

## Subcutaneous ("S /C") Injections

—also called hypodermic, are made into the tissue under the skin;
a drug commonly given in this way is insulin. Absorption is fairly
rapid except in the case of preparations in insoluble form, the
effect of which is intended to be prolonged, e.g. insulin zinc suspensions. Large volumes, e.g. 250 or 500 ml, are also given by subcutaneous injection (or "infusion") when the intravenous route
presents difficulty; a full description of the routine is given on
page 47.

## Intramuscular ("I /M") Injections

—are given deep into a muscle, e.g. the gluteal muscle; this route
is much employed. Absorption is normally quick, but again certain
drugs are so formulated as to be slowly released from the muscle,
e.g. the so-called "depot" preparations.

## Intravenous ("I /V") Injections

—are given into a vein in the arm or leg; this route is also widely
used. In this country it is customary for the insertion of a needle
or cannula (a tube inserted with the aid of an incision or needle)
into the vein to be performed only by a doctor. Small volumes,
e.g. from 1 ml to 50 ml are given by means of a syringe and
needle, but if large, e.g. from the usual $\frac{1}{2}$ litre or 1 litre bottle
(or plastic container), this is hung up well above and connected
to the needle or cannula in the patient by plastic tubing (which
has generally replaced rubber), the rate of flow being controlled
by a screw clip above a glass drip-chamber. Injections of large
volume are usually called intravenous "infusions" or "drips". The
intravenous route provides rapid effect as it introduces the drug
directly into the blood stream.

It can happen that when an intravenous drip has been set up
and commenced, a rapid initial response to the drug may be vital;
this may be achieved by injecting a full dose into the tubing of

the giving set, i.e. into the running infusion. This is termed a **bolus** injection, and an instance of this technique will be found under Lignocaine on p. 63.

### Intra-arterial Injections
—are made (by a doctor only) directly into an artery, and are occasionally used for introducing cytotoxic drugs as near as possible to the site of a malignant growth (see page 204).

### Intrathecal ("I /T") Injections
—are made (by a doctor only) into the theca, the sheath, composed of the meninges, which encloses the spinal cord. They are used to introduce spinal anaesthetics, and also in the treatment of meningitis should the drug concerned not be able to pass the blood /brain barrier to reach the affected meninges when given by other injection routes. **Epidural** injections, which are a modification of the intrathecal injection, are now used far more frequently in spinal anaesthesia; these are referred to more fully on page 123.

### Intra-articular Injections
—are made directly into joints, such as those of the knee or elbow, for their local effect, an example being the use of steroid drugs in long-acting "depot" form (see page 190).

### Sub-Conjunctival Injections
—are made into the inner surface of the lower eyelid, usually in the treatment of severe infections (see p. 213).

The term "parenteral" is sometimes used to describe the injection route, but refers only to injections such as those mentioned above, i.e. given into a tissue or blood vessel; it does not include injections given per rectum.

## THE RECTAL ROUTE
—is used for the administration of a large number of drugs. The form chiefly used in the **suppository**; this is prepared with a base of either cocoa-butter fat (or synthetic equivalent), or glycerine and gelatine, and is solid and suitably shaped for use. It is inserted into the rectum, where it melts at the body temperature and releases the drug. **Enemas** of various liquid preparations are also employed.

Drugs are frequently given per rectum for local effect in a wide range of conditions, e.g. in relieving constipation, the pain of haemorrhoids and the inflammation of ulcerative colitis, and in the preparation of the bowel pre-operatively; these uses are discussed in the appropriate Chapters. However, systemic effect also may be achieved by the rectal route, on account of the fact that the rectal mucosa is capable of absorbing drugs into the circulation; examples are the use of suppositories containing aminophylline to relieve distressed respiration (p. 87), and the induction of sleep by rectal paraldehyde (p. 93). The use of suppositories to administer drugs for systemic effect is assuming major importance due to the fact that many of the newer drugs have the disadvantage of causing gastro-intestinal upset when taken orally (e.g. indomethacin, see page 117).

## OTHER ROUTES

The oral, injection and rectal routes discussed have been concerned in the main with the introduction of drugs systematically, i.e. into the circulation. Other methods of achieving this are also occasionally used. Thus, drugs may be administered by the surgical implantation of a tablet into the tissues; this is described more fully on page 201. They may also be absorbed into the circulation via the nasal mucosa and the alveoli (the tiny air sacs of the lungs); these routes are referred to on pages 37 and 52 respectively.

Drugs are also used for their *local* effect in a number of sites in the body, e.g. the eyes, ears, vagina, etc.; this is dealt with in Chapter 20.

### To note

**Bioavailability** is a word covering broadly the degree of absorption, and hence effectiveness, of a drug taken orally. It has assumed especial importance since work on the preparation of tablets of digoxin has emphasised that the potency of a tablet may depend to a significant extent on the manufacturing process concerned, i.e. tablets may vary significantly in effect from one maker to another, although each may contain the exact amount of the drug, e.g. 250 micrograms in the case of digoxin. The important criterion is the degree and speed of absorption, i.e. the "bioavailability".

Tablets of differing activity are of potential concern in the case of drugs like digoxin which patients take daily, and on the unvarying effect of which they depend. Hence, common agreed standards of manufacture have become an essential requirement to be implemented, so that if a different "make" of any drug preparation happens to be dispensed, the effect will not vary on that account.

### Strip Packaging

—has become established as a method of dispensing tablets and capsules in the commercial and hospital fields, and this type of sealed individual cellophane or plastic enclosure has several advantages. Thus, each item is untouched by hand until opened for administration; it facilitates counting when checking, etc.; and it makes for economy in that tablets or capsules can be taken back into stock and re-issued with confidence. It is envisaged that in time liquid medicines also may be dispensed in single-dose "sachets" in strip form or in single-dose plastic cups; the use of strip sachets is already established in the case of some antiseptics (p. 173).

# CHAPTER 2

# THE METRIC SYSTEM

The Metric System is now established and in effective operation in Medicine; it has replaced the previous combination of systems which comprised the complex Imperial System.

The Metric System has three pronounced advantages. Firstly, it brings this country into line with those on the Continent, thus making a contribution to the desirable free interchange of medical knowledge and practice. Secondly, it is easy to operate and is relatively free of the mysterious and often confusing symbols of the previous system. Lastly, calculations are straightforward and need merely a knowledge of the Decimal System together with relatively elementary arithmetic.

### The Decimal System

It should be clearly understood that accuracy depends very greatly on the correct use of the decimal point; this is vital, for if it is wrongly placed, or its position misinterpreted, then serious consequences can result, such as doses being given which are ten times too much—or ten times too little. The student must also be clear regarding the basic rule, which is that figures to the left of the point represent *whole numbers,* and figures to the right *fractions*—either tenths (the first figure after the point) or hundredths (the first two figures after the point). The first three figures after the point represent thousandths, but rarely need to be used by the student nurse. Thus:—

$$1 \cdot 0 \ = 1 \qquad\qquad 0 \cdot 25 = \frac{25}{100} \text{ (or } \tfrac{1}{4})$$

$$0 \cdot 1 \ = \frac{1}{10} \qquad\qquad 0 \cdot 5 \ = \frac{5}{10} \text{ (or } \tfrac{1}{2})$$

$$0 \cdot 01 = \frac{1}{100} \qquad\qquad 0 \cdot 75 = \frac{75}{100} \text{ (or } \tfrac{3}{4})$$

If the decimal point is moved one place to the *left*, the figure is *divided* by ten.

Thus:—

1·0 becomes 0·1 $\left(\dfrac{1}{10}\right)$        0·5 becomes 0·05 $\left(\dfrac{5}{100} \text{ or } \dfrac{1}{20}\right)$

0·1 becomes 0·01 $\left(\dfrac{1}{100}\right)$        2·0 becomes 0·2 $\left(\dfrac{2}{10} \text{ or } \dfrac{1}{5}\right)$

Conversely, if it is moved one place to the *right,* the figure is *multiplied* by ten.

Thus:—

| | |
|---|---|
| 1·0 becomes 10·0 | 2·5 becomes  25·0 |
| 0·1 becomes  1·0 | 10·0 becomes 100·0 |

An important rule is that the decimal point should never be left "naked" before a figure less than 1.

Thus:— ·25 should be written 0·25.

This is a safeguard against missing the decimal point, when the figure in this case would become 25 (i.e. 100 times too much).

**Now to proceed to the Metric System itself:—**

### Weights

Four units only are in general use in Medicine; they are:—

| Unit | Symbol or Abbreviation |
|---|---|
| Microgram | μg or mcg (but preferably written in full to avoid mistaking for mg) |
| Milligram (= 1 000 micrograms) | mg |
| Gram     (= 1 000 mg) | g |
| Kilogram (= 1 000 g) | kg |

The microgram is extremely minute, as may be gathered by the fact that 5 grams (e.g. an average teaspoonful of sugar) contains 5 million micrograms. However, the microgram is of practical value, for it caters for the very small doses used of potent drugs, e.g. 50 micrograms of thyroxine (which is better expressed in that way as a whole number of micrograms than as "0·05 mg"), and 25 micrograms of digoxin (this is better and safer than "0·025 mg", which has been the cause of infant fatalities due to 0·25 mg having been given in error).

Thus, weights up to 1 mg should be expressed as micrograms, e.g. 100 micrograms (not 0·1 mg), 250 micrograms (not 0·25 mg), and 500 micrograms (not 0·5 mg). Likewise, weights from 1 mg up to 1 gram are expressed as milligrams, e.g. 300 mg (not 0·3 g) and 500 mg (not 0·5 g). Note how the use of the decimal point is avoided by these general rulings.

Weights above 1 gram are expressed in terms of grams and parts of a gram, in the decimal system, e.g. 1·25 g and 2·5 g.

### Volume

Two units only are in general use, the smaller being the millilitre, which is equivalent to the cubic-centimetre, or cc.

| Unit | Symbol or Abbreviation |
|------|------------------------|
| Millilitre | ml or mil or cc |
| | (Note—ml is favoured) |
| Litre (= 1 000 ml) | l |

Note the abbreviation for the *plural* of "ml" remains as ml (i.e. without an "s"); thus, 1 000 ml, not 1 000 mls.

### Length

Here, three units only will be of general concern to the nurse-in-training. These are

| Unit | Symbol or Abbreviation |
|------|------------------------|
| Millimetre | mm |
| Centimetre (= 10 mm) | cm |
| Metre (= 100 cm) | m |

An idea of what these lengths mean may be gauged by the fact that—

1 Centimetre = approx. 0·4 (i.e. 2/5) of an inch.

1 Metre is slightly more than $3\frac{1}{4}$ feet.

The above units of length are included here because measurements in millimetres and centimetres are often met in surgery, e.g. in the case of needles and sutures, and instruments, etc.

Note also that 1 square metre is an area equal to that of a square with sides of 1 metre long. This is mentioned because dosage of certain potent drugs, e.g. some of the cytotoxics, *is based on the surface area of the body*; this especially in the case of children, e.g. procarbazine therapy (p. 206) is maintained at "100 mg per square metre of body surface". The height and weight of the patient are lined up on a special set of tables, and this leads to a figure corresponding to the surface area in terms of square metres; this is known as a **nomogram**.

With regard to the figures used to denote whole numbers, the Arabic (i.e. 1, 2, 3, 4, 5, etc.) is generally preferred to the Roman, as being clearer and with less risk of misinterpretation; thus "5 grams" is preferred to "grams V".

Dosage of fluid medicines in the Metric System is officially based on *5 ml* and *10 ml*, but if a very thick mixture is concerned the volume of the dose may have to be diluted by the Pharmacist to 20 ml in order to make it pourable. Suitable metric measures are employed for ward use, together with accurate 5 ml plastic spoons for medicines which are taken neat, such as linctuses and children's mixtures. The 5 ml spoons are essential also for out-patients, because the domestic "teaspoon" may hold anything from 3–6 ml.

Calculations in the Metric System are discussed in Chapter 25.

Certain units in the old system of weights and measures may still be encountered; the following are two likely examples—

1 stone           = approx. $6\frac{1}{3}$ (6·3) kg
1 pint            = approx. 560 ml

Note also that—

1 kg              = approx. 2·2 ($2\frac{1}{5}$) lbs
1 litre (1 000 ml) = approx. 35 fl. ounces ($1\frac{3}{4}$ pints).

# CHAPTER 3

# ANTACIDS AND GASTRIC SEDATIVES
## with Carminatives; Emetics; Anti-emetics

**Antacids** are drugs or preparations which neutralise acid, in this case the hydrochloric acid normally present in the gastric juice which is released, or "secreted", into the stomach to take part in the process of digestion. If acid production is excessive, or the stomach or duodenal lining unduly tender, pain may result; this will be severe if an ulcer is present. Antacids fall broadly into two groups; the first is employed for occasional and relatively mild gastric discomfort, and the second for the longer-term treatment and healing of gastric or duodenal ulcer.

The short-term antacids have long been based largely on carbonates and bicarbonates. The carbonates mainly concerned are **Calcium Carbonate** and **Magnesium Carbonate,** and the bicarbonate is **Sodium Bicarbonate**; all have a direct effect and neutralise acid speedily—as may be observed by adding sodium bicarbonate powder to an acid liquid, which will then effervesce, with evolution of carbon dioxide gas, before becoming still. **Bismuth Carbonate** has also long been used in "indigestion" mixtures and powders, but has been largely superseded by **Magnesium Trisilicate**, which is cheaper and equally effective; both are mild antacids with fairly prolonged action, and in addition provide a soothing protective coating to the lining of the stomach.

A number of mixtures and powders based on the antacids mentioned are in use for the treatment of gastric discomfort; an example is the B.N.F. Magnesium Trisilicate Mixture which also contains magnesium carbonate and sodium bicarbonate. Commercial tablets and powders are available in a great variety of similar combinations. An antacid which has an additional laxative action is **Magnesium Hydroxide**, which is also included in the B.N.F. in mixture form.

The carbonate and bicarbonate antacids are preferably reserved for short-term use, because their rapid action can result in a "rebound" secretion (production) of still more acid; furthermore, the carbon dioxide gas, which is produced during their neutralising action, itself has a stimulating effect on acid secretion.

A distinct approach to flatulence and gastric discomfort is the use of **Polymethylsiloxane**, a compound derived from silicone which has an "anti-foam" effect and so prevents the formation of gaseous bubbles in the stomach, often the cause of painful distension: it is also said to exert a protective, lining effect on the stomach and duodenal mucosa. The formulae employed usually contain, in addition, antacids such as aluminium hydroxide (see later) and magnesium oxide, and typical examples of brand preparations are 'Asilone' and 'Polycrol Forte', both in the form of tablets and suspension (dose 5–10 ml); normally taken before meals and at bed-time.

In the more serious and painful condition of a highly inflamed gastric or duodenal mucosa (lining), or an actual ulcer itself, the alternating periods of marked acidity and alkalinity which occur during treatment with the quick-acting antacids mentioned above do not encourage the healing process; the need is, therefore, for mild and prolonged neutralisation of gastric acid, and a drug successfully used for many years is **Aluminium Hydroxide**. This is a white powder, which is commonly used in the form of a "gel" or suspension, the Aluminium Hydroxide Mixture of the B.N.F.; a normal dose is 5 to 10 ml (after well shaking the bottle) before and/or after meals. A commercial form is 'Aludrox', which is available also in tablet form. Preparations of aluminium hydroxide have two especial advantages. Firstly, due to its steady and prolonged action, and non-production of carbon dioxide, the rebound secretion of further acid is not stimulated. Secondly, the insoluble aluminium compound acts as a protective coating to the tender mucosa of the stomach and duodenum, and by virtue of an astringent or "shrinking" effect it also tends to reduce the secretion of acid-containing gastric juice. A minor disadvantage of its astringent action later upon the intestinal wall, however, is that it impedes peristalsis, and thus constipation may result and the patient need a laxative to correct this.

### Anticholinergic drugs

The antacids discussed so far have been those which directly neutralise the acid of the gastric juice present in the stomach. Another group of drugs has what might be termed an "indirect" antacid effect in the treatment of conditions of gastric and duodenal spasm and ulcer; these are the anticholinergic drugs. The term "anticholinergic" is also used when discussing the action of drugs employed in other conditions and deserves a brief explanation at this stage.

The autonomic nervous system (A.N.S.), which is involuntary in action, i.e. self regulating and independent of conscious control, is composed of two sections, the sympathetic and the parasympathetic. The function of these two sections is the control of the activity of the internal organs, and, broadly, each balances the effect of the other. Thus, if one has a stimulating effect upon a particular organ, the effect of the other on that organ will be inhibitory, or restraining. In regard to the gastro-intestinal tract, the parasympathetic section of the A.N.S. acts as a *stimulant*; the impulses which produce this effect are conveyed along its nerve fibres to the organs concerned, i.e. the stomach and intestines, which are activated as a result (e.g. into peristaltic movement); likewise the secretion of gastric juice is also stimulated.

Now in the *parasympathetic* system, the arrival of the impulse at the nerve fibre ending, i.e. where it meets the muscle of the organ concerned, leads to the release of the substance *acetylcholine,* and it is this agency which activates the organ(s) concerned—this is termed the *cholinergic* effect; in the case of the gastro-intestinal system there is stimulation, as already described.

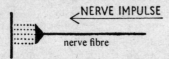

Fig. 1. Illustrating release of acetyl-choline at meeting point of para-sympathetic nerve ending and tissue concerned.

Hence the important role of acetylcholine will be apparent, and also the fact that if its action is blocked at the nerve endings the organ concerned will not receive the impulses and will thus remain unaffected. This explains the effect of the *anti*cholinergic drugs— they inhibit the action of acetylcholine at the nerve fibre endings. In the case of the gastro-intestinal tract, the stimulating impulses are blocked and the result is a reduction in the flow of gastric juice (and in turn the hydrochloric acid it contains), together with inactiva-tion (and hence relaxation) of the stomach and duodenal wall— which may have been in the painful spasm so often present in the condition of ulcer. Thus, the action is not only one of reducing acid secretion, but is also sedative, i.e. antispasmodic (sometimes termed spasmolytic). The sympathetic section of the A.N.S. differs from the parasympathetic in its chemistry of function, and this is explained on page 55.

**Belladonna**

—is an anticholinergic drug which has long been in use; it is of plant origin—the common deadly-nightshade, the black berries of which are so dangerous to children. Belladonna is used as the green-coloured tincture (av. dose 0·6 ml), which is often combined with antacid mixtures, e.g. the Magnesium Trisilicate and Belladonna Mixture of the B.N.F. **Atropine** is the chief active principle of belladonna (i.e. the constituent, or ingredient, mainly responsible for its action), and is sometimes used in preparations for its sedative effect on the gastro-intestinal tract. In pyloric stenosis, a form of spasm in infants which hinders the passage of food through the pyloric opening between the stomach and duodenum, a solution of atropine methonitrate ('Eumydrin') is given before each feed, an average dose being 2–4 drops (0·4–0·8 mg).

The side-effects which may follow the blocking of acetylcholine activity during normal dosage of belladonna or atropine (i.e. the anticholinergic effect) include dry mouth and throat and trouble in swallowing, difficulty in passing urine, constipation, and the typical dilated pupils (mydriasis—see page 212) resulting in blurred vision. In toxic overdosage, e.g. poisoning by belladonna berries, there is very rapid pulse and delirium followed by drowsiness; in addition to gastric lavage (stomach washout), sedation and catheterisation, injections are given of the specific antagonist, neostigmine (p. 108).

The discomfort of the side-effects normal to the use of belladonna have led to the introduction of several synthetic drugs which are said to have similar anticholinergic action but less of the disadvantages; a prominent example is **Propantheline**, tablets of which are taken three times a day and at night.

Propantheline-'Probanthine'-av. dose 15 mg

## Cimetidine

—presents a new and distinct approach to the treatment of gastric and duodenal ulcer. A principal cause of this condition is the hydrochloric acid contained in the gastric juice, and cimetidine acts, not by a neutralising effect as do the antacids, but by actually blocking production of the acid. The tablets of 200 mg ('Tagamet') are taken with each meal and at bedtime, and syrup and injection forms are used where necessary.

## Carbenoxolone

—is also employed in the treatment of gastric ulcer; it is in tablet form ('Biogastrone'), is taken before each meal, and a course lasts for four weeks or longer. This drug is derived from liquorice, and has pronounced anti-inflammatory and healing properties. For the treatment of duodenal ulcer, carbenoxolone is available as a capsule ('Duogastrone') which is taken 15–30 minutes before meals; this interval allows just enough time for the capsule to swell and soften sufficiently to burst when being passed under pressure through the pylorus, thus enabling the release of the carbenoxolone in concentrated form into the duodenum where it is needed.

## CARMINATIVES

—are preparations which induce a feeling of warmth in the stomach and relieve distension by stimulating eructation, i.e. the bringing up of gas, or "wind". Thus, after an excessive or indigestible meal, flatulence may increase the sense of fullness in the stomach, and the taking of a carminative will afford relief. A useful preparation is the liqueur taken after a meal, but in the hospital ward the cheaper and just as effective equivalent is **Peppermint Water** (Aqua Menth. Pip.), 30 ml of which soon alleviates discomfort; peppermint is also usefully employed as a flavouring agent—as in Magnesium Trisilicate Mixture and other antacid and indigestion remedies. For children, an excellent carminative is **Dill Water**, occasionally used to flavour paediatric mixtures and an ingredient of the time-honoured 'Woodward's Gripe Water'.

## EMETICS

—are substances which induce emesis, or vomiting, and are occasionally used in the treatment of certain cases of poisoning, where emptying of the stomach is an immediate need; they are sometimes useful also in helping to clear the air passages in young children.

An emetic can be a factor in saving life, and it is useful to bear in mind that in extreme emergency two common examples, normally available in the home, are **Salt** and **Mustard**; both act by irritant effect, and their use is described on page 264.

**Ipecacuanha** is a drug of plant origin which is used as the tincture in expectorant mixtures (p. 83). In larger dosage it has a strongly emetic action, is very safe in use and is much favoured for children (av. dose 10 ml), for whom it may be preferred to the use of gastric washouts, which carry the risk of the stomach contents being aspirated (i.e. sucked) into the lungs by inhalation, e.g. should a child be distressed. There is normally full awareness of this dangerous possibility.

The most effective emetic known is **Apomorphine**, which is made from morphine; it is given by subcutaneous or intramuscular injection in dosage of up to 8 mg, and acts by stimulating the vomiting centre in the brain, from which powerful impulses reach the stomach and cause certain expulsion of its contents a few minutes later. Apomorphine is of value in appropriate and carefully supervised cases where emetics cannot be given by mouth, or the stomach emptied by other means. It is sometimes asked why it is not included in the Controlled Drugs list, being so closely related to morphine, but the answer is that a drug which causes violent vomiting is hardly likely to become one of addiction.

It needs to be stressed that not all cases of poisoning are suitable for the use of emetics; for example, in cases of corrosive poisoning where extensive damage to the oesophagus and stomach may have already been caused, the use of an emetic can well lead to perforation, with even more serious results. Likewise, emetics may also carry the hazard of vomit being aspirated (see earlier) in patients who are not fully alert.

## ANTI-EMETICS

—are used to prevent or reduce vomiting in conditions where it is common or may be expected, e.g. post-operatively, during pregnancy, and following deep X-Ray therapy or the drug treatment of cancer.

Post-operative vomiting is reduced by including in the premedication an intramuscular injection of either an antihistamine such as **Promethazine** ('Phenergan') or a tranquillizer of the phenothiazine type such as **Promazine** ('Sparine'), for one of the actions of several drugs in these two groups is depression, i.e. subdual, of the vomiting centre in the brain. Two further phenothiazine drugs with particular anti-emetic effect are **Thiethylperazine** ('Torecan') and **Prochlorperazine** ('Stemetil'); the latter is often effective in the vomiting and vertigo (giddiness) associated with the condition of the inner ear known as Ménière's disease, in which the antihistamine **Cinnarizine** ('Stugeron') is also employed.

**Metoclopramide** ('Maxolon') is a distinct drug, i.e. it is unrelated chemically to other anti-emetics; it differs also in acting not only by depressing the emetic centre in the brain, but also locally by its sedative effect on the nerve endings in the stomach. It is available as tablets, syrup and injection, and an average dose is 10 mg.

The above drugs are also employed to alleviate the distressing nausea and vomiting following treatment with deep X-Ray or the cytotoxic drugs that sometimes replace it; this is referred to in Chapter 19.

The vomiting of pregnancy is occasionally treated with certain drugs of the phenothiazine or antihistamine type such as **Trifluoperazine** ('Stelazine') and **Meclozine** ('Ancolan'). **Pyridoxine** (vitamin $B_6$) is also used in various combinations. A point that is borne in mind and merits stressing is the possibility of teratogenic effect, i.e. induced abnormality of the foetus, when certain drugs are administered during pregnancy, and this imposes caution in prescribing. Here the sedative effect of simple antacid preparations is safer and often of some value.

Travel sickness is inevitably an increasing problem, and much used in this connection are the antihistamines **Cyclizline** ('Marzine') and **Dimenhydrinate** ('Dramamine'), both as 50 mg tablets. **Hyoscine** (p. 93) is also effective on account of its depressant effect on the brain, including the vomiting centre; it is contained in certain commercial preparations, e.g. 'Kwells'.

The antihistamines and phenothiazines are described in more detail in Chapter 11, and pyridoxine on page 79.

### Pancreatin

The pancreas, in addition to housing the source of insulin (i.e. the islets of Langerhans, p. 181), also supplies the pancreatic juice to the duodenum via the pancreatic duct. The pancreatic juice contains the enzymes trypsin, lipase and amylase, which are essential to the digestion of protein, fat and carbohydrate, respectively. Lack of pancreatic juice may occur as a result of pancreatitis (inflammation of the pancreas), and especially in cystic fibrosis, should this damaging condition affect the tissue of the pancreas. There is then failure of digestion of protein, fat and carbohydrate, due to lack of the enzymes already mentioned; bulky, fatty stools are a particular feature. Treatment of this condition is based on *replacement* by the administration of preparations of pancreatin, a pale buff-coloured powder of meaty odour obtained from animal pancreas. Pancreatin contains the pancreatic enzymes, and is given several times daily as powders; or one of the several commercial preparations may be employed, e.g. the 'Pancrex' range which includes powder, granules (coated so as to delay disintegration until the duodenum is reached), capsules, and tablets (also similarly coated). 'Pancrex V' is a form of pancreatin which is five times the normal strength.

Pancreatin powder is affected by air and moisture, hence if dispensed in separate folded powders these are usually double-wrapped, the inner wrapping being of parchment paper to ensure fullest protection; it is likewise important that during storage on the ward *bulk* containers of the powder are kept well closed to prevent possible access of moist air.

# CHAPTER 4

# LAXATIVES AND ANTIDIARRHOEAL DRUGS

Laxatives are drugs and preparations which induce or aid evacuation of the bowel. They may be termed purgatives if the action is powerful and drastic, often due to heavy dosage; thus a mild dose of senna will have a laxative (or aperient) effect, whereas a heavy dose may well act as a purge. Several types of laxatives are available, and they exert their action in differing ways.

## The Lubricating Laxatives

**Liquid Paraffin** is a thick, clear mineral oil which is not digested and absorbed, hence it softens the bowel contents, lubricates the intestinal channel, and encourages a smooth painless movement. An average dose is 15 ml, taken at night or in divided doses with meals, but the amount should be regulated until just sufficient. Too much can over-soften the bowel contents and thus so reduce pressure against the intestinal wall as to lessen the peristaltic response which ensures movement of food and residue along the intestinal tract; furthermore, leakage per anus can occur, which is inconvenient to the patient and may cause soiling of underclothing and bed linen. It is said against the regular taking of liquid paraffin that it will dissolve certain essential food factors such as the fat-soluble vitamins and thus withhold their absorption. It is probable that liquid paraffin is now used rather less than in former years.

Liquid paraffin separates immediately when mixed with water, but if emulsified (see page 2) a thick white permanent cream results, in which it is finely dispersed. These emulsions are flavoured and are more palatable than the plain oil; an average dose is 30 ml. Liquid paraffin emulsions may also contain **Agar**, a substance derived from seaweed; this has the property of swelling when it meets the moisture of the gastro-intestinal tract, and the bulk so formed encourages peristaltic movement by pressure against the bowel wall. A further addition to certain liquid paraffin emulsions is **Phenolphthalein**, a substance which is a direct stimulant to bowel activity. Commercial preparations of these emulsions are 'Agarol' and 'Petrolagar', which are available with or without phenolphthalein.

### Bulk-producing Laxatives

These preparations, by their filling effect in the intestine, exert pressure on the bowel wall. Several types are available. Some are produced from certain plant sources and are available as granules, a teaspoonful of which is taken with a glass of water and swells into a thick mucilage which stimulates bowel activity; an example is 'Isogel'. Another, 'Celevac', is based on methylcellulose, and is available in tablet or granule form; it is taken, and acts, in a similar way to 'Isogel'.

A further useful function of these bulk-producing laxatives is that they produce a firm, well-formed stool if taken with a minimum of liquid, and this can be a boon to patients in colostomy control. Another use, distinct from laxative effect, is in the treatment of obesity, or overweight, when a few tablets of 'Celevac', for example, taken with a small amount of water between and before meal-times, will help to alleviate intense hunger by filling the stomach and deceiving the appetite.

'Fybogel' is a newer member in this section; it is prepared from seed husks, and is distinct as presented in one-dose sachets which are taken in water as a pleasant effervescent drink.

### Saline Laxatives

Here the word "saline" indicates certain compounds of sodium and magnesium. The best example is **Magnesium Sulphate**, commonly known as Epsom salts, a white crystalline substance with an unpleasant taste, which, taken dissolved in water (and well diluted) before breakfast, produces an evacuation of the bowel a few hours later; it is greatly helped if the dose is followed by a hot drink. Saline laxatives act by osmotic effect (p. 28), retaining water in the bowel and thus producing a copious watery stool. An average dose of magnesium sulphate is one teaspoonful (about 5 g), but up to 15 g can be taken, which would be termed a saline purge. The B.N.F. Mixture of Magnesium Sulphate is a long-used laxative, and is also known as "Mist. Alba" ("White Mixture").

Magnesium Hydroxide Mixture, the use of which as an antacid is described on page 12, is also employed as a laxative, especially for children, and the combination Emulsion of Liquid Paraffin and Magnesium Hydroxide B.P.C. is also much prescribed.

Another saline laxative is **Sodium Sulphate**, known as Glauber's salt, which is also a white crystalline substance and of similar dosage and action to magnesium sulphate. Further use is made of the osmotic action of various other sodium compounds in certain commercial enemas described later.

It is of interest to note also the use of the osmotic effect of magnesium sulphate in the "paste" commonly applied to wounds, etc., where it withdraws fluid by its self-diluting action; a further instance is the introduction per rectum as a retention enema of a 25% or 50% solution of magnesium sulphate, in order to relieve intra-cranial pressure by osmotic attraction of water.

## Stimulant Laxatives of Vegetable Origin

Plant life provides many laxatives, and the best known is **Senna**. The time-honoured senna tea is prepared by pouring boiling water into a cup containing a dozen or so of the fruit pods, or a larger number of the leaves, and allowing to infuse until cool; the pods or leaves are then strained off and the liquid provides a very efficient laxative, preferably taken first thing in the morning because of its urgent and powerful action. A widely used commercial preparation of senna is 'Senokot', which is available as tablets (average dose 2–4) or flavoured granules or elixir (average dose 1–2 teaspoonfuls); it is said to be without griping action and can be taken at night with greater safety. Senna preparations act by irritating the muscular coat of the large bowel, thus stimulating peristalsis. Compound Syrup of Figs also contains senna and is a pleasant laxative for children, an average dose being 5 ml.

'X-Prep' is a pleasant tasting liquid preparation of senna with powerful effect; it is used as an adjunct in radiography. The whole of a bottle of 71 ml is taken between 2 and 4 p.m. on the day before an X-Ray examination of gastro-intestinal or urological involvement; a light meal is taken before the draught, and the patient is warned to expect the required purging bowel action. Effective removal of flatus and faecal content lessens the possibility of picture distortion and misleading shadow.

**Cascara** and **Aloes** are two further drugs of vegetable origin used as laxatives, mainly in tablet form; the liquid extract of cascara is efficient, but has a very unpleasant taste. The still popular "vegetable laxative" tablet is also a combination of drugs of plant origin, which all act on the large bowel.

Note that these drugs (with the possible exception of senna tea, as explained) are normally given at bed-time, thus allowing eight to ten hours for the large bowel to be reached and stimulated into action the following morning.

## Synthetic Laxatives

These are not of natural origin, as are senna and cascara, etc., but are artificially produced, i.e. synthetic. **Phenolphthalein** has already been referred to as being sometimes included in liquid paraffin emulsions, and this laxative is also used commercially in chewing gum and chocolate form, as well as in the "teething powders" given to infants.

**Bisacodyl** ('Dulcolax') is a well established synthetic laxative which is taken as small tablets which pass through the stomach into the duodenum before disintegrating; it is also used in suppository form (see later). Bisacodyl is one of the most certain evacuants; it is completely unabsorbed and stimulates the intestine progressively, with final powerful effect on the large bowel, hence it is also employed in the preparation of this organ before X-Ray investigation.

Another group of laxatives combines a peristaltic stimulant, similar in effect to senna, with a softening agent of detergent-like action which "seeps" through the contents of the bowel; this softens the stool and helps to avoid impacted faeces, and is thus particularly useful in geriatric wards (i.e. for long-stay elderly patients). A popular example is 'Dorbanex', average dose 5–10 ml, also available in capsule form.

## Castor Oil

This vegetable oil acts on the *small* bowel, where it is broken down to substances which irritate the wall into vigorous peristalsis; hence its value in cases of poisoning where it is essential to clear the intestinal tract of its contents as soon as possible. An average dose is 15 ml, and as it has a nauseating taste it is usually taken floating on fruit juice.

The use of castor oil as a laxative has greatly diminished. It is useful to mention that its once popular administration to relieve "stomach-ache" in children can be fraught with danger, e.g. if the cause is an impending appendicitis. This applies also to the indiscriminate giving of *any* powerful aperient if severe abdominal pain is present.

## Enemas

—are liquid preparations which are given by injection per rectum (p. 5), the action being prompt and effective. The following are examples of traditional types which are still used:—

**Soap Enema**—usually green soft soap, 30 g, dissolved in water and made up to 600 ml: the addition of 30 ml of turpentine oil stimulates the expulsion of flatus and is occasionally used to relieve distension. It is worth noting that **plain water**, given warm likewise and in the same volume, is said to be as effective as soap enema, and has superseded it in a number of hospital centres.

**Olive Oil**—now usually used is **Arachis Oil**, which is a cheaper equivalent; it promotes smooth action.

**Glycerin**—is also highly lubricant and gentle.

Commercial disposable units are now available, comprising a plastic bag with a long tube which is inserted high into the rectum after heating the bag to body temperature in warm water; the bag is then gently squeezed to eject the contents and the enema retained until bowel action takes place. Three "Fletcher" types are available, the one mainly used containing sodium compounds, which act similarly to the saline laxatives (see Page 20), the other two being of arachis oil and a 50% solution of magnesium sulphate, the latter for withdrawal of water from the system to reduce intra-cranial pressure as mentioned earlier (page 21).

## Suppositories

These are also for use per rectum (see page 5) and several types are available, most popular being the plain "Glycerin" type—made of glycerin and gelatine, which act in two ways; firstly the insertion of a bulky object into the rectum may itself induce a commencement of peristaltic action, and secondly, as they melt, they provide lubrication, which is of value in constipation of several days' standing. Glycerin suppositories are available in infant's, child's and adult's sizes, 1, 2, and 4 ml, respectively.

Other suppositories used for laxative effect may contain a drug which is released and then stimulates peristalsis, an example being bisacodyl ('Dulcolax'), which irritates the rectal and colon walls into activity; its bulk in the rectum is likewise a stimulant. 'Beogex' suppositories are distinct in mode of action, and appear to be favoured in Obstetric Units. They contain two sodium compounds, one acidic in reaction and the other alkaline, and when they become moist within the rectum, these ingredients react to liberate carbon dioxide, which inflates the colon and induces peristalsis. Sizes are available for adults and children.

## Peristaltic Stimulation by Parenteral Injection

Occasionally, in the event of intestinal atony (lack of muscle power) post-operatively, normal laxative treatment and other measures may be ineffective. **Neostigmine** is used by subcutaneous or intramuscular injection in such cases, and by its anticholinesterase effect (p. 107) it increases the availability of acetylcholine (p. 14) to the intestinal muscles and so stimulates peristalsis. **Carbachol** (p. 108) is also used similarly (and as tablets by mouth), but its action is directly related to that of acetylcholine, although it is more prolonged.

A study of the differing actions of the various types of laxatives described will not be unrewarding, particularly as it concerns the hospital ward, where, although, ideally, the doctor should prescribe, the choice of a laxative may on occasion have to be left to the nursing staff. Factors to be borne in mind include the timing and the amount of the dose, the danger of vigorous peristalsis in certain cases, and the especial need for gentle action in others (e.g. following the removal of haemorrhoids); it is also probable that laxatives are sometimes administered more often than is actually necessary.

Finally, and as a generalisation, sight should not be lost of the value to the gastro-intestinal tract of a naturally bulky diet (unless contra-indicated); the inclusion of wholemeal bread (preferably not fresh)—and a bran cereal if necessary, plus adequate fruit and vegetables, these are valuable contributions to the common-sense diet which is so relevant to this section of the Chapter.

## ANTIDIARRHOEAL DRUGS

—are used in the treatment of diarrhoea; this can be of varied origin.

Firstly, the simple loose bowel occasionally met in the hospital ward, possibly caused by nervous reaction or change in diet and routine, etc. **Kaolin**, an aluminium compound, is the drug commonly used in conditions of this type. This is a light, off-white, insoluble powder, of which a tablespoonful can be given, mixed to a thin cream with water, several times a day; more often used is 10–20 ml of the B.N.F. Kaolin Mixture, which also contains antacid ingredients. Kaolin is thought to act by providing bulk, so improving the form of the stools, and also by absorbing irritant toxins which may be present in the bowel. Kaolin and Morphine Mixture contains a little morphine, which has a constipating effect and is thus of further value in diarrhoea.

**Chalk** (Calcium Carbonate) has similar effect to kaolin, and is employed as Chalk Mixture for young children and Chalk and Opium Mixture for adults; the latter contains opium tincture which, in turn, contains morphine, hence, again, the enhanced sedative effect on bowel activity.

Codeine is another active principle of opium, and likewise has an anti-peristaltic effect; this continues to be made use of in treating diarrhoeas for which there appears to be no specific cause. It is employed as **Codeine phosphate**, and average dosage is one 30 mg tablet three or four times daily.

**Diphenoxylate** ('Lomotil', tablets and liquid) and **Loperamide** ('Imodium', capsules and syrup) are synthetic drugs which are taken three or four times daily in both chronic and acute diarrhoeas; they reduce peristaltic activity, and 'Lomotil' contains also atropine for its further sedative effect on the bowel.

The second type of diarrhoea is more powerful and persistent and is caused by an organism; it is termed infective diarrhoea, and by its nature, can spread rapidly. It may originate from a food or water source, and/or human agency; in particular, inefficient personal hygiene and post-toilet routine can be contributory factors. The organism concerned will survive the stomach acid and digestive processes, and reach the bowel, to multiply rapidly and produce toxins which irritate the nerve endings in the intestinal wall, resulting in the violent contractions of severe diarrhoea. Whilst kaolin preparations are useful, effective treatment is based on appropriate bowel antiseptics, which can deal with the foreign organism and restore the bowel picture to normal. These mainly comprise certain members of the sulphonamides and antibiotics, which, when taken by mouth, are not absorbed from the gastro-intestinal tract, and thus continue to exert their anti-bacterial effect along the entire gut.

The non-absorbed sulphonamides used are **Succinylsulphathiazole**, **Phthalylsulphathiazole** and **Sulphaguanidine**, usually in tablet form (500 mg); dosage varies, but may safely be liberal, for minimal absorption ensures that the possibility of side-effects can be disregarded.

Succinylsulphathiazole—'Sulfasuxidine'—average dose 5–10 g daily in divided dosage.

Phthalylsulphathiazole—'Thalazole'—average dose 3 to 5 g daily in divided dosage.

The diarrhoea which is a symptom of ulcerative colitis resolves during treatment of the condition with a partially absorbed sulphonamide, **Sulphasalazine**: this is a specific drug in this condition, and is discussed on page 130.

**Streptomycin** and **Neomycin** are antibiotics which are used as bowel antiseptics. Streptomycin is not absorbed when given orally, hence its use in infective diarrhoeas in 1 gram doses several times daily. Neomycin is also not absorbed from the gastro-intestinal tract, and is generally the more popular, being effective against a wider range of organisms; two 500 mg tablets 3 or 4 times daily is normal dosage, and liquid preparations are available for children. Again it should be noted that antibiotics given orally for antiseptic effect in the bowel are free from toxic side-effects, due to their not being absorbed.

Several combinations of non-absorbed sulphonamides and antibiotics are available, often with kaolin and mainly in the form of creams or suspensions; examples are—

'Cremomycin'—succinylsulphathiazole, neomycin and kaolin

'Guanimycin'—sulphaguanidine, streptomycin and kaolin

'Ivax'—contains only neomycin and kaolin

The non-absorbed sulphonamides and antibiotics are also given in short courses before colon surgery, the aim being to reduce the bacterial number in the gut to the minimum and so ensure as aseptic a field as possible for the operation. The routine is full dosage by mouth, frequently supplemented by giving a suspension of the drug (or solution if neomycin) daily as a retention enema, thus treating the large bowel from both directions.

Several other antibiotics are available which are also poorly absorbed by the oral route, but these are reserved for use in bowel infections which are resistant to the drugs already mentioned. **Nystatin** is a prominent example; it is used in bowel infections which are caused by organisms of the yeast type and which may occur during treatment with the broad-spectrum antibiotics such as the tetracyclines—this is fully explained on page 139.

# CHAPTER 5

# DIURETICS

*and other drugs acting on the urinary system*
*—drugs and procedures used in kidney failure*
*—drugs used in retention of urine—antidiuretics*
*—drugs used in enuresis*

Diuretics increase the output of urine.

The importance attached to urinary output has increased greatly during recent years, particularly as it concerns the treatment of conditions such as heart disease, hypertension and acute poisoning by certain drugs. In order to fully appreciate the pharmacology of this interesting group of drugs it is worth recalling the elementary facts of kidney function. Each kidney is composed of a million or more units, called the nephrons; each of these consists of a

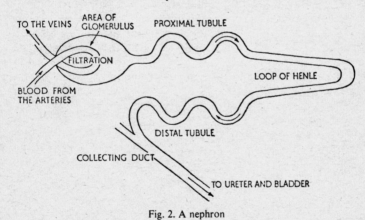

Fig. 2. A nephron

filter, the glomerulus, leading to a coiled (i.e. twisted) tube, the proximal tubule, then to a U-shaped tube, the loop of Henle, and finally to a further coiled tube, the distal tubule. During circulation, the water content of the blood, with its soluble constituents, filters through the glomerulus and passes on to the rest of the nephron until it leaves the distal tubule to reach the ureter, which conveys it to the bladder and thence to the urethra, to be finally excreted as urine. During its passage through the nephron the major part of the water is reabsorbed and there also occur exchange processes involving electrolytes—sodium (particularly), potassium, chloride, bicarbonate, etc.; these processes are designed to maintain the fluid volume and delicate balance of electrolytes in the blood and body tissues which are essential to health. A governing factor in this process is osmosis, and a brief explanation of this term will enable a clearer understanding of many aspects of Pharmacology.

## Osmosis

The Greek word osmos means "pull", and osmosis refers to the power of a solution of certain substances to attract water through a membrane (of what is called a semi-permeable type) from a solution of lower concentration. Thus, if a solution of sodium chloride (salt) lies on one side of such a membrane, and water, or a weaker solution of sodium chloride, lies on the other, then water will be pulled through the membrane by osmotic attraction, i.e. the stronger solution of sodium chloride will dilute itself; sodium chloride may also tend to transfer in the reverse direction, *but very much more slowly.* The process will then continue until the solutions on both sides are in equilibrium, i.e. of the same strength. Typical such membranes are those of the cells and tissues of the body. The other electrolytes (p. 40), and also dissolved substances such as dextrose and other sugars, and urea, etc., have similar osmotic effect, and this factor will be found of importance during discussion in other Chapters. However, it should be clearly understood that sodium is by far the major electrolyte present, and thus becomes the focal point of water distribution in the body. Whenever there

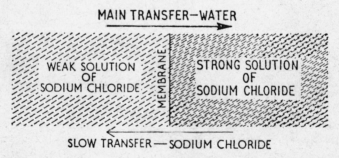

Fig. 3. Illustrating osmosis. Note the osmotic "pull" of the stronger solution and the resultant transfer of water from the weaker solution; also the very slow transfer of sodium chloride in the opposite direction. Transfer (mainly of water) continues until both sides are at equal concentration.

is retention of sodium there is retention of water, and, conversely, if sodium is eliminated, water is eliminated too, and this is the background to the action of several of the important drugs, and to the diseases concerned, which are mentioned in this Chapter.

Diuretics comprise several types; each is distinct in various respects, and will now be discussed in turn.

## The Saline Diuretics

These are mainly sodium and potassium compounds, as are sodium and magnesium compounds in the case of the saline purgatives (p. 20), and the one chiefly used is **Potassium Citrate**—as the B.N.F. Mixture (3 g in 10 ml); taken well diluted three or four times a day, it produces an improved urinary flow. This can be helpful in simple cystitis (inflammation of the bladder), particularly as potassium citrate makes the urine alkaline and so discourages the growth of certain organisms which are a factor in aggravating the condition. Potassium citrate is also of value in the prevention of crystalluria and, in turn, haematuria (blood in the urine) when patients are on systemic sulphonamide treatment (p. 128). Sodium citrate has a similar diuretic effect. The citrate diuretics are excreted as the alkaline bicarbonate, e.g. potassium citrate is converted in the liver to potassium bicarbonate, and their action is due to an osmotic effect which retains water in the renal tubules, thus reducing its re-absorption, and, in turn, increasing the volume of urinary output. It should be noted that the citrates are relatively mild diuretics, and their main value lies in their alkalising effect on the urine.

## Digitalis

—can be termed a cardiac diuretic, for by its tonic effect on heart action it improves the blood flow in the circulation and hence to the kidneys; this results in improved function of these organs, a raised level of filtration, and a higher output of urine. This effect is of great value in conditions where the heart is failing (see page 51).

## Aminophylline

The tea leaf contains caffeine, hence the diuretic value of "tea", not only for its fluid volume but also because caffeine reduces reabsorption of water in the kidneys. It is rarely used in treatment, but a related compound, also found in tea but now synthetically manufactured, is theophylline, which holds an important place in medicine. Theophylline is used either as the compound aminophylline, or as commercial tablets, e.g. of choline theophyllinate, which are said to be less irritant to the stomach. In addition to its diuretic action aminophylline relaxes the bronchi and makes breathing easier, and also improves heart action by dilating the coronary vessels and increasing blood supply to the heart muscle (see pages 87 and 53).

Aminophylline                  —av. dose 100-200 mg
Choline theophyllinate-'Choledyl'— ,,    ,,    100-200 mg

Now to be discussed are diuretics of greater potency, which are chosen in conditions where a profound increase in urinary output is required.

## Mersalyl

—is a compound containing mercury and theophylline, and although now seldom used is a powerful diuretic with prolonged effect lasting several days; it is given by i/m injection, and ammonium chloride (2 g) is usually given by mouth beforehand to acidify the urine, which improves its action. 'Neptal' is a similar brand (trade) preparation.

## The Newer Oral Diuretics

A disadvantage of mersalyl is that it has to be given by injection, and it also carries the risk of toxic side-effects; a number of drugs have now been introduced which are safer and which can be taken by mouth with similar powerful diuretic effect. The first was **Acetazolamide**, which, taken in the morning, induces diuresis over about 12 hours. Acetazolamide is a carbonic-anhydrase-inhibitor (p. 95) and causes the elimination of bicarbonate in the urine as sodium and potassium bicarbonate; these bicarbonates retain water in the kidney tubules and hence there is increased diuresis. Unfortunately, the diuretic effect tends to diminish in use, hence it is now mainly employed in epilepsy (p. 95) and glaucoma (p. 216), where it appears to act by relieving internal tension in the organs affected.

Thus the first real diuretic advance was the introduction of **Chlorothiazide**, which is given in varying dosage—e.g. one 500 mg tablet twice a day or two on alternate days; an intravenous injection is also available. Chlorothiazide acts by preventing the reabsorption of sodium and other electrolytes from the proximal tubules in the kidneys during the normal exchange processes mentioned earlier; the sodium (mainly) retains water with it (see under "Osmosis", p. 28) and the urinary volume is greatly increased. As with all new drugs, many derivatives have been produced, all claimed to have advantages—smaller dosage and less side-effects, etc.; examples are listed below. Bendrofluazide is probably the drug most often used in this group.

Chlorothiazide      —'Saluric'      —av. dose 1 g
also I/V      — „    „    500 mg
Hydrochlorothiazide—'Hydrosaluric' — „    „    50 mg
Hydroflumethiazide —'Hydrenox'     — „    „    50 mg
Bendrofluazide      —'Aprinox'     } — „    „    5 mg
                  'Neo-Naclex'
Polythiazide      —'Nephril'      — „    „    1 mg

A disadvantage of the thiazide diuretics is that they cause rejection, and thus loss, of *potassium* as well as sodium, and this can be serious, for, unlike sodium, potassium is not present in quantity in the diet, being limited mainly to such sources as bananas, oranges, tomatoes and meat. Hence, because adequate levels of potassium are essential to muscular activity and cardiac function, and also because patients with heart disease are more prone to the side-effects of digitalis if they are short of potassium (p. 51), treatment with thiazide diuretics is usually accompanied by potassium orally in order to forestall such deficiency; a note on potassium therapy will be found on page 33. Alternatively, the loss itself of potassium may be greatly minimised by the use of amiloride (p 33).

Many other new powerful diuretics have been introduced, all of which act by preventing the reabsorption of sodium at some site in the nephron, varying from the proximal tubule and the loop of Henle to the distal tubule. Amongst the most important are **Frusemide, Ethacrynic Acid** and **Bumetanide**; all three are available in tablet and injection form. Their action is relatively short, which is an advantage in treatment control, but is dramatic. Thus 7 litres of urine may be produced in 24 hours on a fluid intake of merely 2 litres, or two stones in weight lost in a matter of days. The oedematous patient, in a waterlogged condition due to congestive heart failure (p. 50), will be enabled to recover, and conditions in which difficult breathing is due to accumulation of fluid in the lungs will be greatly improved, the action being striking in pulmonary oedema. These drugs likewise cause loss of potassium, which thus has to be replaced.

Frusemide      —'Lasix'    —av. dose 20–40 mg
by injection — „    „     20 mg
Ethacrynic Acid—'Edecrin'— „    „     50 mg
by injection — „    „     50 mg
Bumetanide      —'Burinex'— „    „     1 mg
by injection — „    „     0·5 mg

Frusemide is also available in high strength tablets (500 mg) and injections (250 mg); these are used in kidney failure of both chronic (of long duration) and acute (of short duration and more severe) nature. Thus, dramatic improvement may be achieved, for example, in shortening the period of oliguria (scanty urinary output) which may follow peritoneal dialysis; reducing the number of dialyses needed; relieving the occasionally stubborn oedema of "waterlogged" patients; overcoming serious uraemia (accumulation of waste products in the blood normally excreted in the urine); and, when kidney failure is imminent following shock, in stimulating production of urine before failure has set in. Dosage may add up to as much as 1-2 grams, or more, daily, and this powerful treatment requires critical judgment in deciding that it is feasible and justified, i.e. that the state of the patient's kidney function will tolerate the demands made upon it; obviously such treatment is confined to the hospital field. Butametanide is likewise available as a high strength injection for use in similar urgency.

Other oral diuretics are **Chlorthalidone** and **Triamterene**, in tablet and capsule form respectively. Chlorthalidone has prolonged effect, and dosage on alternate days or twice weekly is normally sufficient; triamterene is milder in action, but does not cause potassium loss and is thus useful in combination with other powerful diuretics.

Chlorthalidone—'Hygroton'—av. dose 100 mg  
Triamterene   —'Dytac'   — „   „   50 mg

## Spironolactone

Occasionally, diuretics of the thiazide type fail to produce the required output of urine, for the following reason. One of the hormones produced by the cortex of the suprarenal glands is aldosterone (p. 193), the essential function of which is to ensure that an adequate sodium level for body needs is maintained by promoting its reabsorption from the *distal* tubule of the nephron as and when necessary, this being done in exchange for potassium which is then excreted in the urine. In patients with failing heart, production of this hormone may increase greatly and result in excessive sodium being reabsorbed, together with water, thus aggravating the already oedematous condition as well as depleting potassium stores. In such cases the thiazide diuretic is unsuccessful because the sodium rejected at the proximal, or near, end is being reabsorbed into the body under the influence of aldosterone at the distal, or far, end. Hence the value of spironolactone, a drug which is given orally and which blocks the action of aldosterone and so ensures diuresis when combined with thiazide therapy.

Spironolactone—'Aldactone'—av. dose 25–100 mg

*Note* that measurement of fluid intake and urine output is a routine often employed to estimate diuretic efficiency.

## Potassium Supplement Therapy

Potassium chloride, whether given as liquid mixture or tablets (even if these do not disintegrate until in the duodenum), can be severely irritant and even caustic to the stomach and duodenal mucosa. Hence, the wide use of potassium chloride tablets which are specially designed to release the drug *gradually* during their passage through the small intestine; examples are 'Slow-K' and 'Leo-K'. Compound tablets of potassium, palatably flavoured, which are dissolved in water and taken as an effervescent drink, are useful for patients who have difficulty in swallowing tablets. Several of the powerful oral diuretics are available *with potassium in the same tablet*, e.g. 'Hydrosaluric-K', 'Neo-Naclex-K' and 'Burinex-K', but in the hospital field *separate* administration of potassium is often preferred as enabling independent adjustment of dosage of both diuretic and potassium.

## Prevention of Potassium loss

A different approach to the maintenance of potassium levels when patients are on oral diuretics (p. 31) is the use of **Amiloride** ('Midamor'). Amiloride acts as a mild diuretic itself by promoting an increased elimination of sodium and chloride (and, in turn, water by osmotic action), but it also has the effect of markedly reducing the excretion of potassium. Hence, one to four 5 mg tablets of amiloride may be given daily to patients who are on any diuretic therapy which involves potassium loss, e.g. frusemide and the thiazides, etc.

It should be noted that amiloride may sometimes cause excessive loss of sodium, resulting in electrolyte imbalance; also that oral potassium supplement, e.g. as 'Slow-K', etc., should not normally be given to patients who are taking amiloride, lest too *high* a potassium level result—which can *also* be serious.

"Moduretic" is a much prescribed tablet incorporating hydrochlorothiazide with amiloride, but, as in the case of potassium supplementation, separate administration of amiloride is more general in hospital prescribing.

The term *"potassium-sparing"* diuretics is sometimes met; this refers to those diuretics which do not cause loss of potassium, e.g. amiloride, triamterene and spironolactone.

## Drugs Used in Urinary Retention

This condition may occur in the post-operative period, and two drugs of specific value are **Carbachol** and **Distigmine**. Carbachol is similar in effect to acetylcholine (p. 14) and stimulates contraction of the bladder muscles and relaxation of the sphincter (opening), therefore facilitating the flow of urine; it is effective orally, but is usually given in urinary retention by subcutaneous or intramuscular injection.

Distigmine acts by antagonising the effect of the enzyme cholinesterase (p. 107), thus allowing the level of acetylcholine activity to rise and stimulate bladder contraction. It is related to neostigmine (p. 107), which is also used to relieve retention of urine, but has a more prolonged action, and may be used post-operatively as an alternative to catheterisation which has its attendant risk of urinary tract infection. Distigmine is given orally and by intramuscular injection.

Carbachol                 —av. dose 2 mg orally
                                         0·25 mg s/c

Distigmine—'Ubretid'— „     „     5 mg orally
                                         0·5 mg s/c

## KIDNEY IMPAIRMENT OR FAILURE

Diuretics are usually contra-indicated when the kidneys are not functioning normally, and two approaches to the serious problem of accumulation of excessive electrolyte levels and of waste products, e.g. urea, are the administration of resins by mouth, and the use of peritoneal dialysis or haemodialysis.

**The Resins**
—are synthetic and resemble fine sand; they are used to treat and prevent hyperkalaemia, a term indicating significantly excessive levels of potassium in the system. '**Resonium-A**' contains sodium, and it releases this in the intestine in exchange for potassium, which is then excreted with the resin in the stool. The potassium removed is mainly that which is taken in the diet and is present in the intestine, some is also removed from the intestinal wall tissue; hence the resin can provide a useful contribution to the treatment of excessive body levels of this electrolyte. The resin is generally taken in water (av. dose 15 g), but can be given per rectum as a retention enema if the oral route is unacceptable; the blood level of potassium is carefully checked lest it gets too low. '**Calcium Resonium**' is a resin which releases *calcium* in exchange for potassium, hence its value in place of 'Resonium-A' when high sodium levels may be considered a danger.

## Peritoneal Dialysis

In kidney failure, there is scanty production of urine or even none at all (anuria); as a result, electrolyte levels become unbalanced and there may be critical overloading with, for example, potassium or sodium, and grave accumulation of end-products of body metabolism, e.g. urea. Such failure may be acute but remediable, or it may become chronic and without expectation of any improvement in kidney function. A measure that can be used with dramatic effect is peritoneal dialysis. The dialysis process resembles osmosis, but with the difference that it is the dissolved solids which cross the membrane and not the water, the latter being prevented from doing so as will be explained. The membrane concerned is the peritoneum, which lines the abdominal and pelvic cavities and has an approximate area (unfolded) in the adult of over 2 sq. yds; this large surface is itself an important factor in the process.

An outline of the routine is as follows. A sterile solution containing the body electrolytes (but usually omitting potassium) is run into the peritoneal cavity, through a previously inserted catheter, from two 1-litre bottles suspended above the patient, and the solution is allowed to remain within for about 45 minutes or less; it is then run out by switching over to a reservoir below or by lowering the empty bottles to the floor. This is repeated hourly (or more frequently) and may be continued for 24 hours or even longer.

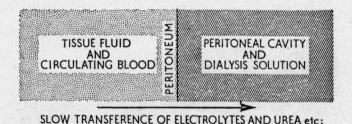

SLOW TRANSFERENCE OF ELECTROLYTES AND UREA etc:

Fig. 4. Illustrating peritoneal dialysis. Note that the presence of dextrose in the dialysis solution withholds the transfer of water, also that regular replacement of the solution is necessary to maintain withdrawal of excess electrolytes and urea, etc.

The electrolytes in the solution are at a concentration similar to that *normally* in the blood, and the effect is to remove *gently* from the tissues on the other side of the peritoneum the electrolytes and urea, etc., which are, as has been explained, in excessive concentration. A point to note now is that the solution also contains dextrose, which, because it does not pass through the peritoneal membrane, raises the osmotic level of the solution to just above that of the blood, and thus retains the water content which would otherwise diffuse through the membrane into the body—contrary to the aim, which is extraction *from* the body of the various substances present in excess.

Potassium is omitted from the solution because in most cases of kidney failure the potassium level in the blood is already high, and the need is therefore to increase the rate of extraction of this electrolyte by omitting it from the solution; in the event of it being necessary, a sterile solution of potassium chloride is added to the solution.

A broad-spectrum antibiotic (e.g. oxytetracycline) is sometimes added to the dialysis solutions to lessen the risk of peritoneal infection.

As already mentioned, the dialysis solutions mainly employed are not intended to withdraw water from the patient to any significant extent, but if this needs to be done, solutions containing a higher concentration of dextrose are used. This increases the osmotic pull, and water also is then extracted across the peritoneum in addition to the excess electrolytes and urea.

Peritoneal dialysis is life-saving in acute kidney failure, and it can be repeated regularly at certain centres; it may also need to be used in severe cases of poisoning by barbiturates and other drugs, in order to reduce the level of the drug in the body by extraction across the peritoneum as described.

### Haemodialysis

In the case of many patients in irreversible kidney failure, the peritoneal dialysis process presents problems of time, equipment and personnel, etc., and use is made of haemodialysis, by which the blood itself is dialysed. In brief, the blood emerges from an artery in the wrist or leg and is fed via tubing through a unit, with suitable membrane walls, which is immersed in a bath of a solution similar to the peritoneal dialysis solution; the blood undergoes the same cleansing and correcting process before returning to a vein near the artery, and so back into the circulation. With suitable equipment the routine can be performed by the patient in his home. The same injection sites may continue to be used, employing a "shunt" unit by which exit and re-entry are controlled by clips, finally sealing off at the end of the dialysis. The process is usually repeated every few days. Haemodialysis is also used in cases of extreme poisoning by barbiturates, etc., as referred to earlier.

It should now be clear that the aim of both peritoneal and haemodialysis is to cleanse the blood and maintain acceptable electrolyte levels; in short, to replace kidney function.

## Forced diuresis

Another method of promoting diuresis is the administration of intravenous solutions, the "forced diuresis" which is often used in the treatment of poisoning by certain drugs, e.g. aspirin and the barbiturates. Various electrolyte solutions are employed, but a substance of specific value in this indication is mannitol; this is a sugar which is not metabolised, like dextrose for example, and hence reaches the kidney tubules in high concentration, retaining water there by osmotic attraction and thus preventing its reabsorption and so increasing the output of urine. Urea solutions are occasionally given by intravenous infusion, when the osmotic effect is of particular value in reducing intra-cranial pressure in cases of severe head injury; it is of special use also during neuro-surgery.

It is of interest to note that forced diuresis is not always applicable in the treatment of poisoning. An example is in the case of 'Mandrax' (p. 92), for heavy overdosage of this drug restricts the ability to urinate, and the use of a forced diuresis regime might then lead to serious results.

# ANTI-DIURETICS

—are used to *decrease* urinary output, a particular example being in diabetes insipidus ("drinking diabetes"), where the patient passes large volumes of urine frequently, and, in turn, is compelled to drink copious amounts of fluid. This is due to failure of the posterior pituitary lobe to secrete (produce) the hormone vasopressin (p. 177) which is a controlling factor in the reabsorption of water from the kidneys following filtration of the blood; the water thus passes on and is excreted as urine. The treatment employed is replacement of the hormone by **Vasopressin**, obtained from cattle, or a synthetic equivalent. Vasopressin is not effective by mouth, and subcutaneous or intramuscular injections are used ('Pitressin'), the effect, however, lasting only a short time. Thus, more usually, preparations of powdered posterior lobe ('Di-Sipidin') containing vasopressin are used to apply to the nasal mucosa; commercial insufflation outfits are available into which capsules of the powder are inserted, making administration easier. Or a nasal spray of the squeezer type ('Syntopressin') containing **Lypressin**, a synthetic equivalent to vasopressin, may be used into each nostril several times daily. The vasopressin, or lypressin, is then absorbed from the nasal mucosa and circulates in the blood to perform its function in the kidneys, reducing diuresis dramatically and making life tolerable for the patient.

A further closely related equivalent to vasopressin is **Desmopressin** ('D.D.A.V.P.') which is administered by injection, or as a solution into the nasal cavity by means of a special plastic catheter. It is claimed that desmopressin has greater and more prolonged anti-diuretic effect than vasopressin, one or two uses daily being normally sufficient.

An interesting addition to the treatment of certain cases of diabetes insipidus is the use of a thiazide diuretic, e.g. chlorothiazide. This may appear puzzling in that a powerful diuretic is being given where a reduction in the output of urine is the requirement. The explanation is that in diabetes insipidus the urine contains very little sodium chloride; consequently this is retained at high levels in the system and creates severe thirst, thus aggravating the condition. The thiazide acts by eliminating sodium chloride (p. 30), thus reducing thirst, and is of proven value where response to vasopressin (or related preparations) alone is not completely satisfactory.

## DRUGS USED IN THE TREATMENT OF ENURESIS

Enuresis or bed-wetting, occurs mainly in childhood, but also occasionally in adolescence and the elderly.

The drugs often employed are those with anticholinergic effect (p. 13), for this induces relaxation of the muscles of the bladder wall and so lessens the strength and frequency of contraction; furthermore the anticholinergic drugs maintain *contraction* of the bladder sphincter (the muscle which controls the opening into the urethra), and this also restricts the forward flow of urine. Thus tincture of **Belladonna** has long been used, commencing with small doses at bedtime and gradually increasing until an effective level is reached. The newer synthetic drugs with equivalent action and fewer side-effects are now more often used, an example being **Propantheline** ('Probanthine', p. 15), which is also taken at bed-time in large dosage.

A different approach to bed-wetting is the use of either **Amphetamine** or **Dexamphetamine**. These drugs are powerful stimulants of the central nervous system (p. 103) and therefore cause insomnia if taken in the evening. However, certain enuretic children are unusually heavy sleepers and thus do not wake in response to the need to pass urine; in such cases the amphetamine is given at bedtime and its stimulant effect results in a lighter plane of sleep and a greater readiness to wake when need calls. The amphetamines are also thought to have some specific effect on the muscle of the bladder wall. Their use in this condition is probably but occasional, and due to the dangers associated with them (p. 104) they are now Controlled Drugs (p. 251).

Other drugs of distinct action are also used in the treatment of enuresis. One approach is to give **Imipramine** or **Amitriptylene** (p. 98) in the evening for their anti-agitative effect. Another is the use of injections of **Desmopressin**, which, by its anti-diuretic action, reduces the volume of urine passed into the bladder. A directly opposite treatment is the ingenious use of the diuretic **Frusemide** (p. 31), which is given in the late afternoon and followed by restriction of fluids; the patient then passes a large volume of urine before bedtime and thus experiences an enforced dry night.

Urinary incontinence in adults and the elderly is generally managed by protective means, but an anticholinergic drug used in this type of case is **Emepronium**, taken in tablet form one hour before bedtime. Emepronium is also used during the period of incontinence which may follow bladder surgery or prostatectomy (removal of the prostate gland).

Emepronium—'Cetiprin'—av. dose 100 mg

It is held that despite the number of drugs of different action employed in the enuresis of childhood, the most successful treatment is still the use of the electric "buzzer". It may be of interest to the student nurse to know how this works. Two rectangular metal foils are positioned in the appropriate area of the bed below the patient; they are separated from each other by a sheet, and the patient lies on a further sheet laid over the top foil. Each foil is connected by a flex to a battery and bell unit at the bedside; this is switched on at bedtime. The bell cannot ring because the foils are separated by the *dry* sheet and thus there is no contact. However, when enuresis occurs, the urine makes contact through the sheet, from foil to foil, and the circuit is completed; the bell then rings and wakes the patient. This is treatment by "training", and has a high rate of success.

# CHAPTER 6

# INTRAVENOUS INFUSIONS

*—types and uses: isotonic solutions: subcutaneous infusions: with a note on the millimole unit*

The body weight is made up by water to the extent of 65–70%, and in an average adult the total fluid volume, including the blood, is about 50 litres. Of this 50 litres (say), 35 litres are contained within the cells (this is called the intracellular fluid). The remaining 15 litres are termed the extracellular fluid, and of these, 12 litres are interstitial (i.e. between the cells), and the remaining 3 litres make up the plasma (the fluid part of the blood). These three fluid "compartments" are separated by semi-permeable membranes (see under "Osmosis", p. 28), through which the exchange processes vital to the functioning of the organs and tissues are continuously taking place. Some fluctuation in total volume obviously occurs following ingestion of fluid, or excretion via urine, faeces, sweat and perspiration, but, basically, the volume is maintained at a broadly consistent level in health by kidney function.

This chapter deals with the means whereby the *intake* of fluid may be augmented, or completely substituted, when the normal oral route cannot be used. Fluid is occasionally given subcutaneously, i.e. into the tissue (this is described on page 47), but the route most commonly used is the intravenous one, whereby fluid is introduced into a vein, i.e. directly into the plasma compartment of the extracellular fluid. The term intravenous "infusion" is used to describe the introduction into the blood stream of these comparatively large volumes of sterile fluid; $\frac{1}{2}$ litre or 1 litre glass bottles or plastic containers are normally used. Such infusions are employed for a number of purposes; these include the restoration and maintenance of fluid volume and electrolyte requirements, establishment of diuresis, and nutrition of the patient.

### Electrolytes

Electrolytes are substances which dissolve to form solutions which are capable of conducting an electric current; in doing so, they dissociate (divide up) into what are termed ions. As considered here, they are metallic compounds, and sodium chloride is a typical example, for when it dissolves in water it dissociates into *sodium* ions and *chloride* ions. The body electrolytes comprise sodium, potassium, calcium and magnesium, in association with chloride, bicarbonate, phosphate and sulphate. They are contained in the body fluid at various concentrations and each plays an important part in body physiology (the function of the organs and tissues referred to earlier). For example, the activity of the heart-beat cycle is greatly dependent on a high level of potassium in the cardiac muscle, and the role of sodium, and chloride, is a controlling factor in the distribution of water by osmotic effect (p. 28). Conditions that can seriously interfere with fluid and electrolyte levels include crises of acute shock and haemorrhage, and severe diarrhoea and vomiting, and in such cases the use of appropriate intravenous infusions is of great value.

**Isotonic Solutions**—the term explained.

The process of osmosis has been described on page 28, and it will· be recalled that if a solution of high osmotic pressure (e.g. a strong solution of sodium chloride) is separated by a semi-permeable membrane from one of lower osmotic pressure (e.g. a weak solution of sodium chloride) then water will pass through the membrane from the weak solution to the strong, until both solutions are at equilibrium, i.e. of the same osmotic strength. Let us consider this in relation to the blood plasma and the red cells. Here, because the wall of the red cell is itself a semi-permeable membrane, the fluid inside the cell must obviously have the same osmotic pressure as the plasma it is circulating in, and there will be no movement of water either way across the cell wall membrane; the fluid inside the cell, and the plasma outside the cell, are thus both at osmotic equilibrium and are said to be **isotonic**. Now this common osmotic pressure (of cell and plasma) is the same as that of a 0·9% solution of sodium chloride—which is thus commonly known as "isotonic saline" or "normal saline" (sometimes also "physiological saline"); and if isotonic saline is infused into the blood (i.e. intravenously) the structure of the blood cells is undisturbed, because there is no passage of water across the cell membrane in either direction. Thus, an isotonic solution can be described as one which has the same osmotic pressure as that of blood plasma.

The term **hypotonic** refers to solutions of weaker strength than isotonic, and it will be clear that if a hypotonic solution were to be infused intravenously, water would pass *from* it *into* the red cells, and they would swell in consequence and might eventually disrupt (this is termed haemolysis). **Hypertonic** solutions, on the other hand, are stronger than isotonic, and if a hypertonic solution were infused intravenously, water would pass *into* it *from* the red cells, and they would shrink and cave inwards; this does not constitute such a danger as the haemolysis caused by hypotonic solutions, for the shrunken red cells resume normal size and shape when the osmotic pressure is subsequently equalised on discontinuation of the infusion.

### "Saline"

The term "intravenous saline" usually refers to "normal saline" (see earlier); it is much employed in hospital routine to restore and maintain fluid volume. However, if normal saline is used too continuously, it is possible for the level of sodium chloride in the tissues to build up gradually until oedema results due to its osmotic retention of water (see p. 28). Hence normal saline may be alternated with solutions of dextrose 4·3% with sodium chloride 0·18%, or dextrose 5% in water, thus reducing the salt intake. These sugar solutions are used to provide calorie value also, and this important point is referred to when discussing intravenous nutrition (p. 45).

Examples of hypotonic solutions of sodium chloride are "half normal" saline, which contains 0·45%, and "1/5th normal" saline which contains 0·18%; examples of hypertonic solutions are "double strength" saline, which contains 1·8%, and the powerful 4·5%. The use of these solutions in intravenous therapy is confined to special need.

### Compound electrolyte solutions

Potassium, magnesium and calcium, and (rarely) phosphate and sulphate, are also included with sodium and chloride in certain compound electrolyte solutions; the need is usually indicated by laboratory report on blood samples. Two standard formulae often used are Hartmann's solution, which contains sodium, calcium, potassium and chloride, and Darrow's solution, from which the calcium is omitted; both solutions also contain sodium lactate, which is converted in the liver to alkaline bicarbonate, as which it circulates in the blood. Solutions containing sodium lactate are thus of particular value in conditions of metabolic acidosis, caused by lowered bicarbonate levels in the body, which occur typically in diabetic coma and aspirin poisoning. Intravenous solutions of sodium bicarbonate itself are sometimes used for their quicker and more direct correction of metabolic acidosis, e.g. in cardiac arrest (p. 63).

It is occasionally necessary to add a solution of an electrolyte (such as potassium chloride) to an intravenous infusion, e.g. to a litre bottle of dextrose/saline. In addition to the aseptic routine necessary during the transfer (including thorough attention to the surface of the closure), it is essential to thoroughly mix by shaking so as to avoid any concentrated solution running into the vein, which may be irritant and cause damage. Antibiotics are also sometimes added, and thorough mixing is equally essential.

It should be noted that increasing attention is being paid to ensuring that additions to intravenous solutions exclude any possibility of harm to the patient. This implies not only a fully aseptic routine and thorough mixing, but also that the drug or substance added is suited to continuous infusion therapy and that there is no possibility of harmful interaction with the ingredients of the solution, e.g. a precipitate of any kind. The range of additives employed is becoming larger and more complex, and it is official intention that instruction on the above points will become a specialised study; the aim being to confine this important phase of ward procedure, as it concerns nursing personnel, only to those who have been properly trained in it and are so designated.

## Forced diuresis

Large volumes of electrolyte solutions are given by intravenous infusion in cases of poisoning, e.g. by barbiturates (p. 92) or aspirin (p. 111); this is termed "forced diuresis" and has been referred to on page 37. Also mentioned there is the intravenous use of strong solutions of mannitol (up to 25%) and urea (up to 30%) to promote diuresis by osmotic effect and so relieve intra-cranial pressure.

### Blood and Plasma

The solutions so far mentioned are normally excreted via the kidneys fairly rapidly, and in cases of urgency other intravenous infusions are used which have particular effect in expanding and maintaining blood volume.

Blood itself, from donors, in half-litre bottles (or plastic bags, as now more usual), is used in emergency, not only for the volume supplied by its liquid base (the plasma) but in particular because it contains electrolytes and other important constituents, including the red cells and their valuable haemoglobin. Occasionally, the need is for the red cells in particular, and not the plasma bulk, and this is met by giving "packed cells" in place; this is prepared by allowing blood to stand and drawing off the yellow plasma after the red cells have settled at the bottom of the container, thus leaving blood from which upwards of 50% of its plasma has been removed. The basic precaution deserves stressing—that the patient who is to be given blood *must* have the correct group, as tested beforehand (or it may be the safe group "O" in emergency), and a double check of the label is imperative.

Donor blood is not plentifully available, and is employed only when considered essential. When the need is not for the red cells but rather for the plasma, then plasma itself may be used. It is issued in the form of a pale buff-coloured powder in a half-litre bottle, which is dissolved in the appropriate amount of Water for Injections for giving by intravenous infusion. Note that although it lacks the red cells, plasma still contains the other valuable constituents of blood. The administration of blood or plasma is of great value in haemorrhage and shock, etc., but a possible serious hazard associated with both is the transmission of a virus which may be present in the blood of a donor and cause hepatitis (inflammation of the liver) and the associated jaundice.

Dried plasma is now giving way in use to Plasma Protein Fraction (P.P.F.), as being a more refined and effective product; a further point in its favour is that during its preparation the organism which causes hepatitis is inactivated by heat. P.P.F. is a clear, straw-coloured liquid, in bottles of 400 ml, and it is required that the solution must be ensured clear and free from deposit by close inspection before use.

A further plasma substitute is the commercial preparation "Haemaccel", a solution of gelatine containing electrolytes and protein; not being of human origin, it has certain advantages over plasma, e.g. possibility of reaction is obviated, also it cannot transmit virus hepatitis and is stable for eight years at room temperature.

### Dextran

The difficulty of obtaining blood and plasma freely, together with the attendant risk of the side-effect mentioned, has led to the use of other solutions by intravenous infusion for restoring blood volume, the so-called plasma expanders. These are solutions of dextran, a substance derived from sugar and the molecules of which (i.e. the basic chemical pattern) are very large. Dextran solutions are not metabolised readily as is the case with solutions of sugars like dextrose, and hence they stay in the circulation for a long period; the time varies according to the molecular size (or "weight") of the grade used. Thus, dextran of a molecular weight described as "40 000" has a duration of effect of about 8 hours only, and is used to encourage the free circulation of blood in the capillaries and thus prevent the "sludging" of blood cells which may accompany stagnant flow. Solutions of a molecular weight of "70 000" maintain their effect as plasma expanders for about 24 hours, and are used in shock accompanied by sudden lowering of blood volume, and also as a prophylactic (preventive) measure in surgery. The effect of heavier or "thicker" solutions of dextran, of a molecular weight of 110 000 or even higher, is prolonged for as long as 48 hours, hence they are employed essentially for stabilising the restoration and maintenance of blood volume in shock following massive haemorrhage or severe burns. Dextran solutions are available in either normal saline or 5% dextrose base. It should be appreciated that they provide merely a mechanical expansion of blood volume and do not confer the other beneficial effects of the constituents contained in blood and plasma. However, dextran solutions do not carry the occasional risk associated with blood and plasma, and, being commercially manufactured, they can be used freely without supply problems.

A possibility associated with the use of solutions of a high molecular weight dextran is the encouragement of blood clot formation. Also, the presence of such solutions in the blood may be a complicating factor in the process of ascertaining the patient's blood group.

### Dextran preparations

| | | | |
|---|---|---|---|
| 'Lomodex 40' 'Rheomacrodex' } | molecular weight | | 40 000 |
| 'Lomodex 70' 'Macrodex' } | ,, | ,, | 70 000 |
| 'Dextraven 110' | ,, | ,, | 110 000 |
| 'Dextraven 150' | ,, | ,, | 150 000 |

## Intravenous Nutrition

—is employed when the patient is too ill to be fed by mouth, e.g. post operatively, or when oral feeding is contra-indicated, as in the case of stomach or bowel operation; it employs a wide range of materials.

The carbohydrate **Dextrose** (also known as glucose) is the sugar present in the blood and which is formed following the intake and digestion of other carbohydrates in the diet. It is extensively employed by the intravenous route. Thus, as a 5% solution or, more often, 4·3% in 0·18% sodium chloride (1/5 normal saline), it provides a ready source of calories (p. xv) and is of value in restoring circulation volume when it is lowered in conditions of extreme dehydration, shock or haemorrhage; both strengths are isotonic (see page 41). Solutions of higher concentration, e.g. 10–20%, are occasionally employed when calorie need is greater. Stronger solutions (up to 50%) are also used, but in this case some of the sugar is not metabolised and is thus excreted in the urine, the volume of which it increases by osmotic effect.

**Fructose**, or laevulose, is fruit sugar and is closely related to dextrose; it is used by the intravenous route at similar strengths to dextrose, and is preferred in certain cases as being less irritant to the venous tissue at the site of injection. An additional advantage is its quicker utilisation compared with dextrose; this is due to the fact that it is not dependent on the action of insulin, as is the case with dextrose.

A high calorie intake can be an urgent requirement, as in the case of severe burns, etc., and this can be provided by the intravenous administration of **fat emulsions**. These are prepared from vegetable oils, e.g. soya-bean oil ('Intralipid'), and have the appearance of thick, creamy milk; they are given by slow drip, providing as many as 1 000 calories per half-litre bottle. Another high-calorie source is **Sorbitol**, a sugar which is occasionally given by intravenous infusion as a 30% solution; like fructose, it does not need insulin for utilisation.

A further essential in prolonged intravenous nutrition is **protein**, and several preparations are available (brand names 'Aminoplex', 'Aminosol', 'Trophysan') in half-litre and one litre bottles. They contain various amino-acids which provide a quickly available source of protein. Certain formulations also incorporate glucose, fructose, or sorbitol for calorie value, and may contain in addition ethanol (alcohol), which provides a further valuable source of calories.

Vitamins are also necessary to complete nutrition, and various combinations may be administered by intravenous injection and infusion during prolonged therapy (p. 80).

The intravenous infusion route is also employed for the quick raising of haemoglobin levels in critical need by giving iron by the Total Dose Infusion ("T.D.I.") technique; this is described on page 66.

An established development in the packaging of commercial intravenous solutions of electrolytes and sugars, etc., is the plastic container in place of the glass bottle, the advantage being that after use it can be disposed of as waste, which avoids the "empties" problem and makes storage easier.

It is timely to emphasise that when putting up *any* intravenous drip (except, of course, in the case of fat emulsions), the bottle or plastic container *must* be examined against strong light for *clarity*, because a flaw in sealing, or a crack or puncture, may result in contamination of the contents, leading to mould or bacterial growth during storage and possibly fatal results if used (see page 239 re 'pyrogens'). Certain commercial intravenous fluids are "vacuum packed", and the label instructs the nurse to turn the bottle upside down and give it a sharp blow with the fist, which should produce a recognisable bell-like sound if the seal is intact. A simple but important point is that in the case of injections, whether in ampoule, multiple-dose vial, bottle or plastic container, once the seal has been broken and the contents exposed to the air, use should commence at once or within a very short time, otherwise the container must be rejected, and the label crossed through accordingly. This is also mentioned elsewhere (p. 240), but no apology is made for repeating it.

It will be clear, too, that if a rubber or plastic closure is to be pierced by a needle or the sharp end of a giving-set cannula, the surface *must* be ensured clean and aseptic by giving it a thorough wipe with a sterile swab impregnated with, e.g., 70% spirit.

## SUBCUTANEOUS INFUSION

It occasionally happens, e.g. in the case of children (particularly) and the elderly, that intravenous infusions may be difficult to administer, due to troublesome movement of limbs or the problem of finding a suitable vein, etc. In this event the subcutaneous route may be employed.

Two needles are inserted into the subcutaneous tissue (e.g. in the thigh) and are connected by a "Y-piece" to the tubing of an administration set leading to the suspended bottle of solution (e.g. normal saline); or one needle only may be used. A problem now is that the rate of infusion is extremely slow by this method, for the fluid tends to stay at the site of injection and accumulates as a swelling. This is due to the presence in the tissue of a substance called hyaluronic acid, which is of a thick, "glue-like" consistency and thus resists the permeation of the infusion solution into the circulation. Hence the wide use of an enzyme, **Hyaluronidase** ('Hyalase'), which is obtained from animal testes and has the property of liquefying (i.e. thinning) hyaluronic acid. When the administration set has been put up as described, and the tubing and needles are filled with fluid from the bottle suspended above, 1 500 units of hyaluronidase (the contents of one ampoule) are dissolved in 1 ml of water and injected through the tubing near the Y-piece and needles; it then proceeds into the tissue and thins and breaks down the hyaluronic acid barrier, thus enabling quick penetration of the fluid.

The use of hyaluronidase makes it possible to give a patient 300 ml of fluid by subcutaneous infusion in as little as 30 minutes, a speed factor which can be of critical importance in the case of children gravely dehydrated in gastro-enteritis, etc. An additional advantage of the subcutaneous route is that there is no risk of vein damage as may occur in intravenous infusions.

Hyaluronidase may also be used by injection to disperse haematomas (swellings filled with blood) and in other procedures, e.g. to enable the quick spread of local anaesthetics.

It is of interest that hyaluronidase has many sources of origin. Thus, it is produced by leeches, to enable easier suction of blood

~ through the tissues; by snakes and bacteria (e.g. the organism causing diphtheria), to promote the quick infiltration of toxin into the tissue; and by the seminal fluid, in order to facilitate the union of the spermatozoon (the male cell of reproduction) with the ovum in the process of fertilisation.

## Millimoles

—is a term now, found on the labels of intravenous infusion and injection solutions (see also "SI", p. xiv), and a simplified explanation will be helpful.

Firstly, and avoiding undue involvement in the chemistry concerned, the basic point to appreciate is that, in general, each of the substances contained in intravenous solutions has its own *molecular weight*; this is a figure, e.g. the molecular weight of sodium chloride is 58·5, and that of dextrose is 180. Now the molecular weight of such a substance in *grams* is termed a **mole** (abbrev. mol), and in *milligrams* it is termed a **millimole** (abbrev. mmol). Thus, a mole of sodium chloride is 58·5 grams, and a millimole is 58·5 milligrams; likewise, a mole of dextrose is 180 grams, and a millimole is 180 milligrams. It will be clear that because there are 1 000 milligrams in 1 gram, there are 1 000 millimoles in a mole. For example, in the case of sodium chloride, there are 1 000 millimoles (of 58·5 mg each) in 1 mole (58·5 g).

Let us now consider a litre bottle of intravenous normal saline; this is labelled as containing 0·9% sodium chloride and also as containing 154 millimoles (mmol) per litre. These two statements tie up quite logically as follows:

0·9% equals 0·9 g in 100 ml
and thus 9 g in 1 000 ml (one litre).

Now 9 g equals 9 000 mg, and we know a millimole of sodium chloride is 58·5 mg, therefore the number of millimoles in a litre of normal saline is 9 000/58·5, i.e. 154 (to the nearest whole number).

Why is this system employed? Firstly, SI is *international*, and thus, as with the Metric System already established in this country, the necessary interchange of scientific expression is greatly facilitated and encouraged. Secondly, the professions involved, e.g. doctors, laboratory personnel, pharmacists and nursing staff, will be using a common system of terminology. Thirdly, both doctor and laboratory personnel will now "talk in millimoles" in respect of intravenous solutions, and it will be clear that actual amounts of substances in injection solutions (expressed in terms of moles or millimoles) have greater meaning and value than mere percentage strength.

# CHAPTER 7

# CARDIOVASCULAR DRUGS

*—digitalis and other drugs acting on the heart*
*—hypotensive drugs—vasodilators—vasoconstrictors*
*—drugs used in cardiac arrhythmias*

Cardiovascular drugs are used to treat conditions of the heart and circulation. A reminder of the main circulatory process is helpful to an understanding of the actions and uses of many of the drugs included under this heading; an outline follows (see also Fig. 5):

A. The heart is composed of four quarter chambers—the right and left atria (or auricles) above the right and left ventricles below. Atrium is the preferred term to auricle; "atria" is the plural.

B. The two atria contract and expand together, the two ventricles likewise but alternating with the atria. Thus, when the atria contract, the ventricles fill, and, in turn, as the ventricles contract, the atria fill.

C. When the left ventricle contracts, blood is pumped into the arteries, thence to the arterioles and finally to the network of capillaries, returning via the veins to fill the right atrium as it expands.

D. As the right atrium contracts, the blood proceeds to the right ventricle, and when this contracts, it passes out via the pulmonary artery to the lungs, where its carbon dioxide is exchanged for oxygen.

E. The blood then returns via the pulmonary vein to fill the left atrium, which, on contracting, sends it forward to the left ventricle and the cycle commences again. The frequency of contraction of the left ventricle is measured when taking the pulse.

## Digitalis
—has been in use for more than 200 years, yet is still unique in effect and is the best known and most used heart drug; its

various preparations originate from the leaves of the common fox-glove plant. The tincture is now seldom prescribed, tablet forms being more stable; these may be of either the dried and powdered leaf itself **(Digitalis Folium)** or the actual active principle (or ingredient) which it contains—**Digitoxin** in the case of the English foxglove, and **Digoxin** in the case of the Austrian species. Where the term digitalis is used in this Chapter, it is intended to cover the use of all three preparations. Digoxin is the most widely used (for reasons explained later), followed by digitoxin, and then digitalis leaf—which is now but little prescribed.

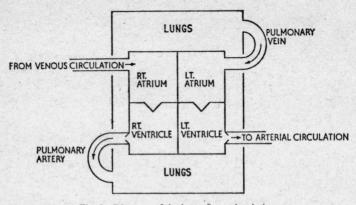

Fig. 5. Diagram of the heart /lung circulation.

Digitalis acts as a cardiac tonic by slowing, regulating and strengthening the heart beat; it prolongs the resting and filling phase (diastole), and stimulates a more powerful contraction (systole), thus sending out an improved flow of blood into the circulation. Its use in congestive heart failure illustrates this action. Here, the cardiac filling and contracting is rapid, weak and shallow, and the overall output is moderate; the poor intake by the right atrium leads to slowing of blood flow returning via the venous system, and the resultant congestion in the circulation gives rise to accumulation of fluid in the tissues, resulting in puffiness (oedema). Likewise, sluggish movement of blood through the pulmonary circulation results in the congested and wet condition of the lungs known as pulmonary oedema. Furthermore, poor blood supply to the kidneys leads to weakened function and there is reduced rate of filtration, so that output of urine is lessened, again aggravating the generalised oedema. Digitalis preparations given in such a condition will slow a rapid pulse, e.g. 100 plus, down to 70, but each contraction of the left ventricle will now be sending out a more powerful supply of blood, and back pressure on the right side will be eased by the more prolonged and complete filling of the right atrium. The more efficient circulation will mobilise and take up surplus tissue fluid and reduce oedema; this will be helped also by a higher urinary output. The distress of wet and oedematous lungs is similarly eased, and breathing improved. The value of additional diuretic therapy in relieving oedema is mentioned on page 31.

Digitalis is also used in atrial fibrillation, where the atria, instead of contracting in alternating unison with the ventricles, twitch haphazardly up to several hundred times a minute, whilst the ventricles contract at perhaps 120 times a minute. Digitalis, by its regulating effect, assists in restoring the rate to normal.

When commencing digitalis therapy, dosage is usually high for the first few days, so as to produce a rapid and effective blood level (i.e. to "digitalise" the patient); this desired level is then maintained by a moderate daily dose.

Digitalis is a cumulative drug, i.e. it may not be "used up" at the same rate as it is taken; this applies more to the English leaf and its active constituent, digitoxin, than to digoxin. It is important to keep its blood level under control, for, if excessive, toxic side-effects can occur. The first signs of overdosage are nausea and sudden vomiting, and possibly diarrhoea; there may be coupling of the heart beat (double systole), and the diuretic effect may be reversed and output of urine reduced. These symptoms occur more readily if there is potassium depletion following the use of diuretics (see page 31). Treatment includes stopping the drug immediately, and ensuring that the patient's potassium level is increased by giving an appropriate preparation by mouth (p. 33) or by slow intravenous injection of potassium chloride.

In the hospital ward, regular taking of the pulse is a protection against it falling below 60, the warning figure, and patients on long-term digitalis treatment are sometimes instructed to omit dosage on one day each week, so as to "use up" possible accumulation. Of the various preparations, digoxin is the most frequently used because of its rapid action and rate of excretion, and the consequent less likelihood of cumulative effects; also, it is available in injection form for intravenous use in emergency, and as a low strength elixir and tablet ("P.G.") which are suitable for paediatric and geriatric use.

| Digitalis folium | —tablets | —av. dose 60 mg |
| | tincture | — ,, ,, 0·6 ml |
| Digitoxin | —tablets | — ,, ,, 100 micrograms |

Digoxin—'Lanoxin'—tablets    — ,,   ,,   0·25 mg
                                             (250 micrograms)
                                        0·125 mg
                                             (125 micrograms)

            —injection      — ,,   ,,   0·5 mg
                                             (500 micrograms)
                                             in 2 ml

            —tablets 'P.G.'— ,,   ,,   0·0625 mg
                                             (62·5 micrograms)

            —elixir 'P.G.'  — ,,   ,,   0·05 mg
                                             (50 micrograms)
                                             in 1 ml

## DRUGS USED IN ANGINA PECTORIS

### The Nitrite/Nitrate group

These drugs are used in angina pectoris, a condition in which the coronary arteries are constricted and unable to dilate, leading to a lessening of blood flow—and thus oxygen supply—to the heart muscle; the result is the typical pain behind the sternum especially during stress of effort or emotion, when the oxygen need is greater and cannot be met. The action of these drugs is to dilate the peripheral (outer) blood vessels, thus lessening resistance, making the flow of blood easier, and reducing the amount of work the heart pump has to perform.

An interesting member of this group is **Amyl Nitrite**, a volatile liquid (i.e. quickly evaporating) contained in thin glass capsules which are enclosed in silk or lint, or lodged in a narrow cardboard tube. In the event of an acute spasm the capsule is snapped within its covering and the vapour inhaled, to be immediately absorbed into the blood stream via the alveoli of the lungs and the pulmonary vein; relief is dramatic but of short duration.

Other members of this group are available in tablet form, the best known being tablets of **Glyceryl Trinitrate** (or **Trinitrin**) which are dissolved under the tongue (sublingually, see page 2) for quicker absorption. **Pentaerythritol tetranitrate** is a related drug which has similar effect, and commercial tablets of both these drugs are also available in long-acting form. Although slower in action than amyl nitrite, tablets are more convenient for frequent use, particularly as a prophylactic (preventive) measure before effort of any kind or at first sign of pain.

Amyl Nitrite                               —capsules of 0·2 and 0·3 ml
Glyceryl Trinitrate—B.N.F.         —tablets, av. dose 0·5 mg
         —'Sustac'         —   ,,   of 2·6 mg and
                 (sustained action)                           6·4 mg

| Pentaerythritol | —'Mycardol' | — | „ | 30 mg |
| tetranitrate | —'Peritrate' | — | „ | 10 mg |
| | —'Peritrate S.A.' | — | „ | 80 mg |
| | (sustained action) | | | |

**Perhexiline** ('Pexid') is used solely for preventing angina pectoris, one or two tablets being taken twice a day; should an attack nevertheless threaten, resort must still be had to a drug such as trinitrin.

**Aminophylline**, in addition to its value as a bronchodilator and diuretic (pp. 87 and 29), has a further useful effect in dilating the coronary arteries, thus making it a cardiac tonic and increasing output; it is occasionally prescribed for routine taking in angina pectoris.

### The Beta-blockers

This group of drugs has assumed major importance in the treatment of several conditions since the introduction of **Propranolol**, the first of the series and still one of the most favoured.

Their action is broadly as follows. Stimulation of the cardiac work rate is promoted by sympathetic nerve impulses which release adrenaline when they reach the heart; this release occurs at points proximal to the *beta-receptor sites* in the heart muscle, and is greatly increased during stress of emotion or effort. The beta-blocker drugs interfere with (or "block") the mechanism of this adrenaline stimulation, hence they lower the cardiac work rate, i.e. they calm the heart, slow the pulse, and reduce the force of blood flow into the circulation. This is made use of in several conditions.

Thus, in angina pectoris, where the lack of the extra blood supply needed for the heart muscle during stress results in the angina pain, the beta-blocker drugs prevent the heart from working harder and so reduce its need for the extra blood supply it cannot get. The sensation of angina does not now occur, or is minimal, and the patient's resort to nitrite medication is far less necessary.

The value of this group of drugs in other conditions will be explained as these are discussed later (pp. 58 & 61).

The beta-blockers have two main side-effects, though these may vary from drug to drug. Firstly, heart rate and function may be unduly lowered—to the point of failure, hence these drugs are used with care where cardiac condition is already weak; and should pulse become critically slow it may be increased again by giving atropine by intravenous injection (p. 63). It is claimed for **oxprenolol** that, whilst slowing the heart rate, it strengthens the contraction, thus lessening the danger of undue reduction of cardiac output. Secondly, some of the beta-blockers have a constricting effect on the bronchi, and this may cause asthmatic distress to "chesty" patients; **Acebutol**, **Atenolol** and **Metoprolol** are among those said not to affect the air passages appreciably, and thus may be preferred for patients with any asthmatic tendency. **Practolol** is similarly cardio-selective (i.e. does not affect the bronchi), but its severe side-effects in the eye, skin, and peritoneal areas now limit its use solely to emergency situations in hospital, and then by injection only.

The following is a representative list of the beta-blocker group. Atenolol is expressly taken once daily, and in the case of several of the others the normal divided daily dosage is sometimes replaced by one larger dose taken in the morning; sustained-action tablets are also being made available, as in the case of oxprenolol ('Slow-Trasicor').

| | | |
|---|---|---|
| Acebutol | —'Sectral' | —capsules, 100 mg |
| | | —injection, 5 mg |
| Atenolol | —'Tenormin' | —tablets, 100 mg |
| Metoprolol | —'Betaloc' | — „ 50 and 100 mg |
| | —'Lopresor' | — „ 50 and 100 mg |
| Oxprenolol | —'Trasicor' | — „ 20, 40, 80 & 160 mg |
| | | —injection, 2 mg |
| Pindolol | —'Visken' | —tablets, 5 mg |
| Practolol | —'Eraldin' | —injection, 5 mg |
| Propranolol | —'Inderal' | —tablets, 10, 40, 80 & 160 mg |
| | | —injection, 1 mg |
| Sotalol | —'Beta-Cardone' | —tablets, 40 and 80 mg |
| | | injection, 10 mg |

## DRUGS USED IN HYPERTENSION

—may be termed anti-hypertensive *or* hypotensive, for their action is to lower the blood pressure where it is abnormally raised. In mild conditions of hypertension of emotional origin, e.g. due to anxiety or agitation, the drugs used may be mild sedatives, such as the barbiturates (p. 91) in small dosage; thus 30 mg of amylobarbitone or phenobarbitone may be given once or twice daily, the effect being one of calming the patient and restoring the blood pressure to a more normal figure.

The more severe hypertension, however, with which this section is mainly concerned, is usually caused by a lack of elasticity in the blood-vessel walls, particularly the arterioles, which, in consequence, do not relax, or "give", to the flow of blood passing through them, the result being raised pressure in the blood vessels, or hypertension. This may lead to serious effects on organs such as the heart, kidneys and brain.

The most powerful hypotensive drugs are the ganglionic-blocking agents. To clarify their action, it should be explained that the sympathetic nervous system exerts a constricting effect on the blood vessels through the release of *noradrenaline* by the nerve impulses when they arrive at the nerve fibre endings (Fig. 6 (b)). During transmission along its nerve fibre, each impulse has to pass through a "relay station", the ganglion (Fig. 6 (a)), and the effect of the ganglionic-blocking agents is to arrest (i.e. block) its further progress at this point. Hence, the impulses do not now reach the blood vessels and, in consequence, noradrenaline is not released, the walls are enabled to relax and "give" to the blood passing through them, and there is a fall in blood pressure. Two examples of these drugs are **Mecamylamine** and **Pentolinium**, both in tablet form. Pentolinium is used in a wide range of dosage, and is of great value by intravenous injection in acute hypertensive crisis.

Mecamylamine—'Inversine'   —av. dose 2·5–10 mg
Pentolinium   —'Ansolysen'  —tablets of 10 mg and 40 mg
       —injection (s/c or i/v) 5 mg per ml

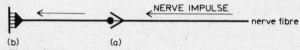

Fig. 6. Illustrating—
   (a) ganglion
   (b) release of noradrenaline at meeting point of sympathetic nerve ending and
      wall of blood vessel.

A disadvantage of the ganglionic-blocking drugs is that in addition to their desired effect upon the sympathetic system they also block the ganglia (plural) of the *para*sympathetic system: this arrests the parasympathetic nerve impulses in like manner and leads to severe constipation, dry mouth and throat with difficulty in swallowing, and blurred vision. Hence the advantage of drugs which are *selective* and act *only* on the sympathetic, examples being guanethidine, bethanidine, debrisoquine, methyldopa, clonidine and prazosin.

**Guanethidine** is normally taken in tablet form, once daily in the morning, and acts by preventing the release at the sympathetic nerve-fibre endings of noradrenaline, which, by its vasoconstrictor action, as mentioned earlier, maintains the tone or strength of the vessels of the circulation. Guanethidine has prolonged action, and as this is exerted only on the sympathetic system, the side-effects of parasympathetic inactivation (see earlier) are absent. However, certain other unpleasant effects can occur, particularly if dosage is high. Firstly, as the sympathetic system is relaxed by the drug, parasympathetic activation increases, and the bowel responds with severe diarrhoea—so powerful as to be termed "explosive". Secondly, giddiness and fainting may occur when rising too abruptly from a sitting or lying-down position; this is called postural hypotension. The explanation is interesting. Normally, when rising upright, the blood vessels in the lower extremities contract, and this mechanism prevents the blood pooling downwards from the brain by gravity. However, the relaxant effect of many of the hypotensive drugs on the blood vessel walls prevents them contracting quickly enough, and this allows blood to pool in the lower limbs sufficiently for the brain to be depleted of blood supply; giddiness and fainting then result. Thus, patients are advised to be sure to rise to their feet slowly and deliberately—so allowing time for the circulatory vessels to adjust to the change of posture.

**Bethanidine,** also in tablet form, is related to guanethidine but has a shorter action of 6 to 8 hours, which makes treatment more controllable; tendency to diarrhoea is also less. Guanethidine and bethanidine are available in injection form for use in emergency, and the former is also used as eye drops to reduce intra-ocular tension.

**Debrisoquine** acts by reducing the release of noradrenaline at the sympathetic nerve fibre endings, thus, again, allowing the blood vessel walls to relax; it is given once or twice daily, dosage being increased if necessary. The only significant side-effect is postural hypotension and, as with the other hypotensive drugs concerned, patients are cautioned on this point, as referred to earlier. Diarrhoea is said to be rarely a complication.

The release of noradrenaline at the sympathetic nerve fibre endings results in what is termed the adrenergic effect, hence drugs such as guanethidine, bethanidine and debrisoquine, etc., which inhibit, variously, the release or effect of noradrenaline, are termed *antiadrenergic.*

**Methyldopa** also blocks noradrenaline action, but is thought to act in the following manner. The process of noradrenaline production depends on the action of a certain enzyme; methyldopa takes up and utilises this enzyme, and is converted by it into a substance similar to noradrenaline but with much weaker effect on blood vessel tone. This substance occupies the place of noradrenaline at the nerve endings, and the blood vessels, now under much weaker control, relax, and blood pressure falls. Methyldopa is available in tablet and injection form and its action is short and its hypotensive effect controllable; postural hypotension is said not to be troublesome, but certain haemolytic blood complications have been reported in occasional patients.

**Clonidine** ('Catapres') is a hypotensive drug the action of which is distinct and possesses certain significant advantages. It appears to act initially by quietening the work-rate of the heart, so reducing the force, and, in turn, the pressure, of the circulation. Subsequently, the response of the peripheral vessels to the stimulating impulses which reach them via the sympathetic system is greatly reduced; the result is a corresponding decrease in blood vessel constriction and a steady prolonged drop in blood pressure. Clonidine is relatively free from the uncomfortable effect of postural hypotension, and may be employed in combination with other hypotensive drugs, e.g. bethadine, methyldopa, etc., particularly if adequate results are not already being obtained.

Clonidine is also used as a low dosage tablet of 25 micrograms ('Dixarit') in the prophylactic (preventive) treatment of migraine; its benefit in this condition relies on its effect of rendering the blood vessels unresponsive to stimulating impulses, thus maintaining a state of equilibrum in the circulation of the area concerned (see also page 60).

**Prazosin** is a hypotensive drug of distinct action, for whilst it directly relaxes arterial muscle, it does not foster pooling of blood in the lower extremities on rising too suddenly; it is thus relatively free of postural hypotension side-effect.

Guanethidine—'Ismelin'   —av. dose 10–25 mg
Bethanidine  —'Esbatal'  — „   „   10–50 mg
Debrisoquine—'Declinax' — „   „   10–20 mg
Methyldopa  —'Aldomet' — „   „   125–500 mg
Clonidine   —'Catapres' — „   „   0·1–0·3 mg
                             (100–300 micrograms)
Prazosin    —'Hypovase'—av. dose 2–5 mg

Guanethidine, methyldopa and clonidine are also used by injection in emergency.

**Reserpine** ('Serpasil'), an active principle of plant origin, has been used for many years as tablets of 0·25 mg in the treatment of mild hypertension. It acts by sedation of the brain and consequent reduction of stimuli which are concerned with the production of noradrenaline in the sympathetic system. A side-effect which can occur is extremely severe depression. Reserpine is of value by intravenous injection (2 mg) in hypertensive crises which are resistant to other drugs.

**Diazoxide** is occasionally used to raise the blood glucose level (p. 187), but it also has a very powerful hypotensive action due to direct relaxation of the muscle of the arterial wall; hence it is given by intravenous injection in cases of acute hypertensive emergency.

The action of the **beta-blockers** in reducing cardiac activity has been explained (p. 53); the result is a decrease in the rate of output of blood into the circulation, and the lowered force of flow eases pressure against the blood vessel walls. This different mode of action does not incur the side-effects associated with so many of the hypotensive drugs, hence the beta-blockers are much employed in the treatment of hypertension, either alone or with other hypotensive drugs. Commencing dosage is moderate, increasing at intervals, e.g. weekly, according to response; similarly, if to be discontinued, this is done by gradual reduction of dosage.

The value of **diuretics** (p. 27) must again be stressed in the case of hypertension. Mild or even moderate cases can be treated with certain oral diuretics alone, e.g. the thiazide group (p. 31), for which some actual effect on blood-vessel wall relaxation has been claimed. The benefit of increased diuresis lies in the fact that it lowers the degree of fluid tension in the body tissues; this, in turn, eases the pressure load on the circulating blood. The addition of a diuretic to the existing treatment regime may oblige the dosage of the hypotensive drug being used to be reduced considerably, even by as much as a half, in order to avoid the risk of blood pressure being lowered too drastically, e.g. to the point of fainting; this is also a decided advantage, because reduction of dosage leads to a similar reduction of side-effects, such as the distressing diarrhoea and postural hypotension referred to earlier.

## OTHER VASODILATORS

The drugs discussed here are used for their more prolonged dilating effect on the peripheral or outer blood vessels, where there is a need to improve the circulation or to relax spasm. A simple example is the use in chilblains of **Nicotinic Acid** (see under Vitamins —page 78), which dilates the blood vessels of the skin and thus improves blood flow and reduces the inflammation; an average dose is 50 mg, and a side-effect is an intense prickling sensation of the skin. Derivatives of nicotinic acid are contained in certain rubefacient preparations (p. 223), which when applied to the skin, are absorbed and improve local blood flow.

**Phenoxybenzamine** and **Tolazoline** are vasodilator drugs of greater power and more prolonged effect, and are used to improve blood flow in severe conditions of vascular spasm (e.g. of arteries) in the extremities, characterised by extreme pain and cramp, as in Raynaud's disease and intermittent claudication, of which lameness may be a feature. Both act by anti-adrenergic effect (see page 56), thus causing relaxation of the walls of the blood vessels affected.

**Nicotinyl alcohol** and **Inositol Nicotinate**, both derivatives of nicotinic acid but with more powerful action, and **Cyclandelate**

and **Isoxsuprine** are other examples of drugs used in peripheral vascular disorders.

| | | | | |
|---|---|---|---|---|
| Phenoxybenzamine | —'Dibenyline' | —av. dose | | 10 mg |
| Tolazoline | —'Priscol' | — „ | „ | 25 mg |
| Nicotinyl alcohol | —'Ronicol' | — „ | „ | 25 mg |
| Inositol Nicotinate | —'Hexopal' | — „ | „ | 200 mg |
| Cyclandelate | —'Cyclospasmol'— | „ | „ | 400 mg |
| Isoxsuprine | —'Duvadilan' | — „ | „ | 10 mg |

It should be explained that the vasodilators described in this section are not used in hypertension or angina pectoris because their action would be too unpredictable, severe or over-prolonged. Also, there is some doubt as to the measure of value of these drugs in the treatment of arterial disease. A vasodilator of specific interest, however, is **Phentolamine** ('Rogitine'), the use of which in diagnosis is described on page 226.

## VASOCONSTRICTORS

—constrict, or narrow, the bore of the blood vessels, and may be used to raise the blood pressure where a fall in volume or force of circulation can be critically serious, as in the acute hypotension which may arise as a result of excessive dilatation of the peripheral vessels following, for example, a spinal anaesthetic. Their action is similar to that of noradrenaline (p. 55), i.e. they increase the tension of the walls of the vessel, and these, in turn, exert greater pressure on the blood passing through, so offsetting collapse and encouraging forward flow.

**Noradrenaline** itself has been employed to raise the blood pressure by its vasoconstrictor effect on the peripheral system; its use as 'Levophed' is referred to on page 188.

**Metaraminol** ('Aramine') is used to treat the hypotension which may accompany such procedures as epidural anaesthesia (p. 123), when it may be given by direct intravenous injection or slow dilute infusion; the effect is prolonged.

The value of using vasoconstrictor drugs in certain situations, e.g. of shock in particular, appears to be losing favour due to the opinion that the constricting of the peripheral vessels can well handicap the objective—which is that of improving capillary flow. Hence, in such episodes, there is increasing employment of **isoprenaline** (p. 63), for this drug stimulates both the strength of heart function and the rate; it also causes dilatation of the peripheral blood vessels, thus making blood flow easier, improving micro-circulation (i.e. in the capillaries), and easing strain on the arterial system. Hence its increasing use in cases of severe haemorrhagic or septicaemic shock, when it is administered as a dilute intravenous infusion, the rate of flow being carefully monitored and adjusted if necessary.

## Ergotamine

—is one of the prominent constituents of ergot; another, ergometrine, is referred to on page 108. Whereas ergometrine is used for its contracting effect on the uterus, the action of ergotamine is mainly one of constricting the peripheral blood vessels, particularly those in the head, and this effect is made use of in migraine headache, in which it often gives relief by suppressing the painful pulsations of the blood vessels concerned. Speed is important in the treatment of this condition, and ergotamine is available as a combination with caffeine (which enhances its effect), the tablets being taken at first sign of an attack, followed by rest in a quiet, darkened room; injections are given in acute conditions, and suppositories are also used. A limit is usually set to the number of doses of ergotamine preparations which may be taken in a day, or week, due to the danger of gangrene developing as a result of the restriction of blood supply to the extremities. An interesting approach to the prevention of migraine is a pocket inhaler ('Medihaler-Ergotamine') which delivers a measured or "metered" dose of ergotamine in each puff, the drug being quickly absorbed from the nasal mucosa.

Ergotamine            —'Femergin'    —av. dose 1 mg
                       by injection— „    „    0·25 mg s/c
                                                 or i/m

Ergotamine 1 mg  }
Caffeine 100 mg  }  —'Cafergot'—two tablets to be taken
                        initially, with a set limit of
                        6 tablets in one day and
                        12 in any one week.

The use of clonidine (as the tablet 'Dixarit') in the treatment of migraine has been referred to (p. 57), and it should be made clear that this drug does not constrict the blood vessels, but instead exerts a quietening effect which prevents them constricting or dilating in response to nerve impulses.

The vasoconstrictors mentioned in this section are those with systemic effect, but certain drugs are also employed for their *local* constricting, or shrinking, action. Thus, the use of adrenaline as a haemostatic by application, and as an ingredient of local anaesthetics, is described on pages 69 and 125, and the action of ephedrine and other "shrinkers" in reducing nasal secretion, on page 216.

## DRUGS USED IN CARDIAC ARRHYTHMIAS

Many such disturbances of heart rhythm may occur. They include tachycardia (abnormally rapid pulse), bradycardia (abnormally slow pulse), heart block, and conditions of fibrillation; the ventricles and/or atria may be involved. The circumstances in which these abnormalities of rhythm appear vary greatly likewise, and include coronary thrombosis, cardiac arrest, and surgical operations, etc. An outline only can be given here of the complex uses and actions of the drugs employed.

**Lignocaine**, the local anaesthetic (p. 124), has a pronounced correcting effect upon excessive heart activity, and is a drug of major importance in this connection; its mode of action is not clearly understood. It is used by intravenous injection in controlling ventricular tachycardia in emergencies where there is danger of development of ventricular fibrillation, a grave condition which can result in failure of heart function; its use in this connection is further referred to later (page 63).

**Procainamide** ('Pronestyl') is a derivative of another local anaesthetic, procaine, and has a direct depressant action on the heart muscle. Thus it is used in conditions of cardiac irritability, such as tachycardia, where it produces a slower and more orderly rhythm. It is given as tablets for prolonged treatment, and also by intramuscular or intravenous injection during surgery and in episodes of paroxysmal tachycardia (extremely rapid and distressing pulse). 'Procainamide Durules' are sustained-action tablets which release the drug gradually along the small intestine, thus maintaining an even blood level.

The bark of the cinchona tree supplies us with two important drugs—the anti-malarial, quinine (p. 157), and quin*id*ine. **Quinidine** prolongs the resting phase between contractions of the heart muscle, hence its employment in the treatment of atrial fibrillation and in both atrial and ventricular tachycardias. It has long been used as the ordinary tablet (200 mg), but again a sustained-release form, 'Kinidin Durules', is available, which provides a prolonged blood level.

**Disopyramide** ('Rythmodan') has specific use in the prevention and treatment of a wide range of cardiac arrhythmias; it acts by slowing the transmission of impulses within the cardiac system and by extending the resting phase of the atria and ventricles. Tablets and intravenous injections are employed, the latter being especially valuable in severe arrhythmias, e.g. as can follow a coronary thrombosis.

**Digoxin** has already been discussed in relation to its regulating action in atrial fibrillation (p. 51). **Propranodol** and other beta-blocker drugs are also used in this condition for their restraining effect on cardiac activity, though they are given with caution to patients with weak heart function lest they slow this unduly and so precipitate failure (see p. 53).

Digoxin and a beta-blocker are occasionally employed together in atrial fibrillation; they make a balanced combination, for the strengthening effect of digoxin compensates for any undue cardiac inactivation resulting from the action of the beta-blocker. **Phenobarbitone** is also frequently used in atrial fibrillation for its general sedative action, which is of value in this condition.

### The use of Isoprenaline in Heart Block

This condition is due to a partial or complete failure of the conduction of nerve impulses along the Bundle of His, the specially adapted strip of tissue which passes from the right atrium to the ventricles. The pulse may fall to 40 or even lower as a result, and in the event of extreme slowness or interruption of ventricular contraction, the acute attack known as the "Stokes-Adams" may occur. Isoprenaline has a powerfully stimulating and quickening effect on the heart rate, and is given by injection in acute heart block, as referred to later (p. 63), but for the long term supportive treatment of *chronic* heart block, tablets are obviously more appropriate.

Tablets of isoprenaline have been dissolved sublingually for their rapid bronchodilating effect in asthma, but in relation to the treatment of heart block their stimulating effect is too brief, and administration several times daily would result in the discomfort of alternating periods of quick and slow pulse. To meet the need for sustained action, tablets have been introduced ('Saventrine') which are composed of numerous small granules of isoprenaline (to a total of 30 mg), each coated to a carefully varied and graded degree of thickness with a substance which commences to dissolve only when it reaches the small intestine; the different thicknesses of coating ensure that the release of isoprenaline is regulated and prolonged during its passage along the intestinal tract, and if these tablets are taken several times daily the heart is kept under constant and steady stimulation without undue fluctuation.

## DRUGS USED IN CARDIAC ARREST

Resuscitation equipment is normally kept readily available in the hospital ward for immediate use in this condition of grave emergency, for speed is vital in recommencing and maintaining respiratory and cardiac function by mechanical ventilation and other supportive measures.

Drugs can play an early and effective part in the subsequent routine, and are usually kept with the resuscitation outfit, together with the necessary syringes, needles, and ampoule files, etc. It will be clear that even though recommencement of heart action be successful, there will have been an interval of drastic disruption of organic function; hence, the disturbances of cardiac rhythm met when the pulse re-starts may vary greatly, and each possibility needs to be provided for. The drugs employed vary between hospitals, but the following are a representative range (according broadly with general opinion) and cater for the eventualities that may occur in the early stages.

**Lignocaine** (previously referred to, see page 61) is used to restore normal rhythm if, for example, ventricular fibrillation has set in. A large dose, of the order of 100 mg, is given by intravenous injection, often conveniently as a bolus (p. 5) into the tubing of an intravenous drip (e.g. dextrose/saline) that may have been set up, and once heart action is stabilised it is then maintained at a steady rate by giving the drug as a slow intravenous drip, e.g. 1 ml per minute of a dilute solution of 1 g (1 000 mg) in 1 litre (1 000 ml) of normal saline or dextrose/saline, i.e. 1 mg per ml.

**Sodium Bicarbonate** is given intravenously as an 8·4% solution to correct the metabolic acidosis which quickly develops due to a sharp fall in levels of the bicarbonate electrolyte. The effect is to enable the action of the heart to pick up more readily and make it less liable to revert to a state of fibrillation.

**Atropine** is given intravenously, 600 micrograms in 1 ml, if there is bradycardia (very slow heart beat). Its anticholinergic action (p. 14) inhibits the effect of the vagus nerve impulses which restrain cardiac activity; the heart is thus freed from this control and the rate and strength of beat are stimulated.

**Adrenaline** is given by intravenous injection, e.g. 5 ml of a 1 in 10 000 solution, if there is asystole (ineffective ventricular contraction). The action is one of direct stimulation of the heart muscle.

**Calcium Chloride** is also given intravenously in asystole, the ampoules usually containing 10 ml of a 20% solution of the "B.P." drug (which is equivalent to 10% of *actual* calcium chloride). The effect is to strengthen the tone of the heart muscle, so enhancing the effect of the injection of adrenaline.

**Isoprenaline** is a powerful cardiac stimulant, as explained earlier, and may be used by intravenous infusion should an acute condition of heart block arise. It is given slowly as a *dilute* solution of 1 mg in 500 ml of 5% dextrose solution.

**Hydrocortisone** is used by intravenous injection should broncho-spasm be associated with the emergency, as in the case of an asthmatic patient. Its action in this respect is referred to on page 190.

The drugs so far mentioned are typical of those which may be used *initially* to correct the arrhythmias that can occur following the recommencement of heart function. A number of other drugs may be used *subsequently* to treat the variety of symptoms that may arise, e.g. frusemide (p. 31) to promote diuresis in congestive conditions, and digoxin (p. 50) for its tonic and regulating effect on the heart. Sedation may be necessary and involve the administration of a barbiturate, e.g. amylobarbitone or phenobarbitone (p. 91), and if respiration has to be maintained with a mechanical ventilator, phenoperidine (p. 115) may be used to depress the patient's own respiratory effort and so prevent it clashing with the regular cycle of the machine.

# CHAPTER 8

# DRUGS WHICH AFFECT THE BLOOD

## —Anti-anaemics—Haemostatics—Anticoagulants.

Drugs used in the anaemias can be separated into two main classes, those used in the treatment of iron-deficiency anaemia, and those used in pernicious anaemia.

It will help the student to be reminded of the processes concerned in the formation of fully matured red blood cells. These originate in the bone marrow as large cells, called megaloblasts; they then become smaller in size (now termed normoblasts), collect haemoglobin, the iron-containing protein in the blood, and are finally released into the circulation as fully matured red blood cells, the erythrocytes. Note that iron is essential for haemoglobin formation.

### Iron-deficiency anaemia

Iron is normally available in sufficient amount in the diet, but should the absorption mechanism in the gastro-intestinal mucosa be disturbed, the intake may become inadequate; other possible causes of iron deficiency are heavy loss of blood during profuse menstruation, excessive haemorrhage following accident or surgery, and even unsuspected gastric bleeding caused by the taking of aspirin (p. 111). In all such cases the iron intake must be increased to produce the necessary level of haemoglobin.

Iron is most commonly prescribed in tablet form; the Latin word for iron is ferrum, hence the term "ferrous". One of the best forms is considered to be **Ferrous Sulphate,** usually taken as a tablet three times a day immediately after food; if taken on an empty stomach it can irritate the mucosa by its astringent, or shrinking, effect and cause nausea or even vomiting. Ferrous sulphate is also available as a mixture for children. A "milder" form of iron is **Ferrous Gluconate,** tablets of which are also taken three times daily after food, and as it is less irritant gastric upset is greatly reduced; a syrup form is acceptable and effective for children. **Ferrous fumarate** is also relatively free of gastro-intestinal side-effects and is taken as tablets or syrup.

| Ferrous Sulphate | —av. dose 200 mg |
| „ Gluconate—'Fergon' | — „   „   300 mg |
| „ Fumarate —'Fersamal'— | „   „   200 mg |

Other side-effects are also common during oral iron therapy. Thus, liquid preparations can stain the teeth, so that use of a drinking straw is of value. The astringent effect on the intestinal tract may cause constipation, leading to need for laxative treatment; incidentally, the stools are invariably a very dark colour, due to unabsorbed iron combining with the sulphur of the bowel to form black iron sulphide.

Several commercial preparations have been introduced, designed to reduce the gastro-intestinal side-effects of oral iron treatment. One is a capsule ('Feospan') containing tiny granules which disintegrate at intervals, thus spreading out the absorption of the ferrous sulphate they contain over several hours. Another is a tablet ('Ferro-Gradumet') made of plastic and impregnated with ferrous sulphate, which is released slowly on its way down the intestinal tract, the plastic body itself being eventually voided in the stool; dosage is also convenient, being once daily before breakfast. The sustained-release tablet 'Slow-Fe' also employs ferrous sulphate.

The B.N.F. Mixture of Iron and Ammonium Citrate is often better tolerated than other oral iron preparations, and the B.N.F. Paediatric Mixture of Ferrous Sulphate contains vitamin C as a stabilising agent; this is also said to aid the utilisation of iron, and is incorporated in certain commercial tablet preparations for this purpose, e.g. 'Ferrograd-C'.

Oral treatment is occasionally ineffective due to poor absorption from the gastro-intestinal mucosa, or if the haemoglobin level is dangerously low it may not produce a sufficiently rapid response. In such cases the complex iron compounds **'Imferon'** and **'Jectofer'** are employed by deep intramuscular injection, commencing with a small dose to check for allergic reaction; a point to note is that care is needed when withdrawing the needle lest any of the solution be released into the superficial tissues and cause permanent staining. The total amount of iron injection needed to raise the haemoglobin level to normal is ascertained by matching up the weight and the haemoglobin level of the patient on a chart issued by the manufacturers; this estimated total dose is then given in 5 to 10 injections at appropriate intervals.

An interesting method of administering 'Imferon' (but *not* 'Jectofer') is by "Total Dose Infusion" ("T.D.I."), the entire amount needed being added to one litre of sterile dextrose 5% solution or normal saline and given *intravenously* over a period of about six hours. This produces a dramatic response and is of special value when the haemoglobin is critically low.

## Iron poisoning

The bright colours of the various iron tablets and capsules make them attractive to young children, and cases frequently occur where a large number has been swallowed in mistake for sweets; care in storing out of reach is vital and should be impressed upon parents.

The effects of such an iron overdose can be serious and even fatal. Symptoms include gastro-intestinal damage, leading to haematemesis (blood-stained vomit) and blood-stained stools; very rapid pulse, followed by cardiovascular collapse; and damage to such organs as the liver caused by high concentrations of the metal.

Successful treatment depends greatly on speed. Firstly, the patient is given an intramuscular injection of **Desferrioxamine** (see next para.), and a gastric lavage with a solution of sodium bicarbonate, which not only removes iron remaining in the stomach but may also reduce possible damage to the gastric wall. A solution of desferrioxamine is then introduced into the stomach and allowed to remain. An intravenous drip is set up, of either normal saline or dextrose in saline and containing additional desferrioxamine, and further intramuscular injections of desferrioxamine may be given at appropriate intervals.

The role played by desferrioxamine is interesting. Ferrioxamine is a compound containing iron, and when treated to remove this iron it becomes *des*ferrioxamine, which is made available sterile in vials ready for dissolving for use. When given, it functions by taking up iron and is thus converted back to the original compound ferrioxamine. Desferrioxamine is not absorbed when taken by mouth, and thus collects all the iron in the gastro-intestinal tract, so preventing further absorption from the stomach and bowel. Given by injection as described, it takes up and removes the iron in the system in the same way, including from the liver and other organs, and is finally excreted in the urine.

Desferrioxamine—'Desferal'—vials of 500 mg

### Pernicious anaemia

Pernicious anaemia differs from iron-deficiency anaemia, in that it is the number of the red blood cells which is reduced and not the level of haemoglobin contained in them. The megaloblast/normoblast/erythrocyte cycle (p. 65) is largely governed by **Cyanocobalamin, Vitamin B$_{12}$,** which is present in the normal diet, e.g. in dairy produce and meat, and is called the *ex*trinsic factor (i.e.

the factor from without). The gastric juice contains the *in*trinsic factor (i.e. the factor from within), and this promotes the absorption of vitamin $B_{12}$, which is then stored in the liver to be called upon when required for the development of normoblasts in the bone marrow. In pernicious anaemia, the gastric juice lacks the intrinsic factor, and the essential vitamin $B_{12}$ is therefore not absorbed.

The discovery that animal liver contains the anti-anaemic factor led to extracts of liver being prepared for injection, but effects were often variable, due to differences in the anti-anaemic factor content of the livers used. Hence the importance of the discovery of the actual active principle in liver, vitamin $B_{12}$, for not only can it be given in pure form, free from the possibility of allergic reaction, but dosage is consistently accurate in effect.

Treatment of pernicious anaemia with vitamin $B_{12}$ commences with a large dose (e.g. 1 000 micrograms), followed by stabilisation on smaller doses at intervals of 3 or 4 weeks; it has to be given by injection (intramuscular) due to the patient's own inability to absorb the vitamin from the gastro-intestinal tract. Preparations containing cyanocobalamin ('Cytacon', tablets and liquid) are available for taking orally, but their employment is reserved for conditions of nutritional deficiency, etc.

**Hydroxocobalamin** (vitamin $B_{12b}$) is closely related to cyano-cobalamin (vit. $B_{12}$), and has the same use in pernicious anaemia. However, hydroxocobalamin has the advantage of providing a higher systemic level of the vitamin and also achieving this more quickly; in addition, the effect is more prolonged, and injections may be spaced out at longer intervals.

A serious factor in pernicious anaemia is damage to the nervous system (termed "sub-acute combined degeneration of the spinal cord"), and this is arrested by vitamin $B_{12}$ therapy in addition to its effect in increasing red cell formation.

Vitamin $B_{12}$ is available in many natural sources. Thus certain organisms present in the human and animal intestine produce a significant amount. But it is of unusual interest that other micro-organisms also do so when grown in suitable solutions, in particular the Streptomyces mould from which streptomycin is obtained, and it is from this latter source that the commercial injections of vitamin $B_{12}$ are prepared.

| | | | |
|---|---|---|---|
| Cyanocobalamin | —'Cytamen' | —ampoules | 250 micrograms |
| (Vitamin $B_{12}$) | | ,, | 1 000      ,, |
| Hydroxocobalamin | —'Neo-Cytamen'— | ,, | 250      ,, |
| (Vitamin $B_{12b}$) | | ,, | 1 000      ,, |

**Folic Acid**

—is a member of the vitamin B group (p. 79) and is also an essential factor in the production of the erythrocytes, the red blood cells. Thus, if it is deficient, the symptoms are closely allied to those of pernicious anaemia. Such deficiency may be caused by a poor diet or may occur in certain conditions, e.g. sprue, associated with malabsorption from the intestine; there is also an increased need of folic acid in pregnancy.

Folic acid is available as the synthetic substance in 5 mg tablets, which are occasionally employed in specific deficiency, but it is chiefly used incorporated in small amounts, e.g. 50 to 100 micrograms, in the iron tablets which are prescribed in ante-natal therapy, e.g. 'Fefol', 'Ferrograd Folic', 'Pregaday' and 'Slow-Fe Folic'.

Although folic acid has a beneficial effect in improving the red cell picture it is of no value in arresting nervous system damage, and is therefore not used in pernicious anaemia.

## THE BLOOD-CLOT SEQUENCE

In order to clarify the two remaining sections of this chapter, it will be valuable to revise the sequence of events which leads to blood clotting. When bleeding commences after an injury, the blood platelets and damaged tissue are involved in the release of the enzyme thromboplastin (also called thrombokinase), which is necessary for the conversion of prothrombin (a soluble protein produced in the liver and already circulating in the blood) into thrombin; calcium must be present for this action to take place. The thrombin then effects the conversion of another soluble protein, fibrinogen, into insoluble fibrin; a sticky mesh is formed, and this, together with red blood cells and platelets, builds up into the clot, which plugs the damaged vessel and stops the bleeding.

## HAEMOSTATICS

—are preparations used to control haemorrhage, i.e. to stop bleeding. In the main they act directly, by application to the bleeding points, but certain drugs can be said to be indirect haemostatics—these will be described later in this section.

**The Direct Haemostatics**

—are those which are used by topical (i.e. local) application. **Adrenaline** (p. 188) is used in strengths of from 1 in 1 000 to 1 in 10 000 during surgery, for its rapid constricting, or closing-up, effect on bleeding vessels, so that operations where bloodless fields are vital, for example on the eye or ear, may be performed safely.

Several direct haemostatics act by encouraging the natural process of blood clot formation. One preparation is powdered cattle **Thrombin** ("Topical Thrombin"), which is dissolved in normal saline before application to the bleeding point on a cotton wool or gauze swab; the value of a concentration of thrombin will be clear.

**Russell viper venom** ('Stypven') is another clot-accelerating application occasionally used in dental surgery, particularly in cases of patients prone to bleed readily, such as the haemophiliac; this haemostatic is also dissolved immediately prior to use.

The blood clot process can be hastened mechanically if a bed or mesh of suitable material is applied; two such preparations are **Oxidised Gauze** ('Oxycel') and **Gelatine Sponge** ('Sterispon'). Oxidised gauze is available as a sterile pad or strip which is valuable for application to deep sites where suturing of bleeding vessels is difficult. The ready-made bed quickly encourages clot formation, and it is of interest to note that the gauze itself is absorbed in a week or two. Gelatine sponge is gelatine which has been whipped into a foam and sterilised, and is available in three sizes; the routine, action and deep-site value are the same as in the case of oxidised gauze, but it is absorbed more slowly. These two mechanical haemostatics are made more effective if soaked in a solution of thrombin before use, thus encouraging clot formation in two ways.

### Indirect Haemostatics

—are described as such here because they assist *indirectly*, in their various ways, in preventing or lessening haemorrhage. They include two vitamins, two drugs which act on the uterus, and three others of distinct type which appear established in the surgical field.

The vitamins concerned are C and K, and are discussed more fully in Chapter 9. **Vitamin C** is an essential factor in the development of healthy cell tissue, and hence in maintaining the strength of the capillary walls. An adequate intake of vitamin C before surgery and during post-operative healing, and prior to dental extraction, is therefore of particular importance. **Vitamin K** is a specific anti-haemorrhagic factor, for it is concerned with the production of prothrombin in the liver and hence with the ability of the blood to clot. Its use in obstetrics (midwifery), and to arrest bleeding due to overdosage with the oral anticoagulants, is described on pages 81 and 73, respectively.

The two drugs which may be said to act as indirect haemostatics by their contracting effect on the uterus are **Oxytocin** and **Ergometrine,** and their use in reducing post-partum haemorrhage in midwifery is described on pp. 108–9. The use of vasopressin to halt bleeding from the oesophageal mucosa (p. 177) should also be noted.

**'Premarin Parenteral'** is a preparation of natural oestrogens (see also p. 198) which is used to control the bleeding that occurs during surgery and in abnormal uterine conditions; it acts by a strengthening effect on the walls of the capillary system, so preventing their breakdown and consequent oozing of blood. It is given by intravenous injection, but in the treatment of uterine bleeding tablets of 5 mg are taken in addition.

**Ethamsylate** ('Dicynene') is a synthetic preparation which also strengthens the walls of the capillaries and is likewise used to control haemorrhage during surgery or if excessive during menstruation, etc.; it is given orally as tablets and by intravenous and intramuscular injection.

**Epsilon-Amino-Caproic Acid** is used in certain conditions in which ineffective coagulation of the blood leads to excessive bleeding. This may occur in thoracic (chest) surgery, prostatectomy (removal of the prostate gland) and other instances, and is due to fibrinolysis, i.e. the breakdown of fibrin, and consequent inability of clot formation. Epsilon-amino-caproic acid ("Epsikapron") prevents this happening and haemorrhage is greatly reduced. It is taken by mouth as an effervescent powder dissolved in water, or as syrup for lower dosage. A compound closely related to epsilon-amino-caproic acid is **Tranexamic acid,** which has a similar action and is occasionally used as 'Cyklokapron' in like conditions.

## Cryoprecipitate

With regard to arresting bleeding in haemophiliacs (e.g. following bruising, etc.), fresh whole blood or fresh-frozen plasma may be used by intravenous infusion; both contain the anti-haemophilic factor normally present but which is missing in the patient's own blood. This factor can be separated from human plasma, together with other anti-haemorrhagic factors, for specific use in such cases; the preparation is a clear solution, known as "Cryoprecipitate", and is superseding fresh blood and plasma for this purpose. The prefix "cryo" refers to the fact that these factors are separated from blood *at cold temperatures*; the final product is stored under deep-freeze conditions and is thawed and warmed to body temperature just before use.

The essential factor itself, referred to above as lacking in haemophiliac blood, is known as Factor VIII. This can be isolated as the pure substance, and is available in vials ('Factorate, 'Hemofil') as a powder which is dissolved in 25 ml of Water for Injections prior to intravenous administration; solution is effected by *gentle* movement of the vial—shaking *must* be avoided—and takes about 5 minutes.

## ANTICOAGULANTS

This group of drugs has the opposite effect to that of haemostatics, and is used both therapeutically (to treat) and prophylacti-cally (to prevent) in conditions in which the formation of blood clots within the circulatory system may be a dangerous factor, for example coronary thrombosis, deep vein thrombosis, thrombo-phlebitis, pulmonary embolism, and in certain types of vascular surgery. Anticoagulants are of two distinct types, differing in both origin and action. **Heparin** is the *natural* anticoagulant of the body which circulates in the blood. It is extracted from animal tissue and made available in 5 ml vials in three strengths, 1 000 units per ml, 5 000 units per ml, and 25 000 units per·ml, and it is extremely important to read the label carefully to avoid error; it is not effective by mouth and must be given by injection—occasionally intra-muscularly, but usually intravenously. Heparin interferes with the conversion of prothrombin to thrombin and thus inhibits blood-clot formation. It will not disperse, or "dissolve", a blood clot, but will prevent it getting larger and also stop others developing. Its action is immediate but of fairly short duration, as it affects only the prothrombin actually circulating in the blood, and thus dosage has to be repeated every six to twelve hours to deal with the further prothrombin being released from the liver. Heparin is non-toxic and non-cumulative. The 5 000 unit/ml and 25 000 unit/ml are the strengths mainly used in treatment, typical dosage being 10 000–12 500 units, whilst the 1 000 unit/ml strength, and occasionally also the 5 000 unit/ml, are employed to prevent blood coagulation in tubing, etc., in such procedures as peritoneal dialysis and haemodialysis, and during use of the heart-lung machine.

The second group of anticoagulants is *synthetic,* and differs also from heparin in being active orally. **Phenindione** and **Warfarin** (particularly) are the ones chiefly used, the former in tablets of three strengths, and the latter in tablets of five, employing different colours for safety of identification; warfarin is also available as an intravenous injection. Both drugs act by reducing the formation of prothrombin *in the liver* and, in turn, its release into the blood stream; this is why they' are slower in initial effect than heparin, for it takes about 24 hours for an effective drop in the level of prothrombin release from the liver to be achieved under their in-fluence. However, their action is more prolonged, and thereafter a single daily dose is sufficient.

Phenindione—'Dindevan'—10, 25 and 50 mg tablets.
Warfarin    —'Marevan' —1, 3, 5, 10 and 20 mg tablets.

Although these two groups of anticoagulants differ in mode of action, they are often employed together when commencing treat-ment; thus, in addition to the initial injection of heparin, the patient is also given one of the oral anticoagulants. The heparin is then discontinued after 24 to 36 hours, having neutralised the circulating prothrombin during the period required by the oral anticoagulant to become effective; if warfarin has been given intravenously the heparin may be stopped after 12 hours. The patient is then maintained on daily doses of the oral anticoagulant alone. Initial dosage of the oral anticoagulants is high, and is then reduced to maintenance levels, but samples of blood are taken regularly to assess prothrombin level, the aim being to adjust the dose so that the clotting time is about $2\frac{1}{2}$ times *longer* than normal.

To sum up, heparin is effective rapidly but is of short duration, whereas the synthetic oral anticoagulants are the drugs of choice for prolonged treatment—patients may be kept on them for life, but always under careful laboratory control.

Symptoms of over-dosage with anticoagulants are spontaneous capillary bleeding (e.g. purpura in the skin), bleeding from the gums, and blood in the urine—haematuria. In such an event, the drug is discontinued or the dose reduced; in addition, both heparin and the oral anticoagulants have specific antidotes.

The antidote to heparin is **Protamine Sulphate,** a substance obtained from fish sperm. It is used if bleeding is heavy, and is given by intravenous injection, 1 mg neutralising 1 mg of heparin (or 100 units). It is interesting to note that protamine is itself an anticoagulant, *but with extremely weak effect*; it acts by taking over the function of heparin in the blood, but as it is far less active it allows the level of prothrombin activity to rise and this corrects the haemorrhagic condition.

Protamine Sulphate—10 ml ampoules of 1% solution
$( = 10$ mg per ml)

The antidote to the oral anticoagulants is **Phytomenadione,** vitamin $K_1$, which has a quicker and more powerful action than the other K vitamins; it is given by mouth as a 10 mg tablet, increasing the dose if necessary, or by slow intravenous injection if bleeding is severe or the oral route not feasible. Vitamin K is essential for the production of prothrombin in the liver (see page 69), and when given as an antidote to the oral anticoagulants (which *lessen* prothrombin release from the liver) it competes successfully with them; the blood prothrombin level then increases and bleeding stops.

Vitamin $K_1$          —'Konakion'—tablets 10 mg
(Phytomenadione)                —injection 10 mg in 1 ml

Certain drugs affect the action of the oral anticoagulants, and dosage of the latter may have to be altered on this account. Thus, for example, lessening of prothrombin production, or effect, is associated with the taking of aspirin, clofibrate (see later), paracetamol, phenylbutazone, the phenothiazine derivatives (e.g. chlorpromazine), broad-spectrum antibiotics and alcohol, all of which, in consequence, potentiate (enhance) anticoagulant action; hence, if a patient is taking any of these drugs, or alcohol, the dosage of phenindione or warfarin may need to be reduced. On the other hand barbiturates reduce the effect of oral anticoagulants; this will increase the prothrombin level and create a need for raised dosage of the anticoagulant. Patients and nursing staff should be aware of this important factor.

### Ancrod

—is an anticoagulant available in 1 ml ampoules ('Arvin') for use by intravenous injection in the treatment of deep vein thrombosis and other related conditions. It acts by reducing the level of fibrinogen in the blood, thus inhibiting clot formation (p. 69). Dosage is based on body weight, the first dose being given by intravenous *drip,* well diluted in normal saline, and subsequent maintenance doses direct from the ampoule by slow intravenous *injection* twice daily. Should its action be excessive and haemorrhage occur during treatment, it is usually sufficient to stop the drug, when normal fibrinogen levels will be resumed in a short time and bleeding then cease; but should haemorrhage cause real concern, 1 ml of a special antidote solution is given intravenously after testing for sensitivity (e.g. reddening of the skin) with a small amount by subcutaneous injection. The unique action of ancrod gives it several advantages, but its use is essentially restricted to the hospital sphere.

### Clofibrate

—is a drug which has an indirect influence on blood coagulation. It would appear that people who have high blood levels of cholesterol, a fatty substance contained in the bile, are more prone to coronary heart disease and other arterial conditions; the bore of the arteries narrows, due, it is thought, to fatty thickening of the walls. Clofibrate ('Atromid S') is given as long-term treatment in such cases, dosage being three or four 500 mg capsules daily, in divided dosage and after food; the effect is to lower blood-cholesterol levels. Clofibrate also reduces the "stickiness" of the blood platelets and the activity of prothrombin in the blood, both of which effects are further factors in lessening the possibility of clots forming in the blood vessels (as in coronary thrombosis); thus it is said to potentiate anticoagulant therapy. For this reason, when clofibrate is added to the treatment of a patient already on anticoagulants, the dosage of the latter is reduced to about half the previous level as a precautionary measure against the risk of spontaneous haemorrhage occurring.

A reference now to the use of **Sodium Citrate** in preventing blood clotting. It will be recalled that calcium is essential for the formation of a blood clot; sodium citrate acts by converting this into calcium citrate, which, being insoluble, becomes ineffective. Hence, sodium citrate solution (usually 3.8%) is used in syringes or bottles when blood samples are taken, and as an irrigation at the same strength following prostatectomy, etc., where the formation of blood clots is undesirable. Sodium acid citrate is an acidic form of sodium citrate which is used by the Blood Transfusion Service to maintain the clot-free condition of donor blood (see page 43).

## Streptokinase

An enzyme is a substance which can effect chemical changes in other bodies without being itself altered in the process. Streptokinase is an enzyme produced by certain streptococci (p. 126), which is purified and made available as 'Kabikinase' or 'Streptase'. Streptokinase possesses the property of inducing changes in a thrombus, or clot, which lead eventually to its breakdown and dissolution (i.e. it is "dissolved"). Hence, streptokinase is used in serious clotting conditions, such as deep vein thrombosis and pulmonary embolism; in such cases the removal of the clot by dissolution may be expected to restore the normal flow of blood. A possible problem is difficulty in controlling dosage.

Streptokinase is issued as a vial of dried powder which is stored in the refrigerator and dissolved for use as required, further diluting to 100 ml or 500 ml for giving by intravenous infusion. The point is worth making, from the handling aspect, that this is one of the most *expensive* drugs in therapy; it can, of course, be life-saving.

# CHAPTER 9

# THE VITAMINS

A vitamin is a special and essential substance, the absence of which from the diet produces symptoms of a deficiency condition. The condition involved may be of a specific nature caused by gross deficiency, due either to inability to absorb the vitamin or to its absence from the diet; or it may be merely the general vitamin lack which can accompany unintelligent diet or loss of appetite, etc. Thus, vitamin therapy may be specific, as when direct replacement need is clearly indicated, or it may be merely supplementary, e.g. during convalescence or in general debility. The range of dosage is, accordingly, very wide.

The vitamins are labelled in alphabetical sequence.

## Vitamin A

—is present in dairy products, e.g. eggs, milk and butter, and in fish-liver oils such as those of cod and halibut; also, carrots and green vegetables contain a substance, carotene, which is converted to vitamin A after absorption. Vitamin A is an essential factor in the development and healthy function of the surface tissue of the skin and the mucous membranes, especially those of organs concerned with the process of secretion, such as the eyes, mouth and bronchi, etc. It is also concerned with the capacity of vision to accommodate itself to poor light conditions, and deficiency of the vitamin may lead to night-blindness, or inability to "see in the dark".

Vitamin A is frequently given with vitamin D in the natural form contained in cod or halibut liver oil for its beneficial effect in growing children; the form used in treatment is mainly synthetic. It is occasionally employed in certain chronic inflammatory eye conditions and in skin diseases, but is rarely indicated as specific replacement in serious deficiency, for this is uncommon in communities enjoying a normal diet.

Vitamin A—'Ro-A-Vit'—tablets

## Vitamin D

—although not in alphabetical order, this vitamin usually follows vitamin A, for both are found associated in many natural sources, such as the dairy products and fish liver oils already mentioned. Another source of vitamin D is the effect of sunlight on the skin; this converts a closely related substance present into the vitamin, which is then stored in the liver, to be called upon as required. The function of vitamin D is to promote the absorption of calcium and phosphorus from the small intestine, for even though the diet be rich in these two factors, which are essential for bone (calcium phosphate) formation, they cannot be ingested unless vitamin D is present in the bowel wall. Lack of calcium and phosphorus absorption leads to poor bone and teeth formation in children, and in severe cases to rickets (now rarely met in the more highly developed countries), hence the description of vitamin D as the anti-rachitic, or "anti-rickets", vitamin.

An interesting point concerns immigrants from sunny climes (e.g. the West Indies). Parents may be unaware of the part played by sunshine in the production of vitamin D in the body (see earlier). Hence they may neglect the special need, in dull areas (as in this country), for their children to have adequate sources of vitamin D in the diet to compensate.

Vitamin D is available in synthetic form as tablets and solutions in oil (it is a fat-soluble vitamin, see later), and is occasionally used in conditions in which calcium absorption is impaired—as in coeliac disease in children, or where a seriously low level of calcium in the blood is due to impaired function of the parathyroid glands, as in tetany (p. 180); in the latter condition, a related compound, dihydrotachysterol, is given orally as a solution in oil (see also page 181). The need for vitamin D intake is heightened during pregnancy and breast feeding; in the elderly it is thought to maintain firmness of bone and may be a factor in preventing development of the brittle condition known as osteoporosis.

Vitamin D—**Calciferol**—tablets and solution in oil
—Dihydrotachysterol—'A.T. 10'

## The Vitamin B Group

—comprises several members, those normally employed in medicine being $B_1$, $B_2$, nicotinic acid, $B_6$, and $B_{12}$; with the exception of the last named, symptoms of serious deficiency are rarely met under normal diet conditions, and thus their use lacks the more specific application of some of the other vitamins.

## Vitamin $B_1$

—is present in yeast, pork, eggs, peas and beans, and wheat germ; it plays an important part in the metabolism of carbohydrates, i.e. sugar, bread and other starchy foods. If it is lacking, the break-down process is halted, and degeneration of nerve tissue may develop and lead to forms of neuritis and mental fatigue. Thus, vitamin $B_1$ can be said to be essential for the health and function of the nervous system.

The vitamin $B_1$ used in medicine is synthetic, and tablets are employed as a dietary supplement where thought necessary; it is contained with other B vitamins in the food products 'Bemax' and 'Marmite'. Vitamin $B_1$ is used in the treatment of certain serious types of neuritis, and, together with other vitamins, is given by i/m or i/v injection as an essential part of nutrition where the oral route is impracticable (see page 80).

Vitamin $B_1$—**Thiamine** (or Aneurine)—'Benerva'

### Vitamin $B_2$

—is a yellow pigment found in liver, yeast and other vegetable and animal sources; it is concerned in the metabolism of carbo-hydrates and is thought to be essential to the proper function of vision. It is available in synthetic form as tablets and injection, and is mainly prescribed in conditions of sore mouth, tongue and lips, and in inflammatory disorders of the eye.

Vitamin $B_2$—**Riboflavine**—'Beflavit'

### Nicotinic Acid

—occurs in liver, cereals, milk and cheese, etc.; it is also an essential factor in the breakdown of carbohydrates, and true deficiency (rarely met) can lead to dermatitis and gastro-intestinal and mental dis-orders. It is available as tablets and injections, and in addition to its use in combination with other vitamins as a supplement, it is employed for improving blood circulation by its dilating effect on the peripheral capillary system, e.g. in such conditions as chil-blains (p. 58). Derivatives such as nicotinyl alcohol and inositol nicotinate are used in the more serious conditions of circulatory spasm, e.g. Raynaud's disease (p. 58).

The uncomfortable prickling sensation of the skin which is a side-effect of treatment with nicotinic acid has been mentioned on page 58; a derivative, **Nicotinamide,** is free of this action and can be used instead, except where vasodilatation is required, in which it is little value.

A natural source of many members of the vitamin B complex exists in the human intestine, where they are produced by micro-organisms normally present. Many of these organisms are destroyed by the broad-spectrum antibiotics, and the administration of compound tablets of thiamine (Tab. Thiamin. Co.) to compensate for this loss is described on page 140.

'Tab. Thiamin. Co.—Vitamins $B_1$ and $B_2$, with Nicotinic Acid
'Becosym' contains Vitamins $B_1$, $B_2$ and $B_6$, with Nicotinamide
'Beplete'          „          Vitamins $B_1$ and $B_2$, with Nicotinamide
'Orovite'          „          Vitamins $B_1$, $B_2$, $B_6$, with Nicotinamide and
Vitamin C

## Vitamin $B_6$

—is found in eggs, peas and beans, and yeast, and also in animal sources, and is an essential factor in the metabolism of protein; it is available as the synthetic substance in tablet and injection form. It has an anti-emetic effect and is mainly employed for alleviating the morning sickness of pregnancy, and also the distressing vomiting which often follows radiotherapy and treatment with the corresponding anti-cancer drugs (see page 203).

Vitamin $B_6$—**Pyridoxine**—'Benadon'

## Vitamin $B_{12}$—Cyanocobalamin (also $B_{12b}$—Hydroxycobalamin)

—is the most important of the essential factors necessary for the production of red blood cells, and its use in the treatment of pernicious anaemia is fully discussed in Chapter 8. It is perhaps the best example of a vitamin used as replacement in specific deficiency.

## Folic Acid

—is a B vitamin, and is an essential factor in the production of red blood cells; it is yellow in colour, and natural sources are green leaves, liver, yeast and milk. Its use in tablet form in certain anaemias (but not in pernicious anaemia) is described on page 69.

## Vitamin C

—is found in fresh fruit, particularly the citrus group (lemons, oranges and limes), rose hips and blackcurrants, and also in green vegetables; it is known as the anti-scorbutic (i.e. anti-scurvy) vitamin, for prolonged absence from the diet results in scurvy (now rarely met), a condition typified by bleeding which occurs in many parts of the body. It is an essential factor in the development of cartilage, teeth and bone formation, etc., and in maintaining a healthy condition of cell tissue; in deficiency, the walls of the capillaries tend to become fragile, and spontaneous bleeding, e.g. of the gums, may occur.

Vitamin C is ascorbic acid (so named from its anti-scorbutic action) and the form mainly used in treatment is synthetic, as tablets and injections; however, the natural vitamin contained in Blackcurrant and Rose-hip Syrups and in Orange Juice is of value, particularly in the case of infants and growing children. This vitamin has a number of applications. Thus, if fruit and vegetables are contra-indicated, as in the restricted diet which may be prescribed for patients with peptic ulcer, tablets of ascorbic acid are taken as a source of vitamin C replacement. Daily intake encourages the healing processes and building up of healthy tissue, and this applies especially following operations and in long-term convalescence. Gums which bleed easily are a further indication for vitamin C therapy.

If vitamin C deficiency is suspected to be a significant factor in certain conditions, the ascorbic acid saturation test is used to confirm (see page 224).

Vitamin C is held to aid resistance to infection, and there is a vogue for the taking of massive doses in effervescent tablet form for the prevention of colds; also, it is now thought that regular daily intake of 1 gram, or even more, is highly beneficial to general health.

Vitamin C—**Ascorbic Acid**—'Redoxon'

**Vitamin E**

—is present in lettuce, dairy products and wheat germ, and is probably concerned with the metabolism of protein and tissue; it is used as the synthetic substance in tablet and injection form. It is claimed to be of benefit in intermittent claudication (p. 58), when it is given in high dosage for several months, but it would appear to be of limited value in the other indications in which it is occasionally employed.

Vitamin E—**Tocopherol**—'Ephynal'

**The parenteral use of vitamin combinations**

In the case of severely ill patients who can be fed only by the injection route, as referred to on page 45, the vitamin preparations used in ampoule form (e.g. 'Parentrovite') comprise the vitamin B group ($B_1$, $B_2$, $B_6$ and nicotinic acid), together with vitamin C. Two types are used, intramuscular and intravenous, and in each case there is a high-potency ampoule for commencing treatment and a maintenance dose for continuation. The B vitamins and vitamin C do not keep well in the same solution, hence they are issued in separate ampoules, which are mixed just before use. The B vitamins in this preparation are also of value in correcting disturbed mental conditions, such as delirium tremens resulting from acute alcoholism (see also chlormethiazole, page 94).

'Multibionta' is an injection solution containing the vitamins A, C and E, with the full B complex; a 10 ml ampoule, added to 500 ml of infusion fluid, is given intravenously once daily.

## Vitamin K

—is referred to in the section dealing with haemostatics (p. 70), and, as stated, it is essential for the production in the liver of prothrombin, which is necessary for the formation of the blood clot; it is thus termed the anti-haemorrhagic vitamin. Vitamin K is found as phytomenadione ($K_1$) in green leaves (especially spinach) and animal sources, but, as with most of the vitamins, synthetic forms are used in treatment; these are usually based on, or related to, menaphthone, and are available as tablets and injections.

Vitamin K is used in deficiency due to impaired absorption from the intestine and in the prevention of bleeding. This vitamin is fat soluble and thus requires the presence of bile in the intestine to ensure its ingestion. Hence it is given by injection when bile is absent, e.g. in obstruction of the bile duct; or a water soluble derivative (e.g. 'Synkavit') may be given by mouth, as it does not need bile for absorption.

The most important use of vitamin K, however, is in the prevention and treatment of bleeding. Phytomenadione, vitamin $K_1$, has a quicker and more powerful action than the menaphthone derivatives, and its use as the specific antidote to overdosage with the oral anticoagulants is discussed on page 73. It may also be given to the mother before childbirth, or administered in a small "neo-natal" dose of 1 mg to the infant itself, to prevent haemorrhagic complications which may be caused by too low an initial blood prothrombin level.

Vitamin K —**Menaphthone** —injection
—**Acetomenaphthone**—tablets
—water soluble —'Synkavit' (tablets and
derivative injection)
Vitamin $K_1$—**Phytomenadione** —'Konakion'

It is sometimes the custom to designate vitamins as being either "fat-soluble" or "water soluble". The fat soluble ones are A, D, E and K, and the water soluble are the B Complex and C. However, there are certain deviations from these groupings, as in the case of the commercial preparation 'Synkavit', a form of vitamin K which is water soluble. A point to note is that the fat-soluble vitamins require the presence of bile in the intestine before they can be absorbed. Also, because they are fat-soluble, they may dissolve in liquid paraffin if this is being taken as a laxative, and hence absorption can be reduced (see page 19).

## TONICS

There is continued faith in the value of tonics in tablet or liquid form, and the greater and more lasting benefit of a healthy mode of living, together with a rational diet, is not sufficiently appreciated. However, in convalescence or "run-down" conditions, tonics have a place. Commercial preparations often contain vitamins, such as A, C and D, with the B Complex, and also iron; for children, particularly, such a combination has undoubted value.

Tonic preparations may also contain glycerophosphate compounds, which are held to be useful in debility, and "bitters", i.e. drugs of plant origin such as gentian, are employed in mixtures taken before meals to improve appetite.

### Compound Vitamin preparations and Tonics

'Abidec'    —Vitamins A, B, C and D—capsules and drops
'Multivite' —Vitamins A, B, C and D—tablets
'Juvel'      —Vitamins A, $B_1$, $B_2$, $B_6$ and C with Nicotinamide
                                        —tablets and elixir
'Minadex' —Vitamins A and D with Iron—syrup
'Metatone'—Vitamin $B_1$ with Glycerophosphates—liquid

Gentian Mixtures (acid or alkaline), B.N.F.

# CHAPTER 10

# DRUGS USED FOR THEIR EFFECT ON THE RESPIRATORY SYSTEM

*—expectorants—sedatives—bronchodilators and antispasmodics—stimulants—oxygen and carbon dioxide*

The respiratory system includes both the upper and lower respiratory tracts, but this Chapter is concerned with the latter only; the drugs and preparations used in conditions of the upper passages, the oral and nasal, etc., are referred to in Chapter 20.

The lungs are concerned with the breathing process (respiration), in which air is inhaled and then exhaled, part of its oxygen content being exchanged for carbon dioxide during its stay in the lung. This "gaseous exchange" takes place through the membranes of the alveoli (the air sacs of the lungs), the blood circulating through them giving up carbon dioxide and receiving oxygen in place; the blood supply concerned is that of the pulmonary circulation referred to on page 49. Many factors disturb the effective functioning of respiration, examples being infection, *smoking*, pulmonary oedema, and depression of the controlling respiratory centre in the brain by drugs or disease. The drugs used in treatment are of a similarly varied pattern.

## EXPECTORANTS

—are used to ease and stimulate the expulsion of bronchial secretion. They provide relief in conditions in which the chest is distressingly "tight", the sputum is viscid (thick and sticky), and the cough is unable to dislodge it and "bring it up". An expectorant mixture taken several times daily in hot water will liquefy or "thin" the bronchial secretion, enabling it to be disengaged more easily; it may also strengthen the cough action so that the sputum is brought up with less difficulty and breathing made more comfortable. Expectorant mixtures may also be useful in unproductive cough, because the liquid secretion which they stimulate acts as a soothing coating to dry bronchial tissue. Amongst the ingredients used in expectorant mixtures are **Ammonium Bicarbonate, Ammonium Chloride, Sodium Bicarbonate, Potassium Iodide** and **Tincture of Ipecacuanha.**

A simple but effective expectorant is the Sodium Chloride Compound Mixture of the B.N.F., which contains sodium bicarbonate and sodium chloride and is flavoured with aniseed; taken (in sips) in a glassful of hot water, it enables the patient to bring up sputum readily and so clear the lungs.

Inhalation of **steam** from the steam-kettle is also of undoubted clearing value in bronchitis in children, and the use of certain additions to steaming water in the Nelson Inhaler is mentioned on page 218.

## Mucolytic Agents

—are also employed in conditions where bronchial secretion is thick, or where it tends to harden and cause obstruction as may occasionally happen in tracheostomy tubes. The method of use is by inhalation as a fine spray or instillation as drops, whichever is appropriate, and the effect is one of thinning the secretion and preventing it from becoming tenacious. A preparation commonly used and which has a wetting/thinning action on mucus is **Superinone** ('Alevaire'), and another of different type is **Acetylcysteine** ('Airbron').

**Bromhexine** ('Bisolvon') is taken orally, and its action in increasing bronchial secretion and reducing viscosity (stickiness) of sputum appears to be established; injections are also available. "Alupent Expectorant" is a mixture which combines the action of bromhexine with the bronchodilating and antispasmodic effect of orciprenaline (p. 85).

## Atropine

Drugs are also used to lessen, or dry up, bronchial secretion. The most prominent example is atropine, and its employment in pre-operative medication is referred to on page 113.

## ◆ COUGH SEDATIVES

—are used to lessen or prevent cough. Those of mild or medium action are employed to treat the cough or "tickle" caused by irritation of the throat or larynx. They are usually in thick syrup or linctus form, to be taken neat and sipped slowly, the main effect being to soothe locally as they pass down; an example of this type is the B.N.F. Linctus Simplex.

The Squill Opiate Linctus of the B.N.F. contains a small amount of morphine, and has a more sedative action; it is well known by its old name of Gee's Linctus. Linctus Codeine and Linctus

Pholcodine are more useful as cough suppressants on account of their subduing effect on the cough centre in the brain. An average dose of these linctuses is 5 ml. Sedative cough mixtures are also prescribed, e.g. the B.N.F. Ipecacuanha and Morphine Mixture, the action again being helped by a small content of morphine. It should be mentioned that cough sedatives may be contra-indicated, or need to be used with discretion, in cases where movement and expulsion of sputum is desirable.

Lung cancer may be associated with a non-productive cough, when the severe pain of effort or spasm is a serious problem; hence the need for a specific sedative which will powerfully depress the cough centre in the brain. Two such preparations are Linctus Heroin (Diamorphine) and Linctus Methadone, both in 5 ml dosage and controlled by the CD Regulations; these drugs are referred to more fully on pp. 113 and 114. Methadone is not well tolerated by children, and safety in dosage of the linctus for paediatric use is usually ensured by its being diluted with seven times its volume of syrup, thus making it one eighth of the strength of that used for adults.

It should be noted that the efficacy of cough sedative preparations often depends on the depressant action on the respiratory centre of active principles derived from opium, e.g. codeine and morphine, and allied drugs such as pholcodine, diamorphine and methadone.

## BRONCHODILATORS AND ANTISPASMODICS

—are used in conditions in which the bronchi are contracted in spasm and breathing is difficult, as in asthma and bronchitis; they provide great relief and are in wide use.

**Ephedrine** has long been used for this purpose, mainly in tablet form (av. dose 30 mg); it is also an ingredient of many commercial remedies used in asthma. Whilst it dilates and relaxes the bronchi, ephedrine has an opposite, shrinking effect when applied to the nasal mucosa (see page 216).

**Adrenaline,** which is described more fully in Chapter 18, is chemically related to ephedrine and the actions of these two drugs are likewise similar, adrenaline being a powerful bronchodilator and antispasmodic. It is, however, not effective by mouth, and is given by slow subcutaneous injection in acute asthma, 0·5 ml of the 1 in 1 000 solution being an average dose; it is now more rarely used for this purpose.

**Orciprenaline** ('Alupent') is related to adrenaline and has similar action in asthma, but differs by being effective *orally*; it is taken as tablets or syrup (note also 'Alupent Expectorant', p. 84), and is also much employed in inhaler form (see later).

The bronchial spasm of asthma can be effectively controlled with drugs by inhalation; thus, 1% solutions of adrenaline can be sprayed into the mouth, the patient inhaling at the same time and thus bringing the drug directly into the bronchi to provide instant relief. The modern approach, however, is the commercial pressurised inhaler, of which many are available. Typical inhalers of this type are the 'Alupent', containing orciprenaline (see earlier), and the 'Medihaler-Iso', containing **isoprenaline**, which is also related to adrenalin and has similar effect. These cleverly designed units are small and convenient to carry, and on finger pressure deliver a fine aerosol, or mist-spray, into the mouth, the patient inhaling simultaneously; many are designed to give an accurately measured, or "metered", dose each time. However, it should be noted that the very ease of use itself can encourage over-indulgence by the asthma patient who seeks relief so anxiously, and grossly excessive use has resulted in fatalities due to the acute stimulation of the heart which is a feature of the action of this type of drug (see isoprenaline, page 62). Hence the need to advise patients to use such pocket inhalers with patience and commonsense.

A pocket inhaler with more prolonged effect is based on **Salbutamol** ('Ventolin'), which also has the decided advantage that it has less tendency to produce palpitations by cardiac stimulation than the other types, and is thus safer in use. Salbutamol is also available in oral form, including the 'Spandet', a sustained-action tablet, and as an injection for use in acute asthmatic spasm.

Awareness of the cardiac risk associated with certain inhaler preparations is leading to the introduction of safer compounds in this form; examples are **Ipratropium** ('Atrovent') and **Terbutaline** ('Bricanyl'). Nevertheless, it deserves repeating that *all* inhaler preparations should be used strictly as directed and with due patience.

A different approach to asthma, i.e. *prevention,* is the use of **Sodium Cromoglycate** ('Intal'), as capsule "cartridges" which are inserted into a special 'Spinhaler' insufflator and the powder inhaled as required. The effect is to block the development of the patient's allergic reaction (p. 101) to his own particular allergen (the cause of the asthma in this case), of which pollen and house-dust are typical examples. Cartridges are also available ('Intal Compound') which include a little isoprenaline to cover any initial spasm caused by the irritant effect of the powder, as may happen in certain sensitive patients. Sodium cromoglycate is also used in the prophylaxis of hayfever (p. 217).

The 'Becotide' metered-dose inhaler contains **Beclomethasone,** a powerful anti-inflammatory steroid compound (p. 188) which is also used in the prophylactic treatment of asthma. It is highly active in the lung at low concentration levels, absorption is claimed to be minimal, and the unpleasant side-effects associated with steroid treatment are thus limited. 'Becotide' inhalation is indicated for supplementing customary bronchodilator treatment if the latter is becoming ineffective; for patients who do not respond to sodium cromoglycate; and, more especially, as total or partial replacement of the *oral* steroids (p. 190) required to control asthma in some patients, with consequent benefit in avoiding or reducing the side-effects referred to earlier. However, patients should still be sure to conserve use within the range of the directions.

**Aminophylline,** in addition to its diuretic and cardiac tonic effect (see pages 29 and 53), has a useful bronchodilating and antispasmodic action. It is contained in many oral combinations and can also be given by intramuscular and intravenous injection, the latter being dramatically successful in acute bronchial spasm, $0.25$ g in 10 ml being given *very slowly*—this is important. A form of aminophylline of great value in patients with dyspnoea (difficulty in breathing) is the suppository, which, inserted per rectum at bedtime, releases the drug slowly into the system via the rectal wall and thus assists in maintaining respiratory comfort throughout the night.

## RESPIRATORY STIMULANTS

—are used in conditions where breathing may be abnormally weak or difficult, as in pneumonia, bronchitis and acute asthma; they act by stimulating the respiratory centre in the brain.

**Nikethamide** is given by subcutaneous or intramuscular injection, or intravenously when rapid effect is essential; in addition to its stimulation of the respiratory centre, it makes this centre more sensitive to carbon dioxide levels in the blood (see page 89).

**Prethcamide** has a direct stimulant effect on the respiratory centre; it is given by intramuscular or intravenous injection, and is also taken as capsules by patients who are subject to hypoventilation, a condition of weakened respiration where there is insufficiency of exchange of stale air for fresh. The strengthened respiration results in an increase in tidal volume (the amount of air inhaled and exhaled during normal breathing) and an improvement in gaseous exchange and oxygenation of the blood.

**Doxapram** is a powerful respiratory stimulant, and is used as $\frac{1}{2}$ litre bottles of dilute solution for intravenous infusion in cases of acute respiratory failure, and as 5 ml ampoules for intravenous injection in supporting weakened respiration—as may occur following surgery or the administration of narcotic analgesics (referred to later).

**Aminophylline,** in addition to its actions as a diuretic, cardiac tonic, and bronchodilator and relaxant, is also said to have a valuable stimulant effect on respiration when given by injection, and is one of the drugs of choice in severe asthma, as mentioned earlier.

Nikethamide (25%) soln.)—'Coramine'—av. dose 5–10 ml
Prethcamide                —'Micoren' — ,,   ,,   225 mg
                                    and as capsules of 400 mg
Doxapram                  —'Dopram' —av. dose 5 ml
                                                (100 mg)

**Nalorphine, Naloxone** and **Levallorphan** are further drugs employed to treat or prevent respiratory weakness. The mode of action of all three lies in their ability to reverse the effects of the narcotic analgesics (p. 113), which include, in particular, *depression of the respiratory centre* (p. 115) and consequent weakness of breathing. Thus, nalorphine and naloxone are used postoperatively should the patient's respiration be weak following the use of a narcotic drug, e.g. papaveretum; narcotic poisoning or overdosage is another indication. Levallorphan is combined with pethidine in the injection 'Pethilorfan', which is much used in obstetrics (midwifery); the pethidine provides the required analgesia and relaxation to the mother, and the danger of respiratory depression in the infant is prevented by the levallorphan component (which passes the placental barrier following administration by injection to the mother). Nalorphine and naloxone are also used in this connection, either by administration to the mother beforehand or to the infant in neo-natal dosage following delivery. Naloxone has additional importance in that it can be used to reverse the adverse effect on respiration of pentazocine; nalorphine and levallorphan are of no value in this event.

Nalorphine      —'Lethidrone' —av. dose 10 mg
                —'Neonatal'    — ,,   ,,   1 mg
Naloxone        —'Narcan'      — ,,   ,,   1 ml (400
                                            micrograms)
                —'Neonatal'    — ,,   ,,   1–1·5 ml (20–30
                                            micrograms)
Levallorphan    —'Lorfan'      — ,,   ,,   1 mg
(with Pethidine—'Pethilorfan')

Pulmonary oedema, infection, and the consequences of excessive smoking have been mentioned at the beginning of this Chapter. In pulmonary oedema, the powerful diuretics, e.g. frusemide, afford relief from respiratory distress by their action in increasing the output of urine and in turn the withdrawal of fluid from the wet and swollen lung tissue (p. 31). The antibacterial drugs (e.g. the sulphonamides and antibiotics) are used in chest infections, such as may supervene in the common cold or influenza and result in pneumonia, and a number are employed in the treatment of tuberculosis; these are dealt with in Chapter 14. The malignant condition of the lung which may result from smoking is sometimes treated with cytotoxic drugs; these are described in Chapter 19.

## OXYGEN AND CARBON DIOXIDE

**Oxygen** is used by inhalation in conditions where respiratory weakness leads to deficiency of its uptake from the lungs by the blood, e.g. pulmonary oedema, pneumonia, emphysema (lack of elasticity of lung tissue), and depression of the respiratory centre in cases of poisoning, etc. It is usually mixed with air so that a known percentage of oxygen is being inhaled; this is achieved with appropriate masks, tents and nasal catheter units—including the oxygen "spectacles".

If the administration is prolonged, e.g. for more than 20 minutes or so, it is usual for the gas to be humidified, or "moistened", by bubbling it through warm water. A useful word of caution is that oxygen can be given *too* freely to "chronic chest" patients, whose strength of respiration may depend not, as is normal, on carbon dioxide levels in the blood (see later), but on the extent of their own intake of oxygen. If oxygen is given too freely to such patients it may actually lead to increased weakness of respiration, hence the value of giving it with due moderation by using the "Ventimask" which will deliver dilutions of oxygen with air, ranging from 24% to 35%.

Points to note are that cylinders containing oxygen are coloured black, with white shoulder, and that the gas is inflammable and explosive; oil is never used to lubricate the reducing-valve assemblies which control the output of gas from the cylinder, for this can be a cause of violent explosion.

**Carbon Dioxide** is given by inhalation as a mixture with oxygen (5–7% of carbon dioxide being usual) in order to strengthen breathing, for a raised level of carbon dioxide in the blood acts as a direct stimulant to the respiratory centre in the brain. In addition to their reinforcing effect, such mixtures may be used to recommence breathing in cases of crisis, as in drowning, and even to initiate it, as in the new-born. A further use is in the Operating Theatre, to stimulate respiration and so enable speedy elimination of the anaesthetic which the patient has been inhaling. Carbon dioxide is not inflammable, and the cylinders containing the pure gas are painted grey. Cylinders containing a mixture of oxygen and carbon dioxide are painted black, with grey and white quarterings on neck and shoulder.

## THE NERVOUS SYSTEM

comprises—

(a) The brain and spinal cord; this is termed the central nervous system ("C.N.S.");

(b) the motor nerves, concerned with activity, which emanate *from* the spinal cord and are under conscious control;

(c) the sensory nerves, which conduct sensation (e.g. pain) *to* the spinal cord and brain;

and (d) the autonomic nervous system ("A.N.S.")—already referred to on pages 13 and 14), which is self-regulating and free of conscious control.

The next three chapters are concerned largely with drugs which act on the nervous system, e.g. by sedative, stimulant, analgesic or anaesthetic effect.

# CHAPTER 11

# HYPNOTICS AND SEDATIVES

*with anticonvulsants: tranquillizers and antidepressants: antihistamines: amphetamines: anorectics: drugs used in Parkinsonism: muscle relaxants: cholinergic drugs: drugs acting on the uterus*

## HYPNOTICS AND SEDATIVES

Hypnotics are used to induce sleep, and the value of a restful night gives this group of drugs a high place in medical treatment. Many of these drugs are also used in low, or "sub-hypnotic" dosage for their sedative effect during the day.

The **Barbiturates** have long been widely used hypnotics, but the prescribing of them is diminishing significantly on account of the associated misuse and danger; they are given orally, some also by injection, and act by depressing the brain. The best known is **Phenobarbitone;** the action of this drug is rather prolonged, and thus it is mainly used for day-time sedation in small dosage, and for its anti-convulsant effect in epilepsy (see page 94). Thus the barbiturates chiefly used as hypnotics are **Amylobarbitone, Butobarbitone, Pentobarbitone** and **Quinalbarbitone,** the action of the first three being of medium onset and duration—about eight hours, and the last (quinalbarbitone) particularly rapid and rather shorter lasting. Amylobarbitone is also favoured for daytime sedation in small dosage. All may be used for their hypnotic effect in pre-operative medication. A capsule combination of amylobarbitone and quinalbarbitone ('Tuinal') is claimed to induce sleep quickly with the quinalbarbitone and maintain it with the longer-acting amylobarbitone.

| | | | | | |
|---|---|---|---|---|---|
| Phenobarbitone | —'Luminal' | —av. hypnotic dose | | | 60 mg |
| | | „ | sedative | „ | 30 mg |
| Amylobarbitone | —'Amytal' | — „ | hypnotic | „ | 100 mg |
| | | „ | sedative | „ | 30 mg |
| Butobarbitone | —'Soneryl' | — „ | hypnotic | „ | 100 mg |
| Pentobarbitone | —'Nembutal' | — „ | „ | „ | 100 mg |
| Quinalbarbitone | —'Seconal' | — „ | „ | „ | 100 mg |

**Thiopentone** and **Methohexitone** are two barbiturates of extremely short action and are employed soley as anaesthetics (see page 120).

It is important to note that the action of the barbiturates is potentiated (i.e. made more powerful) by alcohol, and it is possible for the taking of a number of alcoholic drinks to convert a high but normally safe hypnotic dose into a fatal one. The barbiturates are generally held to be non-addictive, but they can easily become habit-forming, and true addiction is not unknown, a condition of gravity equalling that of narcotic addiction. They are governed by the Scheduled-Poisons Regulations, and many hospitals employ the excellent routine of recording the administration of each dose and balancing ward stocks.

A not uncommon side-effect of barbiturate hypnotics is a "hang-over" feeling for some hours after waking the following morning, and this is particularly noticeable as mental confusion and dizziness in the elderly patient.

Massive overdosage is a common form of suicide attempt. In such an event the patient will be in a coma, reflex action will be absent, and there will be retention of urine; the principal effect, however, is profound depression of the respiratory centre, and death may result from paralysis of this centre or from the broncho-pneumonia which can supervene following a lengthy period of weak and shallow breathing. Treatment may include gastric lavage (stomach washout) if the drug has been taken within the previous few hours, and the use of forced diuresis, involving the intravenous infusion of large volumes of fluid (p. 37), in order to increase excretion of the barbiturate in the urine; the patient then emerges very slowly on his own from the deep plane of sleep, an antibiotic, e.g. penicillin, being given if there appears risk of development of pneumonia. In severe cases involving extreme overdosage, or when kidney function is suspect, resort may be had to peritoneal dialysis or even haemodialysis, routines which are discussed on pages 35 and 36.

## Other hypnotics

The established place of hypnotics, and the frequency of misuse of the barbiturates, has led to the introduction of several tablet alternatives claimed to offer advantages. Four that are quite distinct are **Glutethimide, Nitrazepam, Flurazepam** and **'Mandrax'**. Nitrazepam and flurazepam are related to the tranquilliser drug diazepam (p. 99), and are said to act not by depressing the brain but by shielding it from external stimuli which interfere with sleep; they are thus claimed to have a great margin of safety. 'Mandrax' is a combination of the antihistamine drug diphenhydramine (p. 103) and the hypnotic methaqualone; the latter component now makes it "CD", i.e. a Controlled Drug (p. 251).

Glutethimide—'Doriden' —tablets,     250 mg
Nitrazepam —'Mogadon'—     „        5 mg
Flurazepam —'Dalmane' —capsules,   15 mg & 30 mg

## Chloral Hydrate

This is one of the oldest hypnotics but is still used; it is a white crystalline substance with a sweet smell but unpleasant taste, and acts by depressing the brain, providing a sound "natural" sleep. The B.N.F. Mixture of Chloral contains 1 gram in 20 ml, flavoured with syrup, an average dose being 10—20 ml for adults, and 2·5—10 ml for children, for whom it is a very suitable hypnotic. Mixtures containing chloral should be well diluted with water due to its caustic effect on the oral and gastric mucosa; note, however, that the Paediatric Chloral *Elixir* of the B.P.C. is given neat, i.e. undiluted. The unpleasant taste has lead to the introduction of chloral derivatives (related drugs) in tablet or capsule form, these being dichloralphenazone ('Welldorm') and triclofos ('Tricloryl'); both are also available as syrups.

## Hyoscine

—also known as scopolamine, is a powerful hypnotic of plant origin (henbane) which acts by depressing the brain. It is usually given by injection as pre-operative medication with morphine, papaveretum or pethidine (p. 113) in order to calm the patient; it also reduces bronchial secretion. The average dose is 0·4—0·6 mg (400—600 micrograms).

Other uses of hyoscine are as eye drops for its dilating action on the pupil (p. 212), and as an anti-emetic in travel sickness (p. 17).

## Paraldehyde

—has been used for many years as a hypnotic. It is a clear liquid with a penetrating and unpleasant smell and taste, and its powerful effect is similar to that of chloral, providing a prolonged and deep sleep. Paraldehyde can be given in three ways—orally (up to 10 ml), in the form of a well-diluted and flavoured draught; per rectum (up to 30 ml), dissolved in normal saline or mixed with three times its volume of olive oil or arachis oil; and by intramuscular injection (5—10 ml), which is the route chiefly employed in the hospital ward. Whichever route is used, the distinctive smell can be detected in the patient's breath, paraldehyde being partially excreted via the lungs.

It should be noted that injections of paraldehyde must be given only with a *glass* syringe, for this drug has a solvent action on plastic and this could be harmful.

## Chlormethiazole

—is manufactured from a component of thiamine (Vitamin $B_1$) which has pronounced sedative properties; it is available as "Heminevrin" in oral form, and as solutions for intravenous injection. Chlormethiazole is used for its calming effect in conditions of acute agitation, such as occur in mania and the delirium tremens which may accompany acute alcoholism and withdrawal treatment in drug addiction. It is occasionally used to control the convulsions of status epilepticus, and as a hypnotic in special cases.

## ANTICONVULSANTS

—are drugs chiefly used in the treatment of epilepsy, a disorder of brain function of generally obscure origin. They fall broadly into two groups, this depending on whether they are used in grand mal epilepsy or in petit mal, though some of the newer drugs provide complete coverage (see later). The grand mal type is associated with the severe convulsant attacks, known as fits, whereas petit mal is characterised by frequent, though fleeting, loss of consciousness, sometimes accompanied by slight muscle contraction, and may lead to grand mal in later years. Other forms of epilepsy also occur, e.g. the psychomotor type which involves disturbances of behaviour, but are mainly treated with the anticonvulsant drugs used in grand mal.

**Phenobarbitone,** the barbiturate hypnotic, is frequently the first drug employed in grand mal, on account of its well established and prolonged sedative action and anticonvulsant effect. Epileptic patients may eventually tend to become insensitive to its hypnotic effect, even in large dosage. However, the problem of controlling the epileptic condition without making the patient heavily drowsed has led to the introduction of a number of anticonvulsant drugs which appear to act selectively on the causative factor in the brain, thus allowing a greater degree of alertness and active existence during the daytime. The following are representative examples; all are taken orally and several are available in liquid form suitable for children.

**Phenytoin** and **Primidone** are largely used in the treatment of grand mal; both have restricted hypnotic effect, but a prominent side-effect of the former in long-term dosage is inflammation and swelling of the gums. Phenytoin is also used by injection in the acute attack, as mentioned later. Primidone is related chemically to the barbiturates, and is often employed in the control of epileptic conditions of severe type.

**Carbamazepine** is related to the antidepressant drug, imipramine, and is claimed to be of additional benefit in the behavioural problems which sometimes accompany epilepsy; it is used as an alternative to, or in combination with, the other drugs employed in grand mal.

**Sulthiame** is an anticonvulsant used in grand mal and similar conditions of seizure type, and has a low incidence of side-effects; as with most drugs in this group its mode of action is uncertain, except that it is known to be a carbonic-anhydrase inhibitor. The diuretic **Acetazolamide** is another carbonic-anhydrase inhibitor used in epilepsy. Carbonic-anhydrase is an enzyme which is essential to the maintenance of bicarbonate levels in the body, and when its action is blocked by inhibitor drugs such as sulthiame and acetazolamide, bicarbonate levels fall and a condition of metabolic acidosis results. It is of interest to note that diets which produce a similar condition of metabolic acidosis are said to be favourable in epilepsy.

Phenobarbitone —av. dose 30–100 mg
Phenytoin —'Epanutin'— „ „ 100 mg
Primidone —'Mysoline'— „ „ 250 mg
Carbamazepine—'Tegretol' — „ „ 200 mg
Sulthiame —'Ospolot' — „ „ 50–200 mg
Acetazolamide —'Diamox' — „ „ 250 mg

**Ethosuximide, Phensuximide** and **Troxidone** are used solely in the treatment of petit mal, the action appearing to be one of relieving tension in the brain. One of the drugs used in petit mal is occasionally added to the treatment of grand mal in cases where it is associated with petit mal also. This addition sometimes results in an increase in frequency of the grand mal attacks, thus illustrating the general difference in action between drugs used in grand mal and petit mal; two exceptions, clonazepam and sodium valproate are discussed later.

Ethosuximide —'Zarontin'—av. dose 250 mg
Phensuximide—'Milontin'— „ „ 250 mg
Troxidone —'Tridione'— „ „ 150–300 mg

Clonazepam and Sodium Valproate are distinct chemically from other drugs used in epilepsy; in addition, they are effective in *all* forms of the disease, i.e. both grand mal and petit mal, *and* the other types.

**Clonazepam** is the first member of the benzodiazepine group (p. 99) to be used in the regular treatment of epilepsy; it is taken three or four times daily, commencing with low dosage and increasing as needed. It is also employed in status epilepticus, but well diluted as an intravenous infusion (see later).

**Sodium Valproate** is normally taken three times daily, commencing with one tablet and increasing if necessary to a daily total of as many as eight or ten. The tablets are swallowed whole with water, but *aerated* drinks of any kind are cautioned against for this purpose.

> Clonazepam —'Rivotril'—tablets 0·5 mg and 2 mg
> —injection 1 mg
> Sodium Valproate—'Epilim' —tablets 200 mg

It is worth noting that sodium valproate breaks down to ketone substances (p. 230), hence this can induce a false reading when the patient's urine is being tested with, e.g. 'Acetest'.

The epileptic patient is usually stabilised on regular daily dosage with one or two, or even three drugs, the routine being carefully assessed by trial, commencing with small dosage in each case and avoiding abrupt increase, or change of drug(s); the combination finally arrived at may vary from dose to dose during the day according to the usual timing of fits. The patient should be equally careful to adhere strictly to the regime, so as to reduce the incidence of attacks. Many of the anticonvulsant drugs possess toxic side-effects, and the necessarily long-term nature of the treatment makes their appearance more possible. These side-effects often differ in type and degree from drug to drug, and combination treatment (as referred to earlier) has the added advantage of enabling the dose of each drug used to be reduced, with a consequent decrease in the level of its side-effects.

The acute condition, known as status epilepticus, in which the convulsive spasms are continuous and may even threaten life, is treated by intramuscular or intravenous injection to obtain speedy control. The drugs which may be employed range from phenobarbitone sodium (the soluble form used for injection), phenytoin sodium and clonazepam to the hypnotic, paraldehyde (p. 93), and the sedatives, chlormethiazole (p. 94) and diazepam (p. 99); muscle relaxants (p. 106) are also used to control the convulsions in severe cases (see page 107). It is useful to note that certain drugs used in tuberculosis carry the possibility of increasing proneness to fits in patients who are epileptic; examples are isoniazid (p. 132) and cycloserine (p. 138).

## TRANQUILLIZERS

—are used in the treatment of various types of mental illness requiring specific sedation. Until their introduction, such conditions were treated largely by day and night sedation, often heavy, of necessity, and employing barbiturates, chloral, and other hypnotic drugs. However, whilst tendency to agitation or violence was suppressed in this way, the patient would often be unable to take an active part, mentally or physically, in the daily life of the community. The availability of the modern tranquillizers has revolutionised treatment, because they can be termed *selective* in effect, appearing to act only on that part of the brain concerned with the condition (and thus with little hypnotic effect), so allowing the patient to live a relatively normal daily life. The drugs employed differ variously in chemical nature and effect, and their use is a highly specialised field, needing expert diagnosis and appropriate choice of treatment.

A major advance in the treatment of mental conditions needing specific sedative control was the introduction of the **Phenothiazine** group of drugs, of which **Chlorpromazine** was the first and still remains the most prominent. Chlorpromazine is available as tablets, syrup, injections and suppositories, and is remarkably effective in controlling mental disturbances of an agitative or aggressive nature, including schizophrenia; thus it may allow the return to normal occupation and family life of patients who might otherwise need to remain within a psychiatric hospital.

Chlorpromazine has several other applications in medicine. Firstly, as with the antihistamine, promethazine (p. 102), to which it is closely related, it has a depressant effect on the vomiting centre in the brain, and thus can be used as an anti-emetic, e.g. to prevent or modify vomiting post-operatively. Secondly, again as with promethazine, it has a potentiating, or enhancing effect on the action of other drugs; thus, the analgesic effect of morphine may be increased if given together with chlorpromazine (see page 114). Chlorpromazine is often used for its calming effect during the day and at night on patients in hospital who are restless or disturbed.

Several other phenothiazine derivatives are used as alternatives to chlorpromazine, or for their more pronounced action in other directions. **Promazine** has a similar tranquillizing action, and the injection is frequently used as pre-medication to prevent post-operative vomiting. **Thioridazine** and **Trifluoperazine** are used mainly for their powerful tranquillizing effect, and **Trimeprazine** frequently for sedation and the pre-operative medication of children and also in dermatology for the relief of pruritus. **Thiethylperazine** and **Prochlorperazine** are used as anti-emetics (p. 17) in conditions where vomiting and vertigo are pronounced, including the sickness which follows radiotherapy and antimitotic treatment, and the giddiness and nausea of Menière's disease.

The phenothiazine drugs are not without significant side-effects, some of the more prominent being symptoms closely allied to those of Parkinson's disease (thus called "drug-induced" parkinsonism—see page 105), occasional serious red blood cell damage (haemolytic anaemia) and jaundice, and sensitivity to sunlight, resulting in skin rash. The skin may be sensitive to chlorpromazine (in particular) and a dermatitis may result; this should be borne in mind when handling the tablets and syrup, and also when giving repeated injections—by changing the site.

| | | |
|---|---|---|
| Chlorpromazine | —'Largactil' —av. dose | 25–50 mg |
| Prochlorperazine | —'Stemetil' — „ „ | 5–25 mg |
| Promazine | —'Sparine' — „ „ | 25–50 mg |
| Thiethylperazine | —'Torecan' — „ „ | 10 mg |
| Thioridazine | —'Melleril' — „ „ | 25–50 mg |
| Trifluoperazine | —'Stelazine'— „ „ | 1–5 mg |
| Trimeprazine | —'Vallergan'— „ „ | 10 mg |

**Fluphenazine** is a phenothiazine compound containing fluorine, which again appears to greatly enhance activity. It is available as 'Moditen' in tablet and injection form, and also as the slightly different 'Modecate' injection. The tablets are used in psychiatric disorders, e.g. of schizophrenic type, but a serious hazard in the more severe cases of this disorder is that the patient may omit to take his tablets if discharged home on oral therapy. Here the injectable form is a positive help, for both 'Moditen' and 'Modecate' are oil-based and thus very slowly released, particularly **'Modecate'**, the effect of one dose of which will last for two to three weeks; the patient may thus be sent home to resume life in the community, arrangements being made for him to receive his regular injection, there being no possibility then of the drug not being taken.

A further drug in long-acting form, **Flupenthixol** ('Depixol'), is used in schizophrenic conditions, especially if accompanied by apathy and lethargy, etc.

A point to note in the case of all *oily* injections is the essential need to aspirate (i.e. withdraw the plunger a very short distance after insertion of the needle) before actually injecting, so as to ensure that a blood vessel has not been entered.

**Haloperidol** is another major tranquillizer. Although differing chemically, it has a powerful effect similar to that of the phenothiazine group, and is used in the treatment of stress/aggression conditions and schizophrenia; its side-effects can be likewise serious, especially in respect of the symptoms of parkinsonism.

Haloperidol—'Serenace'—av. dose 1·5 mg

The pronounced action and side-effects of the major tranquillizers so far discussed, the phenothiazines and haloperidol, have created a need for a calming drug which is moderate in action and with but mild, if any, side-effects; such a drug is **Chlordiazepoxide,** a prominent minor tranquillizer, which is widely prescribed in hospital and general practice. It is available in oral and injection form, and has a remarkable sedative action in anxiety and agitation; this is illustrated by the fact that aggressive animals can become docile under its influence.

**Diazepam** is a drug closely related to chlordiazepoxide and is also available in oral and injection form. It is given orally in a wide variety of mild conditions needing sedation, such as anxiety neurosis, but the injection has a very dramatic and rapid effect, of particular value in such serious conditions as status epilepticus (p. 96) and tetanus.

Chlordiazepoxide—'Librium'—av. dose 5–10 mg
Diazepam         —'Valium' — „   „    2–5 mg
                            by injection, 10 mg

Chlordiazepoxide and diazepam belong to the **benzodiazepine** group, other members of which, with similar tranquillising effect in anxiety tension conditions, etc., are **Lorazepam** ('Ativan'), **Oxazepam** ('Serenid D') and **Potassium clorazepate** ('Tranxene').

**Meprobramate** ('Miltown', 'Equanil') is a further mild tranquillizer in tablet form, of short action and relatively free of serious side-effects. It is employed for minor conditions of tension (e.g. pre-menstrual) and anxiety; an average dose is 400 mg.

### Antidepressants
—are used in the treatment of depression, and comprise several distinct groups and compounds.

The **Tricyclic** group, so termed from its chemical structure, is used, generally, in the type of depression which is accompanied by marked agitation; this it reduces by its selective, sedative effect on the central nervous system. **Amitriptyline** and **Imipramine** are two members prominently used, not only for their specific action in severe conditions but also in moderate dosage for their balancing effect in less serious cases. A point of interest is that it takes from ten to twenty days for treatment to take effect.

**Clomipramine** is closely related to imipramine, and is likewise used as an anti-depressant. However, it has a more powerful action, and in severe cases of depression which require urgent treatment it may be given well diluted by slow intravenous injection.

**Dothiepin** is also a tricyclic compound used in depression; the incidence of side-effects is claimed to be less than with other members of this group.

| Amitriptylene—'Tryptizol' | —av. dose 25 mg |
| Imipramine —'Tofranil' | — „ „ 25 mg |
| Clomipramine—'Anafranil' | — „ „ 25 mg |
| Dothiepin —'Prothiaden'— | „ „ 25 mg |

**Maprotiline, Mianserin** and **Viloxazine** are distinct from the tricyclics and are claimed to cover more widely the varied symptoms which may be associated with "depression"; each is given in three divided doses daily, but in the case of maprotiline, the full daily dose may be taken in one amount at night. Mianserin and maprotiline are employed with caution in epileptic patients, and the dosage of the anticonvulsant drugs being taken may need to be increased; likewise the ability to drive or operate machinery may be affected.

| Maprotiline—'Ludiomil'—av. dose 75 mg daily. |
| Mianserin —'Bolvidon'— „ „ 10 mg |
| Viloxazine —'Vivalan' — „ „ 50 mg |

**Flupenthixol** (see earlier) is also of value *in low dosage* in conditions of depression, anxiety neurosis and "lack of drive"; the tablets ('Fluanxol', 0·5 mg) are taken morning and mid-day, but not later than 4 p.m., because of the animating effect of the drug.

The action of some of the antidepressant drugs so far mentioned may appear similar in certain respects to that of the tranquillisers discussed earlier, and there may seem to be a degree of overlapping of action and use between the two, especially as some are occasionally combined in treatment. Factors involved, however, include variation in mode and degree of action and in side-effects, together with the complexities of the conditions concerned, and thus both sections of drugs have a defined place in treatment.

**Lithium** is a metal which, as the carbonate compound, is effective in the treatment of the type of depression which is accompanied by irrational behaviour; it does not affect mental and physical alertness, and is chiefly employed for its value in preventing attacks. Dosage is carefully assessed so as to avoid side-effects, these may include nausea, diarrhoea, hand tremor, weight gain, and thirst with high output of urine. An adequate intake of salt is essential in order to ensure elimination of lithium and so prevent toxic accumulation, hence salt-free diets are contraindicated. Lithium carbonate is taken as a normal tablet or in sustained-release form ("Phasal", "Priadel") which provides more prolonged effect.

The **Monoamine-Oxidase inhibitors** (often shortened to M.A.O. inhibitors) are employed in severe depressive conditions, and the background to their action is interesting. Certain amines produced in the body, of which noradrenaline and serotonin are important examples, are essential to the nutrition and activity of brain tissue, and the level of these amines is kept under safe control by an enzyme called monoamine-oxidase. The M.A.O. *inhibitors* block the action of this enzyme, thus allowing raised levels of the amines to become available to the brain; the resultant stimulation and elevation of mood is employed to reverse depression. Suitability of patient for this treatment is essential. Prominent M.A.O. inhibitors are **Isocarboxazid, Phenelzine** and **Tranylcypromine.**

Isocarboxazid —'Marplan'—av dose 10 mg
Phenelzine —'Nardil' — ,, ,, 15 mg
Tranylcypromine—'Parnate' — ,, ,, 10 mg

Several points concerning M.A.O.-inhibitor treatment are important to note. Firstly, if the patient takes foods which are rich in certain amines, the M.A.O. inhibitor may prevent their normal breakdown by the enzyme and allow a toxic level to build up; this may so stimulate the central nervous system as to create a serious hypertensive crisis. Cheese has been incriminated as a direct cause of actual fatalities, and other items of diet which the patient is warned against indulging in are broad beans, 'Bovril', 'Marmite' and beer. Secondly, other anti-depressant drugs, e.g. imipramine and amitryptyline, must not be given at the same time as the M.A.O. inhibitors; furthermore, after stopping treatment with the latter, an interval of several weeks must be allowed before changing over to imipramine or amitriptyline, etc. Also contra-indicated during treatment with M.A.O. inhibitors is a great variety of drugs such as adrenaline and the amphetamines (both on account of hypertensive risk), the antihistamines, and analgesics such as pethidine and morphine, the action of all of which may be potentiated to a dangerous level.

## ANTIHISTAMINES

Histamine is a substance which occurs widely in animal and plant tissue; it is occasionally used by injection to aid diagnosis (p. 225). When an injection of histamine is given, a red flare (erythema) usually develops at the needle site, often followed by a swelling and finally a wheal, this being due to its effect of liberating fluid from the blood into the adjacent tissue. This typical effect is the underlying cause of the symptoms of many types of allergy, or sensitivity. Thus, when body tissue is in contact with a substance (e.g. a protein) to which it is allergic, it responds by producing histamine; the result is the distressing symptoms so commonly met. The patient may be allergic to something eaten, and suffer an acute urticarial skin reaction with widespread swelling of the wheal type. Or the allergen (the initial causative factor) may be certain pollens or house dust, which, when inhaled, cause an asthma (of the allergic type) due to an inflammatory response in the lungs; or the nose and eyes may be affected, as in hay fever. Mere contact with certain materials or plants, e.g. pyrethrum, may even cause a skin reaction. Hence the value of the group of drugs known as the antihistamines, which, as a broad generalisation, block the effect of histamine. It should be noted, however, that allergic asthmas frequently do not respond to antihistamine treatment.

A large number of antihistamines of various types are available in the form of tablets or capsules, syrups, injections, nasal sprays, eye drops, and creams for application. Duration of action varies greatly, some needing to be taken several times daily, others once only; certain long-acting preparations are also available which are released slowly along the gastro-intestinal tract. The following is a representative selection:—

| | | | | |
|---|---|---|---|---|
| Chlorpheniramine | —'Piriton' | — av. dose | | 4 mg |
| Cinnarizine | —'Stugeron' | — „ | „ | 15 mg |
| Cyclizine | —'Marzine' | — „ | „ | 50 mg |
| Diphenhydramine | —'Benadryl' | — „ | „ | 50 mg |
| Diphenylpyraline | —'Histryl' | — „ | „ | 5 mg (long acting) |
| Mepyramine | —'Anthisan' | — „ | „ | 50 mg |
| Phenindamine | —'Thephorin' | — „ | „ | 25 mg |
| Promethazine | —'Phenergan' | — „ | „ | 25 mg |
| Triprolidine | —'Actidil' | — „ | „ | 2·5 mg |

In addition to their use in allergic conditions the antihistamines are employed in several other indications. Thus, several have a depressant effect on the emetic centre in the brain and thus prevent vomiting, examples being the use of promethazine by injection pre-operatively and tablets of cyclizine before travelling (p. 17). Cinnarizine is claimed to be unusually selective in action on the labyrinth (the cavities of the inner ear) and is used for its sedative and stabilising action in the vertigo and vomiting of Ménière's disease.

The antihistamines are widely used in the treatment of skin conditions, for they not only reduce irritation when taken orally, but are also employed externally as creams, etc.; the indiscriminate use of such applications, however, is said to be unwise due to the possibility of their aggravating the condition or even actually inducing a dermatitis. The sedative effect, mentioned later, is also of value in calming the patient and making him less conscious of skin irritation.

A marked effect of most of the antihistamines is drowsiness, which, although of benefit in certain conditions, can be a source of danger, and thus patients should be routinely warned against cycling, driving, or working machinery after taking these drugs. Diphenhydramine has particularly powerful hypnotic action and is contained in the tablet 'Mandrax' (p. 92). Phenindamine is one of the few antihistamines which are relatively free from hypnotic effect.

The antihistamines are widely advocated for the relief of the symptoms of the common cold, especially the running nose, but there is some doubt as to whether such use is justified, except in special need, for it can aggravate the feeling of congestion in the head, the cold itself can be prolonged, and there is always the associated risk of drowsiness in dangerous situations.

## THE AMPHETAMINES

This group of drugs comprises **Amphetamine** and **Dexamphetamine,** both given orally, and **Methylamphetamine,** which is given orally and by injection. All have a powerful stimulating effect on the central nervous system; in addition, they induce a pronounced sense of well-being (euphoria) and confidence, which can easily make them drugs of dependence and then addiction. The amphetamines are thus designated "C.D.", i.e. they are fully controlled under the Misuse of Drugs Act (p. 251).

| | |
|---|---|
| Amphetamine | —av. dose 5 mg |
| Dexamphetamine    —'Dexedrine'— | „    „    5 mg |
| Methylamphetamine | —av. oral dose 5 mg |
| | —by injection, 10–30 mg |

The employment of the amphetamines is diminishing greatly due to the dangers associated with them, but they may still be occasionally prescribed in certain conditions of depression assessed as likely to respond to their elevating effect. A further use has been in weight reduction, where the action is said to be two-fold, the patient being stimulated into energetic activity, and the secretion of gastric juice reduced at the same time, thus lessening appetite and intake of food. Used in the above conditions the amphetamines are normally taken morning and mid-day, but not later, for otherwise the stimulant effect of the drug may cause a sleepless night; or a sustained-action preparation may be employed (see later). An unusual use of the amphetamines at bedtime, however, is in the treatment of enuresis, or bed-wetting; this is described on page

38. A still further interesting use in the treatment of hyperkinesia in children, where the patient is continually restless and "on the move", and cannot settle down to anything; here the stimulating effect of the amphetamine on certain centres of the brain enables the child to concentrate and apply himself more normally to projects or study, etc. The amphetamines are also of value in narcolepsy, a condition in which the patient has an uncontrollable desire for sleep.

The amphetamines are also available in commercial preparations of various types and combinations. Some contain a small amount of a barbiturate (e.g. amylobarbitone in 'Drinamyl'), which is intended to offset undue stimulation but is probably of little value in this respect. A useful preparation is the sustained-action capsule ('Dexedrine Spansule', 'Durophet') containing the equivalent of a high dose of the amphetamine, this is taken first thing in the morning and exerts its effect for most of the day due to the slow release of the drug along the gastro-intestinal tract; the unduly stimulating level of amphetamine at normal morning and mid-day dosage is thus avoided.

There are two especial fields for misuse of the amphetamines. Firstly in sport, where their energy-stimulating effect can be an attraction to athletes—in field events and cycling for example; here the danger is of work load exceeding cardiac endurance, and many deaths from collapse have occurred. Saliva tests are often routine, as in the Olympic Games. More serious is the attraction these drugs have for many classes of society (the adolescent in particular) on account of the vivacity and sense of importance which they induce; dependence is soon developed and may easily lead to addiction, when as many as 50 or more 5 mg tablets may be taken in a day. The great decrease in prescribing, together with strict 'CD' control and increased security against illegal obtaining and distribution, should do much to correct the picture.

### Anorectics

—are drugs which lessen appetite and are thus used to reduce weight in obesity. Caution in the use of the amphetamines in this connection has been referred to, but related drugs are available which have similar appetite suppressing action, but with less potential danger; nevertheless, these are still obtainable only on medical prescription. The anorectics are said to be of value where obesity is of serious medical concern and reduction of weight is difficult to achieve by other means. The anorectics mentioned here act via the C.N.S., and may effect changes in the mood, e.g. by stimulation or depression, hence the care with which they, too, are employed.

Examples are—

Phentermine        —'Duromine'        —capsules
Fenfluramine       —'Ponderax'        —tablets
                   'Ponderax' 'P.A.'  —sustained-action capsules
Diethylpropionate—'Tenuate'           —tablets
                   —'Tenuate Dospan'—sustained-action tablets

## DRUGS USED IN THE TREATMENT OF PARKINSON'S DISEASE

Parkinsonism is the term applied to a syndrome (or collection of symptoms) which includes the typical tremor, muscle spasm and ridigity (involving also the "mask-like" countenance), loss of power of action, excessive salivation, and generalised weakness. It arises from damage or degeneration of part of the nervous matter of the brain; this may follow a virus infection of the brain (it is then called post-encephalitic parkinsonism) or it may be of more obscure origin. The syndrome can also result following prolonged taking, or very high dosage, of certain drugs such as the phenothiazines, e.g. chlorpromazine; in this case the condition is termed "drug-induced" parkinsonism and differs from "true" parkinsonism in being reversible when the drug concerned is discontinued or the dose reduced.

Various preparations of belladonna have been used for many years in the treatment of parkinsonism, the anticholinergic (and hence antispasmodic) action (p. 14) being the effective factor. However, the disadvantage of unpleasant side-effects (p. 15) has stimulated the production of synthetic drugs with improved action and reduced incidence of side-effects.

**Benzhexol, Benztropine** and **Orphenadrine** are widely used. All are in tablet form, and the action in each case is specifically anticholinergic, but with less side-effects than occur when using belladonna. However, dryness of mouth and throat, blurring of vision, giddiness, constipation and difficulty in passing urine, all can still occur, and it is usual to commence treatment with small dosage, gradually increasing to as effective a level as possible within the limits of the patient's tolerance. Likewise, if treatment has to be stopped for any reason, it is tailed off gradually, for abrupt cessation may give rise to an increased severity of the symptoms.

Benzhexol     —'Artane'    —2 & 5 mg tablets
Benztropine   —'Cogentin'—2 mg tablets
Orphenadrine—'Disipal'   —50 mg tablets

**Levodopa** (also called L-dopa) is a major drug in the treatment of Parkinson's disease. It is taken orally, and following absorption it is converted in the brain to dopamine, a substance which is deficient in the brain tissue of patients with this disease; dopamine counterbalances the activity of acetylcholine, hence probably its beneficial effect, as in the case of the anticholinergic drugs described above. Treatment may commence with 125–250 mg four times daily, increasing very gradually until symptoms are well controlled— at perhaps 8 to 10 tablets (4–5 g) daily; tablets are normally scored in quarters (of 125 mg) to facilitate gradual change of dose. Dosage is assessed carefully to minimise the unpleasant side-effects that may occur, such as nausea, vomiting, "difficult" irritability, and hallucinations; constant chewing, with licking of the lips, is often also a feature. One of the anticholinergic drugs referred to earlier is often combined with levodopa in treatment.

A disadvantage of employing plain levodopa is that part of the dose is used up in the system and does not reach the brain, hence the value of two drugs, carbidopa and benserazide, either of which incorporated in the tablet ensures that *all* the levodopa reaches the brain tissue; this means that the patient can be controlled with a smaller dose of levodopa and side-effects are likewise reduced.

| | | | | | |
|---|---|---|---|---|---|
| Levodopa | —'Larodopa'—tablets, 500 mg | | | | |
| 'Sinemet–275' | —levodopa 250 mg plus carbidopa | | 25 mg | | |
| 'Sinemet–110'— | „ | 100 mg | „ | „ | 10 mg |
| 'Madopar 250'— | „ | 200 mg | „ | benserazide 50 mg | |
| 'Madopar 125'— | „ | 100 mg | „ | „ | 25 mg |

It is worth noting that pyridoxine (p. 79) antagonises the effect of levodopa, hence multi-vitamin preparations containing pyridoxine should not be taken by patients who are on levodopa therapy.

A further drug employed in Parkinsonism is **Amantadine** ('Symmetrel'), dosage being normally one capsule daily for a week, then twice daily; it is employed alone or in conjunction with levodopa. Amantadine was first introduced as an anti-viral drug, and is sometimes used as a prophylactic during periods of influenza risk.

## MUSCLE RELAXANTS

The main important use of this group of drugs is in surgery, where muscle relaxation is an especial factor in enabling ease of intubation (introduction of the endotracheal tube) and also in the subsequent smooth performance of the operation itself; thus, for example, the relaxation and consequent absence of muscle rigidity allows greater ease of access to the abdominal cavity. In addition, muscle relaxation reduces the depth of anaesthesia necessary, and the patient will thus require less of the anaesthetic and recovery will be more rapid.

The muscle relaxants chiefly used are **Tubocurarine, Alcuronium** and **Pancuronium,** which are related to curare– the poison once used on arrow-heads in South America, and **Gallamine** and **Suxamethonium,** which are entirely synthetic in origin. All are given by injection. Although the mode of action of the first four mentioned differs from that of suxamethonium, the end-effect of all these drugs is the same, i.e. the transmission of nerve impulses to the muscles is blocked and relaxation follows as a natural consequence. Two points to note about suxamethonium are, firstly, that unlike the curare-related relaxants and gallamine, its action cannot be reversed by the anticholinesterase neostigmine—as referred to in the next section; and secondly, it deteriorates at warm temperatures and should be stored in the refrigerator.

Tubocurarine —'Tubarine'
Alcuronium —'Alloferin'
Pancuronium —'Pavulon'
Gallamine —'Flaxedil'
Suxamethonium—'Anectine'

Tubocurarine, pancuronium and alcuronium, are used for their powerful relaxant effect in the control of the convulsions of tetanus and status epilepticus (p. 96); they also enable the patient to "accept" (i.e. accommodate himself to) the respirator with greater ease in these and similar conditions when artificial ventilation may need to be prolonged.

## CHOLINERGIC DRUGS

Whereas anticholinergic drugs block the production of acetylcholine (p. 14), other drugs are available which have the opposite *(cholinergic)* effect, i.e. they *increase* the availability of acetylcholine; these are the **Anticholinesterases.** Cholinesterase is an enzyme which controls the level and activity of acetylcholine by destroying it after it has completed its function at the nerve ending (p. 14). The action of *anti*cholinesterase drugs is to block the action of cholinesterase and thus allow acetylcholine levels to rise and so exert increased effect.

A naturally occurring anticholinesterase, of plant origin, is **Physostigmine,** also known as **Eserine,** which is directly opposite in effect to the anticholinergic drug atropine, e.g. its action on the eye is miotic (contracts the pupil), compared with the mydriatic (dilating) effect of atropine (see page 213). The drug mainly employed as an anticholinesterase, however, is the synthetic compound **Neostig-**

mine, which has a chemical structure similar to that of physostigmine, and is available in tablet, injection and eye-drop forms.

Tablets of neostigmine are taken in the condition known as myasthenia gravis, in which there is pronounced muscle weakness, typical symptoms being difficulty in swallowing, in forming words clearly, and in keeping the eyelids open. The action of the drug in increasing the availability of acetylcholine leads to a strengthening of muscle activity. Neostigmine eye-drops are used for their miotic effect, and the injection is employed as an antidote in belladonna poisoning (p. 15), and also occasionally in acute inability of bowel movement (p. 23) and in urine retention (p. 34) where it stimulates muscle activity in the bowel and bladder, respectively, by increasing the level of acetylcholine effect. Neostigmine is used by injection in the Operating Theatre to counteract the excessive relaxation that may be produced by the anticholinergic action of certain of the muscle relaxants used, as mentioned in the preceding section.

Neostigmine—'Prostigmin'—tablets of 15 mg
injection, 0·5 mg per ml and
2·5 mg per ml

**Pyridostigmine** ('Mestinon') and **Distigmine** ('Ubretid') are two further drugs of the neostigmine type. The former is also used in myasthenia gravis and has a more prolonged action. Distigmine has a specific use in urinary retention (p. 34).

**Edrophonium** ('Tensilon') is an anticholinesterase used in the diagnosis of myasthenia gravis, and is referred to on page 225.

### Carbachol

—is a drug closely related chemically to acetylcholine, and has a similar action though more prolonged; it is given either as tablets or by subcutaneous injection, and through its cholinergic (i.e. acetylcholine-like) action, it stimulates the intestinal and bladder muscles and is of value in post-operative bowel apathy and urine retention (pages 23 and 34).

## DRUGS ACTING ON THE UTERUS

Two drugs of importance here, ergometrine and oxytocin, have been referred to briefly in the section dealing with haemostatics (p. 70); both stimulate contraction of the uterus.

**Ergometrine** is obtained from ergot, a fungus which grows on the head of the cereal, rye; it is available as tablets, and solutions for injection, an average dose in each case being 0·5 mg. Ergometrine is given intramuscularly or intravenously following delivery of the foetus or the subsequent expulsion of the placenta; if given before, or during the event, the uterine contractions it produces may be so vigorous as to be a possible danger to the child. The contracting effect of the drug constricts the bleeding points involved and so reduces the risk of excessive post-partum haemorrhage (bleeding following delivery); in addition it helps to ensure complete expulsion of the placenta and membranes. Tablets of ergometrine are sometimes given for this latter purpose.

**Oxytocin** is one of the hormones produced by the posterior lobe of the pituitary gland (page 177); it can be obtained from cattle sources but the synthetic form ('Syntocinon') is mainly used. It is destroyed by the digestive action of the stomach, and is thus used as an injection containing 2 to 10 units; a tablet is employed for buccal absorption, this is mentioned later. Oxytocin has a smoother and more predictable action than ergometrine, hence it can be used with safety before and during labour, as well as after. If there is a lack of uterine activity, and labour needs to be induced, oxytocin is given by injection—often in the form of a weak intravenous drip (2·5 units in 1 litre). The action of oxytocin ensures effective completion of labour, and, as with ergometrine, greatly reduces post-partum bleeding.

As referred to earlier, oxytocin is available as a high strength tablet ('Pitocin'), which the patient lodges in the buccal cavity, between the cheek and gum; absorption is then effected via the mucosa, so avoiding the need to give the drug by injection. There is also direct control of action by this route, for the tablet can be easily dislodged from the mouth and the contractions will then lessen.

Ergometrine and oxytocin are also available in one intramuscular injection ('Syntometrine'), which, again due to its ergometrine content, is usually not administered until the stage of crowning of the head or birth of the anterior (foremost) shoulder.

Oxytocin is known to play a further role in the release of milk from the breast during suckling of the infant, and in cases where flow is considered insufficient—as may occur during a period of tension or anxiety, etc.—improvement may be effected by its use as 'Syntocinon' nasal spray; this is done 2–5 minutes beforehand, which gives time for the hormone to be absorbed and exert effect.

## The Prostaglandins

—are a group of over a dozen compounds which are found in the prostate gland and the seminal fluid. They also occur widely in minute amounts throughout body tissue and, it is thought, may serve as agents within the cell which are essential to its effective response to nerve stimuli. It is of interest that sources of prostaglandin compounds exist in certain deposits of sea coral, but those preparations now being used in medicine, and others in course of evaluation, are all of synthetic manufacture.

The prostaglandins exert a wide range of effects, and these may vary from one to another, even to being directly opposite in some instances. The use of those at present available is confined to their stimulating action on smooth muscle, with particular relation to uterine contraction and hence for induction of labour and termination (therapeutic) of pregnancy.

**Dinoprostone** ('Prostin E.2.') is equivalent to the natural prostaglandin, type E.2., and is used to induce and complete labour, either as a dilute solution by slow intravenous drip, or as tablets or solution taken orally—in a small glass of water in each case; it is essential to use a glass syringe to measure the oral solution, as it reacts with plastic and this can be dangerous. It is claimed to be superior to oxytocin (p. 109) in that far from causing water retention, as may happen with the latter, it does, in fact, act as a mild diuretic. In the termination of pregnancy, dinoprostone is again given by slow intravenous drip, but may also be administered by instilling 1–2 ml of a stronger solution through a Foley's balloon catheter (12 or 14 French gauge) into the extra-ovular space, and repeating at intervals of one or two hours.

**Dinoprost** ('Prostin F.2 Alpha') is another synthetic prostaglandin which is used in a similar way to dinoprostone, and in similar conditions.

Other effects of the prostaglandins are generally (and, in some cases, varyingly—see earlier) as follows. They lower blood pressure; reduce the secretion of gastric juice and also the ability of blood platelets to clump: cause shrinking of the nasal mucosa and dilatation of the bronchi (though some constrict the latter); act as sedatives when introduced into the brain; and have miotic action (p. 213) when injected into the eye. Hence, it is possible that the prostaglandins may constitute a major drug source for employment in a wide range of conditions in the future.

Prostaglandin substances are thought to play a role in sensitising the tissues to pain, and the action of many analgesic drugs (Ch. 12), e.g. aspirin, paracetamol, and ibuprofen and other anti-rheumatoids, is held to be one of inhibiting prostaglandin activity.

In contrast to the contracting effect of oxytocin, ergometrine and the prostaglandins, **Ritodrine** ('Yutopar') has a *relaxant* action on the uterus, and is used to control premature labour and so prolong pregnancy; three routes are used in turn, firstly an intravenous infusion, then intramuscular injections, and finally oral tablets which are taken as long as considered necessary. Ritodrine is also used in *actual* labour to relax the uterine contractions in cases where these may constitute a danger to the child through possibility of asphyxia.

# CHAPTER 12

# ANALGESICS

## with antirheumatic drugs

### Analgesics

—are drugs which relieve pain. Some have relatively mild effect and are used in simple conditions, others are of powerful action and are employed in the severe pain of serious illness; a few are also available which are intermediate in action. The antirheumatic drugs are also largely analgesic, and are dealt with later in this chapter.

### The Mild Analgesics

Typical conditions in which these are employed are headache, dysmenorrhoea, influenza and simple rheumatic pains. The most commonly used is **Aspirin** (acetylsalicylic acid), and the beneficial effect of two 300 mg tablets taken with a hot drink is well established. An excellent form of aspirin is the soluble tablet ('Disprin', 'Solprin') which can be dissolved in water to make a palatable draught. Paediatric tablets, flavoured and of quarter or half the adult strength, are also available.

Side-effects of normal dosage of aspirin can include dizziness, tinnitus (ringing in the ears) and stomach irritation. Bleeding from the gastric mucosa may cause haematemesis (vomiting of blood) or melaena (dark, tarry stools), but can be often unsuspected; if this occurs over a long period, an iron-deficiency anaemia (p. 65) may result. The symptoms of gross overdosage, as in attempted suicide, include coma, weak and rapid pulse, and acute respiratory depression.

Treatment of aspirin poisoning includes stomach lavage with a solution of sodium bicarbonate (which is antacid), together with forced diuresis (see page 37) employing intravenous solutions containing either sodium bicarbonate alone or electrolytes together with sodium lactate (which is metabolised and converted into sodium bicarbonate), the aim being a raised output of alkaline urine which induces increased excretion of the aspirin in the form of salicylates. Mannitol is often included in these intravenous solutions for its powerful osmotic/diuretic effect (p. 37). In severe cases, resort may be had to peritoneal dialysis or haemodialysis (see pages 35 and 36).

**Phenacetin** is a mild analgesic, but prolonged use can cause serious blood conditions and kidney damage, and it is now little employed. A derivative of phenacetin is **Paracetamol**, and this compound is available as tablets ('Panadol') which are being increasingly used as both safer than phenacetin and useful where aspirin is not well tolerated; an average dose is one or two 500 mg tablets.

The ready availability of paracetamol to the public by purchase has made it a drug of significance in suicide attempt, and as few as 20–30 tablets may cause severe liver damage. In cases of overdosage, a stomach wash-out is given if in time, i.e. if soon after the tablets have been taken, but treatment of severer conditions will depend on factors such as the time lapse since the overdose, the plasma level of the drug, and the possibility of liver damage already commenced; measures taken may involve the administration of an amino-acid, e.g. methionine, intravenous fluids containing dextrose, electrolytes and vitamin K, or, in the last resort, the employment of haemodialysis (p. 36).

Various combinations of aspirin and paracetamol are available, and in some the analgesic effect is strengthened by a small amount of codeine, a constituent of opium which depresses the pain centre. One such preparation, long established, is the Compound Tablet of Codeine ('Veganin').

In addition to their analgesic effect, aspirin and paracetamol are antipyretic, that is they may help to lower the temperature when it is raised in illness, e.g. in influenza. Despite their long use, the mode of action of these mild analgesics is not completely understood, though in the case of aspirin it is thought possibly associated with inhibition of the normal production of prostaglandin substances (p. 109) in the body tissues.

### Analgesics with Intermediate Effect

Two drugs of more pronounced action in relieving pain are dextropropoxyphene and mefenamic acid.

**Dextropropoxyphene** is a synthetic drug which bears some relation chemically to the narcotic drugs; it has a useful analgesic effect but is non-addictive. It is available as capsules and in a variety of formulations, but is more commonly used in combination with paracetamol (above) as the distinctively shaped tablet 'Distalgesic', of which two are taken up to four times daily.

**Mefenamic Acid** ('Ponstan') is taken as capsules of 250 mg, and is employed in many conditions, especially pain of joint and bone origin, etc.; it is said to be of value also in dysmenorrhoea.

**The powerful analgesics**

The analgesics so far mentioned are of little value in the severe pain of post-operative conditions and terminal disease such as cancer, where the absolute need is for drugs which powerfully block pain sensation. Originally such drugs were derived entirely from opium, but there are now also available a number of synthetic compounds, which have broadly equivalent effect and are claimed to be an improvement in certain respects.

**Opium** is the dried juice of an Eastern poppy, and from it are prepared a number of powerful analgesics which act by depressing the pain centre in the brain; they are also termed narcotics, for they induce deep sleep. **Tincture of opium**, once commonly known as laudanum, is occasionally used (av. dose 1 ml) in mixture form. **'Nepenthe'** is a preparation closely similar to tincture of opium but is slightly weaker in strength; as well as also being used (av. dose 1 ml) in oral mixtures, it is frequently given by subcutaneous injection to infants and young children, 0·06 ml per year of age (i.e. 6 × $\frac{1}{100}$ ml divisions on a tuberculin syringe).

**Morphine** is the chief active constituent of opium, and is mainly given by subcutaneous injection; it is one of the most widely used powerful analgesics. Morphine is frequently given with hyoscine as pre-operative medication, the combination making the patient sleepy, indifferent and free from anxiety; the hyoscine also helps to reduce bronchial secretion. Atropine is frequently used in place of hyoscine in this combination for its especial effectiveness in reducing secretions and maintaining the heart rate (p. 63). Morphine is also available as injections ('Cyclimorph') which contain, in addition, the antihistamine, cyclizine; this, by its anti-emetic effect (p. 17), reduces the tendency to nausea and vomiting which is referred to later as a side-effect associated with many of the narcotic drugs.

**Papaveretum** is a concentrated preparation of opium, containing all its active constituents, and is mainly used by subcutaneous injection; it is useful to note that papaveretum contains half its weight of morphine, thus 20 mg contains 10 mg of morphine. Papaveretum is also combined with hyoscine in an injection widely used for premedication.

**Diamorphine (Heroin)** is made from morphine, and is a more powerful analgesic; it is particularly depressant to the respiratory centre in the brain, hence its use as a linctus to suppress cough in serious lung conditions (see page 85).

A very useful combination much employed in the pain of terminal conditions is the "Brompton Cocktail" mixture, which contains either morphine or heroin, together with cocaine and a little honey and gin (or other spirit) to flavour. Here the analgesic effect of the morphine or heroin is combined with the elevation of mood provided by the cocaine. The B.N.F. contains two elixirs based on the "Brompton" mixture, these are Morphine and Cocaine Elixir, and Diamorphine and Cocaine Elixir. These are strengthened in two further B.N.F. elixirs by the addition of chlorpromazine (p. 97), which enhances the effect of the morphine and diamorphine in cases where pain is particularly difficult to control.

Morphine —av. dose 15 mg
Papaveretum—'Omnopon' — „ „ 20 mg
Heroin —Diamorphine— „ „ 10 mg

**Dihydrocodeine** is prepared from codeine, and is available in tablet, elixir and injection form; it is a powerful sedative to the pain centre in the brain, and an advantage in ward routine is that the tablet and elixir forms are *not* subject to the full Controlled Drugs Regulations—note, however, that the injection form *is* C.D., i.e. a fully Controlled Drug (p. 251).

Dihydrocodeine—'D.F. 118'—tablets, 30 mg
—elixir, 10 mg in 5 ml
—injection, 50 mg in 1 ml

A disadvantage of the opium-derived analgesics is that they may cause nausea and vomiting, and also constipation, even when given by injection; in addition they may exert an undesirable hypnotic effect during the daytime. Hence synthetic drugs have been introduced which are claimed to be superior in action and/or freer of side-effects; all act similarly by depressing the pain centre in the brain.

The best known of these powerful synthetic analgesics is **Pethidine**, which is available as tablets but is more usually given by injection. It is said to be less hypnotic and less depressant to respiration, to cause minimal nausea and vomiting, and to be more antispasmodic than morphine; this makes it an ideal analgesic during labour—its combination with levallorphan ('Pethilorfan') is mentioned on page 88).

Other examples of synthetic narcotic drugs are levorphanol, methadone and dipipanone. **Levorphanol** is said to have less pronounced hypnotic effect, hence patients are more alert during the daytime. **Methadone**, like heroin, is particularly useful in linctus form as a pain and cough suppressant (p. 85). **Dipipanone** is used only in tablet form; this also contains the antihistamine, cyclizine, which, as in the case of "Cyclimorph" injections (see earlier), prevents the nausea and vomiting possible with narcotic drugs.

Pethidine —tab. & inj.—av. dose 50–100 mg
Levorphanol—'Dromoran' — „ „ — „ „ 2 mg

Methadone —'Physeptone'—tab. & inj.—av. dose 5–10 mg
Dipipanone —'Diconal'    —tablets   — „   „   10 mg
               (with cyclizine)

Further narcotic drugs of special interest are phenoperidine, fentanyl and dextromoramide. **Phenoperidine** is a powerful analgesic which is more strongly depressant to the respiratory centre than is any other drug in this section; it is this very feature that makes it the analgesic of choice in cases where breathing has to be controlled by a mechanical respirator, because the suppression of the patient's own respiratory activity ensures that inspiration and expiration (breathing in and out) proceeds smoothly and regularly under the sole control of the respirator. In addition, the resulting lack of muscle activation in the bronchi can be a factor in encouraging healing where there has been bronchial trauma of the "stove-in-chest" type following car accidents.

Phenoperidine—'Operidine'—av. dose 1 mg i/m or i/v

**Fentanyl** ('Sublimaze') is an extremely potent analgesic, for the maximum dose is 600 micrograms (0·6 mg). It may be given alone, but is often combined with droperidol ('Droleptan'), a tranquillizing drug which is also strongly depressant to the vomiting centre in the brain. This combination is known as 'Thalamonal' and is given not only in the relief of pain but also as a valuable form of premedication, providing analgesia, mental indifference, and reduced risk of post-operative sickness. In cases where full general anaesthesia is contraindicated, certain operations may be performed with the aid of 'Thalamonal' plus the light administration of nitrous oxide and oxygen.

Fentanyl                —'Sublimaze' —dose up to 600
                                 micrograms i/m or i/v
Fentanyl plus droperidol—'Thalamonal'—av. dose 1–2 ml
                                 i/m or i/v

**Dextromoramide** has similar analgesic effect to morphine, and in addition to tablets and injections there is a suppository ('Palfium') which releases the drug for systemic absorption via the rectal mucosa; this form of administration is convenient in certain conditions of severe pain where the oral or injection route is impracticable for some reason.

The signs and symptoms of overdosage of morphine and the other preparations obtained from opium apply also to all the synthetic narcotics; they include absence of reflex action, contracted ("pinpoint") pupils and depressed respiration. Nalorphine ('Lethidrone') and naloxone ('Narcan') are specific antagonists to the action of the narcotic drugs (see page 88) and are given intravenously as an antidote; they are used in the Operating Theatre should the patient exhibit signs of undue sensitivity to morphine, pethidine or other narcotic drug which may have been given.

The powerful narcotic analgesics induce profound euphoria (sense of well-being and pleasure), and are thus drugs of addiction governed by the Controlled Drugs Regulations (pp. 251–3). Furthermore, patients can gradually become resistant to their effect and dosage need to be increased, for example it is not unknown for patients with terminal cancer to require 100 mg or more of heroin or morphine for relief to be obtained, compared with the normal dose of 10 and 15 mg respectively.

The risk of addiction associated with narcotic drugs (which may involve even members of the professions which prescribe and administer them, for these drugs are no respecters of persons) creates a need for analgesics with equivalent effect but without this disadvantage. Dihydrocodeine *tablets and elixir* are a step in this direction, and another notable advance is **Pentazocine**, in oral, injection and suppository form, which is claimed to provide powerful analgesia without risk of addiction. More of this type of safer drug may well follow.

Pentazocine—'Fortral'—av. oral dose 25–50 mg
by injection 30–60 mg
suppository 50 mg

## ANTIRHEUMATIC DRUGS

—are used in the treatment of minor rheumatism, rheumatoid arthritis, rheumatic fever and gout; many of those discussed here cover more than one of these conditions.

### Drugs used in minor Rheumatism

In this group of less severe rheumatic conditions, e.g. slight aches, stiffness, simple fibrositis, etc., the mild analgesics, aspirin and paracetamol, and the various combinations of these drugs, some with the addition of dextropropoxyphene or codeine, etc. (see p. 112), all have value. Another drug related chemically to aspirin, **sodium salicylate**, has a similar analgesic effect and is used as the B.N.F. Mixture. In these simple conditions, *external* salicylate preparations are also beneficial, in cream or liniment form, one being methyl salicylate (oil of wintergreen), which has a penetrating odour; it is often used in combination with other rubefacient drugs such as camphor and menthol (p. 223) for their warming effect and stimulation of local circulation.

## Drugs used in Rheumatoid Arthritis

Treatment of this condition is usually long-term due to its chronic nature, and several distinct drugs are employed.

The analgesics used for simple rheumatism also apply in this condition, but dosage is usually fuller, more frequent and regular, as, for example, aspirin 900 mg, four times daily.

A very widely used drug is **Phenylbutazone**, the mode of action of which also remains uncertain. Injections are available, but the drug is usually taken in tablet form, dosage being kept at a moderate level due to the possibility of side-effects, which can be severe and may include liver damage and agranulocytosis, a serious condition in which certain of the important white blood cells are greatly reduced in number, and there is consequent failure of the defence mechanism of the body against infection. Peptic ulcer, an increase in weight and oedema are also occasional problems associated with phenylbutazone therapy. Oedema is due to retention of sodium and chloride, and, in turn, water, and patients may be advised to restrict salt in the diet and reduce fluid intake. Suppositories are also available, the drug being absorbed from the rectal mucosa, thus avoiding the irritant effect of the drug on the gastro-intestinal tract.

Several other drugs have been evolved which are specific in the treatment of rheumatoid arthritis. **Indomethacin** is available in capsule and suppository form, its analgesic and anti-inflammatory effect being comparable with that of phenylbutazone; in particular, great relief is obtained from the suppository inserted at night, for the slow absorption, and prolonged effect, markedly reduces early morning stiffness, as well as avoiding gastric irritation. **Ibuprofen**, **Fenoprofen**, **Ketoprofen** and **Naproxen** are also widely employed, but again are not without risk of significant side-effects. **Benorylate** is distinct in being an oral suspension, well tolerated and non-irritant, which breaks down to salicylate and paracetamol *in the blood stream.*

| | | | |
|---|---|---|---|
| Phenylbutazone | —'Butazolidine' | —av. dose | 100 mg |
| Indomethacin | —'Indocid' | — ,, ,, | 25 mg |
| Ibuprofen | —'Brufen' | — ,, ,, | 200 mg |
| Fenoprofen | —'Fenopron' | — ,, ,, | 300 mg |
| Ketoprofen | —'Alrheumat', 'Orudis'— | ,, ,, | 50 mg |
| Naproxen | —'Naprosyn' | — ,, ,, | 250 mg |
| Benorylate | —'Benoral' | — ,, ,, | 5–10 ml |

The **Corticosteroids**, together with **Corticotrophin** (A.C.T.H.), will be discussed in Chapter 18, but it is of interest to mention that the value of the drug cortisone—which introduced the corticosteroid era of therapy—was discovered by the physician in control of a large rheumatoid clinic in America. The initial theory that cortisone was a *cure* for rheumatoid arthritis was soon realised to be unfounded, but the corticosteroids (and A.C.T.H.) are much prescribed as helpful treatment in this condition. Small maintenance doses of a corticosteroid such as prednisolone, even as low as 2·5 mg daily, are of value in controlling the symptoms, due to the powerful anti-inflammatory action of this group of drugs. A.C.T.H. injections are occasionally used instead of the corticosteroids, because they stimulate the patient's adrenal cortex to produce a larger amount of its natural corticosteroids (p. 178). A specific application of corticosteroid treatment is by intra-articular injection for local effect. Thus, in painful conditions of bursitis (e.g. "tennis elbow"), a "depot" injection of an insoluble suspension (e.g. 'Depo-Medrone') is given at the site; absorption is slow, and the local anti-inflammatory action is thus prolonged—as is required.

Gold therapy is employed occasionally in severe cases of rheumatoid arthritis. The drug is given by injection in the form of a complex compound, **Sodium Aurothiomalate** ('Myocrisin'), commencing with a small test dose, and following, in the absence of any untoward reaction (e.g. skin rashes), with a course of treatment in progressive dosage over a long period and to a total amount of approximately 1 gram. The side-effects of gold therapy can be severe, in particular there may be kidney damage, and it is often customary to test the urine for albumen before each injection in order to check if such damage is occurring.

Certain anti-malarial drugs based on **Chloroquine** also have a place in the treatment of rheumatoid arthritis; examples are chloroquine sulphate ('Nivaquine') and hydroxychloroquine sulphate ('Plaquenil'). A serious side-effect which may result following prolonged treatment is damage to the retina (the inner lining of the eye), which may be irreversible.

**Penicillamine** ('Distamine') is prepared from penicillin and is available as tablets of 125 and 250 mg; little is known of its mode of action in rheumatoid conditions, but it is of proven value in certain severe cases which have not responded to the drugs more commonly employed. Dosage commences at up to 250 mg daily for the first few weeks, increasing by a similar amount at intervals of two to four weeks until the patient is stabilised on perhaps 750 mg daily, or more if necessary. This is maintained for 6–12 months, when it is gradually reduced at intervals of two to three months until final discontinuation; further courses are usually required. Treatment with penicillamine is closely controlled due to the side-effects which may occur; these include nausea and vomiting, loss of appetite, and fever, but, more seriously, blood complications such as agranulocytosis (p. 117).

An interesting feature of penicillamine is that it is a *chelating* agent, i.e. it attracts, or "gathers" to it, heavy metals such as lead and copper, hence it is used in the treatment of lead poisoning and also Wilson's disease, in which defective metabolism leads to an accumulation of copper in the body; in each case the penicillamine is excreted via the urine, and takes with it the lead, or copper, it has collected.

## Drugs used in Rheumatic Fever

This severe condition, associated with infection, is also termed acute rheumatism, and the drugs employed include phenylbutazone, the salicylates (aspirin and sodium salicylate), and the cortico-steroids and A.C.T.H. This is an acute rather than a chronic condition, and dosage is therefore on a high scale, e.g. as much as 8 grams of aspirin may be given daily in divided doses. Response to the drug used is indicated by a reduction of swelling, pain and temperature. A point to note is the subsequent long-term use, usually orally, of antibiotics such as penicillin as a prophylactic (preventive) measure against the development of common infections such as sore throat, etc., which can initiate danger of a resumption of the associated endocarditis (inflammation of the membrane lining the heart).

### Drugs used in the treatment of Gout

Certain of the drugs already mentioned as used for various rheu-matoid diseases are also employed in this painful condition. Thus, in the treatment of an acute attack, phenylbutazone or indomethacin may be used in high dosage for the short course which is usually adequate to subdue the inflammation. **Colchicine**, an active con-stituent of the autumn crocus, is still often employed, the common routine being to give one tablet of 0·5 mg every two hours up to a maximum total of six to twelve; vomiting is the chief side-effect.

Several drugs are used in moderate daily dosage as prophylactic treatment, together with a diet avoiding those foods and drinks which encourage high uric acid levels in the body. Some act by increasing the output of uric acid via the urine, the so-called "uricosuric" effect, and examples are **Sulphinpyrazone** and **Probenecid**. **Allopur-inol** has an entirely different action in that it blocks the production of uric acid, but an interesting point is that it can actually precipitate a short attack of gout at the commencement of treatment, this being usually controlled by giving colchicine.

```
Sulphinpyrazone—'Anturan'—av. dose 100 mg
Probenecid      —'Benemid'— „    „   500 mg
Allopurinol     —'Zyloric' — „    „   100 mg
```

# CHAPTER 13

# ANAESTHETICS
## —general—local

Anaesthetics are used to produce insensitivity to pain. The *general* anaesthetics produce complete loss of consciousness and are mainly used in the Operating Theatre. The *local* anaesthetics act only on the sensory nerves leading from the required site, thus confining the action to a relatively small area or region and leaving the patient fully conscious (the sensory nerves are those which convey impressions, e.g. sense of pain, to the brain or spinal cord).

## GENERAL ANAESTHETICS

These are of several types, varying not only chemically and physically but also in duration of action; some are used to maintain general anaesthesia for any length of time necessary, and others solely for short periods. We commence with the latter.

The barbiturate compound **Thiopentone** ('Pentothal', see page 92) may be given by intravenous injection to provide general anaesthesia for operations of short duration, such as joint manipulation, the effect lasting only a few minutes, but its chief use is to induce loss of consciousness before the patient is conveyed into the Operating Theatre, where it is maintained with other general anaesthetics which are discussed later. The action of thiopentone is almost instantaneous. Thiopentone is also given per rectum as a solution or suppository; this is very suitable for inducing anaesthesia in children. **Methohexitone** ('Brietal') is also a short-acting barbiturate; it is used similarly to thiopentone and is claimed to allow patients to recover normal alertness more quickly.

**Propanidid** ('Epontol') is a non-barbiturate drug which is likewise used intravenously both for short operative procedures and for induction, as mentioned under thiopentone; its duration of effect is particularly brief, and recovery to alertness equally rapid, both factors in its increasing use.

**'Althesin'** is an intravenous anaesthetic of steroid structure (p. 188), which induces loss of consciousness in about 30 seconds, this then lasts for 5–10 minutes. As with the other members of this group, it is used for surgical procedures of short duration and to induce anaesthesia. It is said to be very safe, and recovery is rapid, but at present its use is not advised in certain situations, e.g. obstetrics and neurosurgery. Storage instructions specify room temperature, *not* refrigerator.

**Ketamine** ('Ketalar') is another general anaesthetic which is given intravenously. Its effect is rapid—within 30 seconds, and lasts for 5–10 minutes; it is likewise used for short procedures, and also for inducing anaesthesia before continuing with other agents. A side-effect of ketamine to be noted is that the patient may experience unpleasant dreams on awakening, hence nursing staff may be particularly requested to see that the patient is not disturbed. Ketamine may also be given intramuscularly, when anaesthesia is slower in onset but more prolonged; this route is particularly useful in the case of children.

**Trichlorethylene** ('Trilene') is a clear, non-inflammable liquid with a typical odour; it is volatile, i.e. it evaporates quickly, and is used by inhalation for inducing light anaesthesia of short duration such as is required in dentistry. Trichlorethylene is a very weak anaesthetic in itself, but produces analgesia (freedom from pain) at concentrations which do not produce loss of consciousness; midwives are therefore allowed to administer the drug by inhalation to relieve distress during labour, this on their own initiative and without supervision, providing an approved vaporiser is used and a doctor has previously given consent.

**Ethyl Chloride** is a powerful anaesthetic, but is far less used than formerly due to the effects of overdosage, which easily occur and may be serious. It is issued as a liquid, under pressure in glass tubes fitted with a nozzle, from which it can be ejected as a *spray* on to a pad placed over the nose and mouth in order to induce rapid general anaesthesia for quick procedures, e.g. dental extraction; this is labelled "general". If directed onto the skin as a *jet* (this type is labelled "local") it provides brief local anaesthesia due to its rapid evaporation, and enables simple suturing, etc., to be performed painlessly.

Now to outline the general anaesthetics which, although some may also be used for brief procedures, are chiefly employed to maintain anaesthesia for as long as is required, following induction (e.g. by thiopentone) as described earlier. They are given by the inhalation route, being either gases such as nitrous oxide, or volatile liquids which are rapidly converted to gases for inhalation.

**Nitrous Oxide** is probably the most commonly used inhalation anaesthetic; it is also known as "laughing gas". When inhaled neat, it produces anaesthesia very rapidly; this lasts less than a minute, and full recovery follows quickly, hence its wide use in dentistry. For use over longer periods it must be mixed with oxygen. Nitrous oxide is a weak anaesthetic, and for the maintenance of prolonged anaesthesia in the Operating Theatre it is generally used, with oxygen, to support the action of other anaesthetics such as halothane and ether; lower concentrations of the latter may then be used. Cylinders containing nitrous oxide are painted blue.

The Entonox apparatus employs a "50/50" mixture of nitrous oxide and oxygen, and is permitted to be used by midwives to relieve pain during labour; it is also employed by Ambulance Units to provide analgesia during transport of patients to hospitals. The Entonox cylinders are painted blue with a half white shoulder.

**Halothane** ('Fluothane') is a general anaesthetic which is very widely used. It is a non-inflammable, colourless, volatile liquid, with an odour like chloroform, and is protected from light by being packed in brown glass bottles. Halothane has a powerful action and is given in very weak concentration with either oxygen, or oxygen and nitrous oxide; it gives adequate relaxation and recovery is rapid.

**Methoxyflurane** ('Penthrane') is a volatile anaesthetic of similar properties and use to halothane; it is said to give equivalent muscle relaxation, but the recovery period is more prolonged.

**Ether** is a clear liquid, very light in weight, and with a characteristic smell; it has been used for many years, and is inhaled as a mixture with air and at a safe concentration. It should be noted that ether is *highly inflammable*, hence the need to avoid the possibility of any naked light or spark about (and this means *anywhere* in the room, Ward or Theatre, etc.) during its use. The anaesthetic grade of ether tends to deteriorate when exposed to light, as does halothane, and it is thus similarly packed in brown glass bottles, is extra-wrapped in dark paper, and is preferably stored under cool conditions. "Solvent ether", or "cleaning ether", is not pure and is thus unsuitable for use as an anaesthetic; it is used frequently for cleansing purposes, and *all* ward personnel *must* be made fully aware of its highly inflammable nature.

**Chloroform** is a heavy, colourless, volatile and non-inflammable liquid, with a sweet smell; it is now very little used, due to the significant risk of damage to such organs as the liver, heart and kidneys.

## LOCAL ANAESTHETICS

These are mainly given by injection. This may be by direct infiltration of the tissues in order to produce anaesthesia of the area by paralysing, or deadening, the local nerve endings. Or the injection(s) may be given at some distance away, with the aim of blocking the sensory nerve paths leading from the desired site; this may be termed nerve block, or regional anaesthesia. An example of regional anaesthesia is "ring block", when injections are given around the normal ring position to produce anaesthesia of the whole finger; toes can be anaesthetised similarly. There are several other modifications of "nerve block", including spinal anaesthesia and epidural anaesthesia; both are now described.

The spinal cord is enclosed by a sheath, the theca, composed of three membranes, or linings; these are the meninges. Spinal anaesthetics (i.e. *intrathecal*) are injected into the space between the two inner linings, and the sensory nerves leading to the spinal cord are paralysed, so preventing the passage along them of the sense of pain from the nerve endings. Various areas of the trunk may be anaesthetised in this way, the desired part being selected by adjusting the site and volume of the injection to correspond. Solutions which are heavier than the spinal fluid are sometimes employed; they tend to sink following injection, and may thus be used to anaesthetise the desired part of the trunk (together with the limbs if need be) by positioning the patient, i.e. by tilting the body accordingly.

*Epidural* anaesthesia is now in considerable use in place of spinal anaesthesia because there are said to be fewer complications. The anaesthetic solution is injected so as to just reach the epidural space which lies outside the outer lining of the spinal cord (i.e. the injection is not as deep as in the case of a spinal anaesthetic, which has to penetrate the theca); it then blocks sensory conduction along the spinal nerves which pass through the epidural space (containing the anaesthetic) to supply the trunk or limbs. The area of anaesthesia again depends on the site of injection and also the amount of local anaesthetic used.

An added advantage of spinal and epidural anaesthetics is that they also block the passage of motor impulses *towards* the anaesthetised area. This results in inactivation of the part affected and, in turn, the desirable depth of relaxation.

Certain local anaesthetics are also effective by application to mucous membranes; this is called surface anaesthesia.

The following are examples of local anaesthetics in general use.

**Cocaine**, obtained from the coca plant, was the first substance to be used as a local anaesthetic, and is the only one of natural origin. It is powerful in action, but has the disadvantage of serious side-effects, together with the danger of addiction—which makes it a Controlled Drug (p. 251). It is mainly used as a surface anaesthetic, particularly in ear, nose and throat operations, in the form of sprays, 2%–10%, and a thick mucilage. Drops of cocaine hydrochloride, 1%–2%, are instilled into the eye to anaesthetise the cornea for removal of foreign bodies; the drug is mydriatic in effect (see page 212) and hence dilates the pupil.

The toxicity and addictive effects associated with cocaine have prompted the introduction of several safer local anaesthetics; all are synthetic.

**Procaine** was the first one brought into wide use; it is employed only by infiltration into the tissue, in strengths varying from 0·5% to 2%, and the action is short. Procaine has no effect as a surface anaesthetic.

**Amethocaine** is far more powerful than procaine, and in addition it is effective by surface application to mucous membranes. It is used by injection in strengths as low as 0·1%, and as sprays at strengths from 0·5% to 2% in ear, nose and throat work. Eye drops (1%) and lozenges are other forms of amethocaine used.

**Cinchocaine** ('Nupercaine') is an extremely powerful local anaesthetic which is effective at very weak dilution. It can be used by tissue infiltration or by surface application, and is employed in spinal anaesthesia; the 0·5% solution is made "heavy" by the incorporation of glucose and is thus used for its property of descending when in the spinal fluid (see earlier). Cinchocaine is an ingredient of certain suppositories and ointments used to relieve the pain of haemorrhoids.

**Lignocaine** is a subsequent introduction and is probably the most widely used local anaesthetic. It is employed in strengths varying from 0·5% to 2% for local infiltration anaesthesia, and for nerve-block procedures, including spinal and epidural injections. A 4% spray or 2% viscous oral sip is used to produce surface anaesthesia of the mouth and throat in painful conditions or prior to examinations, and also before bronchoscopy (the introduction of a telescope into the lung via the mouth, throat and trachea). The discomfort of oesophagoscopy (the passing of a telescope into the oesophagus) may be similarly avoided by sucking lozenges containing lignocaine. Lignocaine is used as a suppository for rectal analgesia and as a 1% or 2% gel (water-miscible jelly) for introduction into the urethra (the outer urinary channel leading to the bladder) prior to passing a catheter or cystoscope (see page 219). A brand name is Xylocaine. The employment of lignocaine as a cardiac steadier and regulator is described on page 61.

**Prilocaine** ('Citanest') is very similar in action to lignocaine, and is claimed to be even safer in use; it has a wide application in surgery and dentistry.

**Bupivacaine** ('Marcain') is four times as powerful as lignocaine, and is issued at strengths of 0·25% and 0·5%; solutions may contain adrenaline, as is referred to later. Bupivacaine has a very prolonged action and is much used in the various nerve-block techniques, e.g. epidural anaesthesia.

Adrenaline is frequently added to local anaesthetics, e.g. procaine and lignocaine, in strengths varying from 1 in 80 000 to 1 in 400 000; this is in order to prolong the anaesthetic effect (as explained on page 188).

CHAPTER 14

# DRUGS USED IN THE TREATMENT OF INFECTION

## —the chemotherapeutic drugs—drugs used in tuberculosis—the antibiotics

This important group comprises broadly two sections, the synthetic chemotherapeutic drugs and the antibiotics; both terms will be explained later. The infections concerned are caused by pathogenic (i.e. disease producing) micro-organisms, made up of a vast number of different types and strains of bacteria, fungi (which include yeasts), and occasionally viruses; it should be noted, however, that very few virus infections may be treated with drug therapy.

The terms used when discussing infections and treatment are often complex, and a few of the more commonly met are worth explaining. Firstly, "*Gram-positive*" and "*Gram-negative*", which are used to describe an infection; these refer to the fact that the bacteria concerned may be of a type that will absorb and *retain* a stain called Gram's stain (when they will be "positive"), or they may not (when they will be "negative"). This is useful during laboratory investigation as a preliminary guide to the type of bacteria involved, and may also be of assistance to the doctor as an early pointer to which drug to use whilst he is waiting for definite information in the laboratory report (see later). Thus, if a Gram-negative infection is found to be involved, penicillin may be of unlikely value as it is often ineffective in such conditions, whereas the tetracyclines (p. 139) may be a more justifiable choice in view of their general activity against both Gram-positive and Gram-negative organisms.

Terms often used to describe an infection are "*streptococcal*" and "*staphylococcal*" (or "strep" and "staph"), and these indicate that a streptococcus or staphylococcus is the organism responsible; a coccus (plural "cocci") is an organism of round shape. Many other names of bacterial origin are also employed to describe infections, such as "E. coli" and "Proteus" (both these organisms are normally found in the colon, but may invade the urethra and cause urinary infections), "Salmonella" (often associated with severe food poisoning), and "Pseudomonas" (infections due to this organism have been commonly called "pyocyanea" or "pyocyaneus" in the past, and this term is still occasionally used to describe them). "Candida" or "Monilia" will refer to a typical yeast infection caused by an organism known both as "Candida albicans" and "Monilia albicans".

It should be noted that there are often many different organisms belonging to the same family; thus there are many distinct types of streptococci and staphylococci, the latter include both Staphylococcus albus (the "staph." common to the skin) and Staphylococcus aureus (a frequent cause of severe infections). Furthermore, there may be different *strains* of an organism, e.g. certain strains of Staph. aureus may be sensitive to penicillin, whereas others may be resistant.

The terms *"bacteriostatic"* and *"bactericidal"* are used to qualify the action of anti-infective drugs. A drug with bacteriostatic action does not directly kill the organism, but blocks, or interferes with, its metabolism and thus weakens it and prevents it multiplying, so enabling the body's natural defence mechanism to overcome it. A bactericidal drug is capable of actually killing the organism. It should be noted that some drugs are bacteriostatic in moderate dosage and bactericidal in high.

The recognition of the organism responsible for an infection is the result of meticulous work by the laboratory technician, and will involve isolating the organism (provided the appropriate specimen of urine, faeces, pus or sputum, for example, is available), growing it speedily in a suitable medium to enable complete microscopic, etc., examination, and finally testing against it the various anti-infective agents available, such as are discussed in this Chapter. His report will then identify the organism and indicate to the doctor the drug, or drugs, best suited to cope with the infection.

Now to discuss the drugs themselves.

## CHEMOTHERAPEUTIC DRUGS

The word chemotherapy is self-explanatory, "chemo" referring to the chemical nature of the drug, and "therapy" meaning treatment; thus chemotherapeutic drugs are chemicals which can be used in the treatment of infection (but see also use in malignant disease, Ch. 19). An important point that needs adding is that, in general, they can be introduced into the system without undue toxic effect upon the patient.

The first prominent group under this heading was the **Sulphonamides**, sometimes called the "sulpha" drugs. Their introduction in 1936 initiated the era of chemotherapy, whereby it became possible for tablets or injections of a drug to be given to the patient, to be then absorbed and carried in the circulation to the site of infection, finally to weaken the organism responsible and so enable the natural defence mechanism of the body to complete the process. Note that the action here is bacteriostatic.

The first sulphonamide was effective mainly in streptococcal and E. coli infections, but others have since been evolved with a wider range of action, e.g. against the pneumococcus which may cause typical pneumonia; they remain drugs of definite value, despite the advent of the antibiotics which have largely superseded them in the treatment of streptococcal and pneumococcal, etc., infections.

### The Systemic Sulphonamides

—are so called because they are absorbed from the gastro-intestinal tract and travel via the blood stream to the site of infection; they may also be given by injection. The one chiefly used is **Sulphadimidine** ('Sulphamezathine'), but two others which may still be occasionally employed are **Sulphadiazine** and **Sulphatriad**, the latter a combination of three sulphonamides. All are given as tablets of 500 mg, commencing e.g. with a loading dose of 2 grams, followed by 1 gram every four hours; flavoured suspensions are used, and sulphadimidine and sulphadiazine are also available as intramuscular and intravenous injections respectively. These systemic sulphonamides can be said to be normally safe and non-toxic, but it is important for the nurse to have a knowledge of such side-effects as can occur and how they may be prevented.

Nausea and vomiting are possible, but can be offset by giving the drug after food, which acts as a buffer; another occasional symptom is cyanosis, the blueish colour of the skin. Patients should avoid sunlight or ultra-violet light (U.V.L.) treatment, to which they can become sensitive and develop a rash. However, the main side-effect of concern commonly possible during sulphonamide therapy is haematuria, or blood in the urine. This is due to the fact that during elimination via the kidneys sulphonamides may tend to deposit as sharp crystals (this is called crystalluria), which injure the lining of the tubules, etc.; if this is allowed to continue, damage to the kidneys can result. This is avoided by ensuring that the patient takes adequate fluid, say up to two or three litres daily, and by giving also Potassium Citrate Mixture (p. 29) several times daily; the resultant high output of alkaline urine ensures that the sulphonamide (which is more soluble in alkaline urine than in acid) remains in solution, and crystalluria and haematuria are thus prevented.

There are also available systemic sulphonamides of which one or two doses only need to be given daily, because excretion via the urine is very slow and this enables an active concentration to be maintained in the body over a long period; in addition, there is the advantage of little or no risk of crystalluria and haematuria developing. Examples are **Sulphamethoxazole** ('Gantanol') and **Sulphamethoxypyridazine** ('Lederkyn'). For acute infections, however, the more effective high levels achieved by frequent doses of the short-acting sulphonamides are preferable. **Sulfametopyrazine** ('Kelfizine W') is an unusually long-acting sulphonamide, for the tablets or suspension are taken just once *weekly*; it is probably little employed in the hospital field.

Sulphamethoxazole is one of the two ingredients of **Cotrimoxazole** tablets ('Bactrim', 'Septrin') which are taken for systemic effect, the other being trimethoprim, a chemical which has a powerful bactericidal effect. These two drugs have what is called a synergistic action, which means that the combined effect is greater than the sum of their individual effects; or, as a simplification, the effect of each drug is enhanced by that of the other. Adult and paediatric tablets and suspensions are available, and dosage is based on two tablets twice daily; two further presentations are the *dispersible* tablet, which disintegrates instantly when stirred in water for taking, and the injection form, which has to be diluted with a specified volume of an appropriate intravenous infusion solution. Advantages of this combination are that it is bactericidal to a wide range of Gram-positive and Gram-negative organisms, including proteus (which is sensitive to few drugs), and that resistance to it is not so easily developed as to many of the antibiotics; side-effects, too, are relatively minimal. Cotrimoxazole is a favoured drug in many common infections, e.g. of the bronchial and urinary systems.

### The Urinary Sulphonamides

The antiseptic effect of the systemic sulphonamides so far mentioned continues during excretion via the kidneys, but if an actual urinary infection is involved two other members of this group, **Sulphafurazole** ('Gantrisin') and **Sulphamethizole** ('Urolucosil') may be preferred. Both are well absorbed and effective against a useful range of bacteria, and they have the additional advantage of being more soluble in urine, hence there is far less risk of the development of crystalluria and haematuria. Sulphamethizole has the further feature of low dosage (200 mg), which makes crystalluria even less possible. Another useful point about these two urinary sulphonamides is that liquid intake need not, indeed *should not*, be as high as when using the systemic sulphonamides mentioned earlier, because their greater solubility permits a lower volume of urinary output, and this results in a higher concentration of the drug in the urine, with consequent increased antiseptic effect.

### Eye Sulphonamides

The main member of this group used in ophthalmic work is

**Sulphacetamide** ('Albucid'), because of its bland and non-irritant nature. It can be used at very high concentration, as eye-drops of from 10% to 30%, and as an eye ointment in strengths of 6% and 10%.

## The Intestinal Sulphonamides

—are distinct from the systemic group in that they are poorly absorbed from the gastro-intestinal tract and are thus of no value in systemic infections; references to their particular use in infective diarrhoeas and prior to bowel surgery has been made on page 25.

## Sulphasalazine

The condition of ulcerative colitis, characterised by diarrhoea and inflammation of the bowel wall, is most often treated medically. In addition to appropriate diet, with avoidance of high residue, etc., drugs that may be used are the corticosteroids (p. 190), and the sulphonamide, sulphasalazine ('Salazopyrin'), which is in the form of brown tablets. When sulphasalazine is taken, part is absorbed from the gastro-intestinal tract and the remainder passes along the bowel, but in each case the drug appears to achieve a significant level in the bowel wall, i.e. from both sides; infection is held to be a factor in the condition, and this explains the benefit of treatment with this sulphonamide, which is usually long-term and in dosage of 4–6 grams daily. Gastric disturbance is sometimes a side-effect, and in such an event tablets ('Salazopyrin EN') are available which pass through the stomach and into the duodenum before disintegration commences. Another useful presentation of sulphasalazine is the suppository, which is inserted per rectum to fortify local effect.

## Metronidazole

—in addition to its use in trichomonas infections (p. 146) and amoebiasis (p. 151) has also been found markedly effective in infections caused by anaerobic bacteria; these organisms are so called because they can grow only in an oxygen-free environment, particular examples being the bacteroides range and certain types of streptococci—there is increasing awareness of the significance of these organisms in infections of the gastro-intestinal and gynaecological fields. Thus, metronidazole is widely used in infections due to such organisms, the tablets being given three times daily, during or after meals; it is also given as a large dose before operations, of gastro-intestinal and gynaecological involvement in particular, followed by moderate dosage three times daily for a week, this as a highly successful prophylactic (preventive) measure. Suppositories and retention enemas are effective supportive therapy, and intravenous injections are additionally coming into use.

## Chemotherapeutic Drugs used in Tuberculosis

Three basic drugs long used in tuberculosis have been P.A.S., isoniazid, and streptomycin. The first two are synthetic chemotherapeutic drugs, and will be discussed here together with others which are now being increasingly employed. Streptomycin is an antibiotic and will be discussed later (p. 137), together with other antibiotics which are likewise used as replacement.

### P.A.S.

—stands for para-amino-salicylic acid, and the form used is the sodium compound, **Sodium Aminosalicylate**, the drug which revolutionised the treatment of tuberculosis, though now giving way markedly to later introductions. It is a white powder with an unpleasant taste, is bacteriostatic to the T.B. organism, and is used in a wide range of tuberculous conditions; it is taken orally, in the order of 12 grams daily. Liquid mixtures may be employed, usually incorporating isoniazid (see later), but can cause nausea and vomiting, and sometimes diarrhoea; they may also deteriorate on keeping, and should therefore be used as freshly made as possible. Nausea and vomiting may be avoided by eating dry food beforehand, and taking the dose in one swallow may help; diarrhoea may be eased with Kaolin Mixture.

Unpleasantness in taking P.A.S. carries with it the risk that the patient may not take the drug regularly and may thus lose ground against the disease—as well as becoming a possible danger to other contacts; hence the additional preference for newer drugs which do not carry this disadvantage.

A normal course of P.A.S. (together with other drugs mentioned later) may last for one to two years or longer, and in favourable response the temperature falls, the pulse rate diminishes and appetite improves. P.A.S. is best taken in the early, active state of the disease, when the body's defence mechanism is still a helpful factor and diffusion of the drug to the site is good. A valuable feature of P.A.S. is that resistance to it on the part of the T.B. organism is slow to develop and this applies likewise to the other drugs given with it as well; such mutual reinforcement is characteristic of the combinations used in tuberculosis.

P.A.S. may also be given by intravenous injection, a routine which has been much used in Switzerland; the full day's dosage of P.A.S. (as high as 24 grams) is contained in 500 ml of sterile solution and given in about two hours; the patient experiences minimal discomfort and there is absence of nausea and vomiting. The very high blood level achieved by this method of administration has proved life-saving in several instances in the author's own hospital experience.

## Isoniazid

Treatment of tuberculosis, as already implied, normally involves the employment of two or more drugs and a prominent one is isoniazid, often abbreviated to I.N.A.H. This drug is available in tablet form and average dosage is 300 mg daily. I.N.A.H. is powerfully bacteriostatic to the T.B. organism, but a disadvantage is that resistance towards it is developed speedily, hence the value of combining it with P.A.S., which delays such resistance—as explained earlier. P.A.S. and I.N.A.H. are conveniently taken together in the same preparation, and, in addition to liquid mixtures, granules ('Inapasade') are available which are taken only twice daily, being poured onto the tongue and swallowed with a cool drink of water; they are tasteless and do not commence to disintegrate until in the duodenum, hence nausea, etc., is avoided.

Isoniazid may be given by injection ('Rimifon'), either intramuscularly or intravenously in the case of severley ill patients, as well as intrathecally in T.B. meningitis; it may also be instilled into the pleural cavity enveloping the lungs.

The important place of isoniazid is illustrated by the fact that it is so often included in the various drug combinations used in treating tuberculosis, e.g. with ethambutol (below) and rifampicin (p. 139).

An interesting feature of the effect of isoniazid is that patients improve in spirits markedly, and investigation of this euphoric effect (sense of well-being) has led to the introduction of related drugs which are used for their anti-depressant effect; these are members of the M.A.O.-inhibitor group and are discussed on page

## Alternative Chemotherapeutic Drugs used in Tuberculosis

The range of synthetic anti-TB drugs has broadened and this allows of variation in the combinations employed, particularly in cases of bacterial resistance or untoward side-effects. **Ethionmide** and **Pyrazinamide** are related chemically and are taken as tablets, usually three times daily. **Ethambutol** is also in tablet form, but is taken only once daily; an unusual side-effect associated with this drug is blurred vision and loss of colour sense. 'Mynah' is a tablet containing ethambutol and isoniazid and issued in several strengths. Ethambutol is a major drug in this group.

> Ethionamide —'Trescatyl'   —av. dose 500–750 mg daily
> Pyrazinamide—'Zinamide'   — ,,    ,,   2–3 g daily
> Ethambutol —'Myambutol'—based on weight of patient

The student is reminded that the treatment of tuberculosis often incorporates streptomycin, or an alternative antibiotic in streptomycin-resistant cases; these drugs are described on pages 138 and

139. Likewise that the combination of at least two drugs (frequently three) is imperative in anti-tuberculosis treatment; development of resistance by the T.B. organism is then checked, and, in addition, the over-all effect of the drugs used is greatly enhanced (see note on synergism, p. 129).

## Other Applications of Chemotherapy

So far chemotherapeutic drugs have been discussed in the generally accepted sense, i.e. in relation to their use as anti-infective agents. However, potent synthetic chemicals are also used in other fields, one of which is the chemotherapy of malignant disease, in which the drugs are used for their effect in inhibiting the development of the cells of cancer tissue; these are discussed in Chapter 19.

## ANTIBIOTICS

—are also substances which possess chemotherapeutic activity, but the difference between them and the synthetic chemotherapeutic drugs already discussed, e.g. the sulphonamides, is that antibiotics are almost entirely derived from *natural* sources. The sources concerned are minute organisms, such as moulds, which abound in nature; a typical example is the green mould which may grow on bread or cheese if kept warm and moist, and which may be related to, or even be, Penicillium notatum, the mould which produces penicillin. An outline of the preparation of penicillin will clarify the background to the antibiotic picture. The Penicillium mould is grown in a nutrient (feed) solution, at a suitable temperature, and during its rapid development it excretes end-products of its metabolism; one of these is the "raw" penicillin. The mould itself is then removed by filtration, and the penicillin is extracted from the solution, purified, and finally presented as a sterile white powder ready for dissolving and administering by injection, and also as various oral preparations, etc. Thus penicillin is *a substance produced by a living micro-organism, which is effective in overcoming infections caused by other micro-organisms;* this is a good definition of an antibiotic. Note, however, that a certain few antibiotics are used specifically in treating malignant disease, as is discussed in Chapter 19.

**Penicillin** was the first antibiotic, an even more valuable discovery than were the sulphonamides, for it is normally non-toxic and without side-effects, and its effective range of action includes staphylococci, against which the sulphonamides are of little value. The first penicillin, still widely used, was benzyl penicillin, or penicillin G ('Crystapen G'); it is given by intramuscular injection and reaches the blood quickly, to be later excreted via the urine. In the early days of penicillin, dosage was low and frequent, maintaining a bacteriostatic level only; the custom now is to give a large dose once or twice daily, e.g. one mega (1 million units), and this provides a more active, bactericidal level. Penicillin G may also be given orally, as tablets and syrup, and is fairly well absorbed if taken at the advised time in relation to meals—as explained later. However, when high peak levels are required, as in acute infections, the injection route is invariably essential.

Penicillin G is effective against many of the bacteria commonly met in infections, such as streptococci, staphylococci and pneumococci, etc., hence its continued use and esteem as a standard antibiotic; resistant strains of some of these organisms are now not infrequently met, however, and this will be discussed later.

Two points should be noted concerning the storage and administration of penicillin preparations. Firstly, penicillin G deteriorates when in solution, expecially if kept at a warm temperature, and stocks of injections which are issued to the ward ready-dissolved should be stored in the refrigerator and used as quickly as possible. Such solutions are usually labelled with the expiry date, and this must be adhered to. In some hospitals it is the custom to dissolve injections on the ward as required. The same dating precaution applies also to the oral syrups which are prepared by adding a specified amount of water and shaking to dissolve; in general, these last for 7 days at room temperature and 14 days if kept in the refrigerator.

Secondly, the activity of penicillin G is affected by conditions of acidity, hence the oral forms, tablets or syrup, are best taken well before meal times, for the acid value of the stomach is then at its lowest and maximum absorption is thus ensured.

## Other preparations of Penicillin

Many derivatives of penicillin G have been introduced with the aim of prolonging the action or achieving higher absorption levels by the oral route.

**Procaine penicillin** ('Depocillin') is an insoluble compound given by injection; it should be shaken before use. It is released slowly, giving prolonged though moderate blood levels, and is suitable for the less severe infections. Other compound preparations with prolonged action (e.g. 'Penidural-AP', 'Triplopen') combine three forms of penicillin, two of the insoluble slow-release type, plus soluble penicillin G for its immediate effect; the prolonged effect of these preparations avoids the need for frequent dosage. In severe infections, however, as previously stated, penicillin G by injection in high dosage daily is usually the penicillin of choice.

**Phenoxymethylpenicillin**, known as penicillin V ('Crystapen V'), is more resistant to gastric acid than is penicillin G, and thus provides higher blood levels at equal dosage; it is accordingly often favoured for oral treatment. It is again best taken before meals, as tablets or syrup, the latter being prepared as is penicillin G syrup and with a similar set date for taking by.

The oral dosage of both penicillins, G and V, is expressed in terms of weight, e.g. 125 mg or 250 mg, whereas injections of penicillin G are in terms of units. 125 mg of penicillin G or V is approximately equivalent to 200 000 units.

## The Semi-Synthetic Penicillins

The forms of penicillin discussed so far have one feature in common—their range of activity is largely identical, i.e. they are effective against the same strains of the same organisms. Duration of action or resistance to gastric acid has certainly been improved by attaching a procaine or phenoxymethyl group, for example, to the original penicillin (see earlier), but it is only by connecting new chemical groups to the actual *core* or *nucleus* of penicillin that its range of action can be extended. The isolation of this "naked" penicillin nucleus was achieved by an English firm, which was therefore enabled to introduce a number of new penicillin compounds of distinct or extended range of activity. Of those produced initially, four were proved of particular importance—methicillin, cloxacillin, ampicillin and carbenicillin. Due to the fact that these new penicillins were evolved in the laboratory by altering the naturally produced penicillin nucleus, they were termed "semi-synthetic".

**Methicillin** and **Cloxacillin** are active against staphylococci which are resistant to other antibiotics, including penicillin G, and it is timely to refer briefly to the problem of resistance. Some organisms are not affected by the action of certain antibiotics and are thus said to be insensitive. However, in a number of cases, organisms which were once sensitive to a particular antibiotic have developed powerfully resistant strains. A notable example is Staphylococcus aureus, many strains of which are now resistant to penicillin G. One reason for this is that when penicillin was freely used in its early years, certain colonies of staphylococci were resistant and survived, due to their ability to produce an enzyme, penicillinase, which inactivates penicillin. Following the continued use of penicillin, particularly in hospitals, these surviving strains have had the "field" left progressively clear to them, and have multiplied sufficiently to produce the extra problem of "resistant staphs." (sometimes called "hospital staphs."); also, resistance can be transferred from one bacterium to another of the same or different type. It is in this field that the value of methicillin and cloxacillin lay initially, for few strains of staphylococci are resistant to them. Methicillin is active only by intramuscular or intravenous injection, whereas cloxacillin may be given intramuscularly but is also effective orally as capsules or syrup; methicillin is now rarely used, having been superseded by cloxacillin and other new derivatives (see later). Again, however, it should be noted that provided the organism is sensitive to penicillin G, the latter continues a highly used and effective penicillin.

The problem of development of resistance is also met in the case of other organisms which have become insensitive to the antibiotics normally effective against them.

**Ampicillin** differs from penicillin G in that it has a broader "spectrum", or range, of activity. The broad-spectrum antibiotics will be described later (p. 139), and it is sufficient to note here that ampicillin is effective against Gram-negative as well as Gram-positive organisms, whereas penicillin is active mainly against Gram-positive organisms. Ampicillin is taken orally and is absorbed more effectively than are the other broad-spectrum antibiotics, e.g. the tetracyclines; gastro-intestinal disturbance is also less of a problem. Good absorption results in high systemic levels, and in the case of ampicillin this applies particularly to the urine, hence its great value in infections of the urinary tract. It is available as capsules, as intramuscular and intravenous injections, and as a syrup for children. Ampicillin has one disadvantage, it is inactivated by the enzyme penicillinase which is produced by resistant staphylococci; this is offset by its being combined with cloxacillin and flucloxacillin (see later) in the 'Ampiclox' and 'Magnapen' series of preparations.

Following the use of so many different antibiotics over a long period, the "resident" bacterial picture in hospitals (particularly) has altered significantly, and infections which were once less common have become more prominent; an example is the pseudomonas (or "pyocyaneus") infections which are now not infrequently met and may be serious. Few antibiotics are effective against this organism, and some of these possess the disadvantage of toxic side-effects. Hence **Carbenicillin** is a drug of great value, for it is virtually non-toxic, is highly effective against pseudomonas, and thus life-saving in acute infection. It is not absorbed orally, being destroyed in the stomach, and is given only by intramuscular injection.

| Methicillin | —'Celbenin'—av. dose 1 g | | |
|---|---|---|---|
| Cloxacillin | —'Orbenin' — „ | „ | 250–500 mg |
| Ampicillin | —'Penbritin'— „ | „ | 250–500 mg |
| Carbenicillin | —'Pyopen' — „ | „ | 3 g (but is often much higher) |

Further semi-synthetic penicillins continue to appear, each said to have an improved or distinct performance. Thus—

**Amoxycillin** is similar to ampicillin in range of activity and freedom from toxicity; likewise it is effective by mouth, but its ready absorption produces blood levels about twice as high. It is available as capsules, syrup and paediatric suspension, and is given only *three* times daily, which is an advantage in ward drug routine.

**Flucloxacillin** is closely similar to cloxacillin, but contains fluorine in its chemical structure. It is also effective against penicillin-resistant staphylococci and is taken orally, but is far more readily absorbed and dosage is lower in consequence. Injections are also available.

**'Magnapen'** is a combination of ampicillin and flucloxacillin, and is claimed to be an improvement on 'Ampiclox' in that the flucloxacillin (see above) it contains is more readily absorbed than is the cloxacillin in 'Ampiclox'.

**Talampicillin** is mainly of interest because following oral taking it is quickly absorbed and is converted in the blood to ampicillin.

**Carfecillin** is likewise converted to carbenicillin following absorption, and because a high level of concentration is achieved in the urine it is especially employed for appropriate urinary infections.

```
Amoxycillin   —'Amoxil'  —av. dose 250 mg
Flucloxacillin—'Floxapen'— „    „    250 mg
Talampicillin —'Talpen'   — „    „    250 mg
Carfecillin   —'Uticillin' — „   „    500 mg
```

## Penicillin sensitivity

Although penicillin is correctly described as free from toxic side-effects, cases of sensitivity are occasionally met. The symptoms may be of simple allergic type, e.g. skin rash, etc., but in severe hypersensitivity (anaphylaxis) acute shock may result. Such sensitivity (as in the case of *any* drug concerned) is carefully recorded in the patient's case notes and is boldly stated on the prescription sheet, for it is possible for a further dose to prove fatal. It should be noted that sensitivity to one penicillin means sensitivity *to all*, and this includes the semi-synthetic group just discussed.

### Streptomycin

The discovery of penicillin made it apparent that in the teeming world of micro-organisms there lay the possibility of other valuable antibiotics being discovered. Continued investigation of soils and manures, etc., has revealed likely moulds and other minute organisms which have been cultured (i.e. grown on), and the excretory products of their metabolism tested for antibiotic or other activity. The first antibiotic to follow penicillin was streptomycin.

**Streptomycin** is issued as a white powder, in 1 g and 5 g bottles, ready for dissolving for injection; it is effective against a more varied range of organisms than is penicillin G, but, in particular, it is active against the bacterium which causes tuberculosis.

Streptomycin is not absorbed from the gastro-intestinal tract, and is given orally solely for infective diarrhoeas (p. 25); thus, in the treatment of tuberculosis it is given by intramuscular injection. The dose is maintained at a moderate level of 0·5 to 1 gram daily, or on alternate days, due to the serious toxic effects possible if dosage is too high, or too frequent over too long a period. Minor side-effects are pains in the joints, and skin rash, the latter making it advisable for the nurse to avoid contact with the solution herself when giving injections, and also spillage on the patient's skin. The most serious side-effect, however, is ototoxicity, or damage to the eighth cranial nerve; this involves the balance and hearing mechanisms, which are located in the labyrinth of the inner ear, and may lead to giddiness and deafness, the latter possibly permanent if dosage is unduly prolonged. Thus, streptomycin is used with extra caution in the elderly, due to possibility of impaired kidney function, or in *any* patient if this is already established, for this could entail lessened excretion of the drug and consequent accumulation and rapid ototoxicity. Likewise, streptomycin is not generally used for conditions other than tuberculosis, except when given with penicillin (as 'Crystamycin') for short (and thus safe) courses of five to seven days; this is a valuable combination because the effect is synergistic (p. 129) and highly bactericidal to a number of common pathogenic organisms.

An important point to note is that if either penicillin or streptomycin is to be given by intrathecal injection—as in cases of meningitis—only the pure powder in the special "intrathecal" ampoule should be used, and this must be dissolved *only* in sterile Water for Injections; if the normal intramuscular solutions are used for this purpose, serious damage can result due to the preservatives, etc., they may contain. This applies similarly to intrathecal injections of *all* antibiotics.

### Alternative Antibiotics to Streptomycin in the treatment of Tuberculosis

Newer antibiotics are employed in place of streptomycin if the infection proves resistant, or if they are considered otherwise more suitable. Two such alternatives are Capreomycin ('Capistat') and **Cycloserine;** the former is a white powder which is dissolved for intramuscular injection, av. dose 1 gram daily, and cycloserine is taken orally as tablets or capsules of 250 mg and is effectively absorbed from the gastro-intestinal tract.

Capreomycin has similar ototoxic effects to streptomycin, and cycloserine may cause a variety of side-effects on the central nervous system, including convulsions and mental confusion, hence both drugs are also used with discretion in relation to length of treatment.

**Rifampicin** ('Rifadin', 'Rimactane') is one of the later antibiotics introduced for the treatment of tuberculosis. It is effective orally and is taken in capsule form once daily, the dose depending on the weight of the patient; it is generally used in combination with other anti-tuberculous drugs. Ototoxicity is absent and side-effects are minimal, a simple one being a reddish coloration of the urine, sputum and tears; it is good nursing procedure to warn T.B. patients of this in the case of sputum. An advantage of rifampicin is that it is bacteri-cidal in effect and is about equal in activity to I.N.A.H., and superior to P.A.S. and streptomycin; it carries less possibility of relapse, and is thus an outstanding drug in this section.

Rifampicin and isoniazid make a particularly powerful combi-nation, and tablets are available which contain both these drugs ('Rifinah' and 'Rimactazid'); the day's single dose is taken before breakfast.

## The Broad-Spectrum Antibiotics

—are so called because they are active against an extended range of organisms, both Gram-positive and Gram-negative (p. 126), com-pared with the mainly Gram-positive activity of penicillin. Ampicillin and amoxycillin have already been alluded to as having a wide range of activity, but the original tetracycline "broad-spectrums", **Chlor-tetracycline, Oxytetracycline** and **Tetracycline** itself, continue to be employed; all three are similar in action and generally interchange-able in use, and are available as a buff-coloured powder in capsule or tablet form, and as syrups, intramuscular and intravenous injections, eye drops, ear drops, ointments and pressurised sprays, etc. In addition to covering a wider range of infections, the tetracyclines are effective against certain viruses, including the one which causes a severe type of "non-typical" pneumonia. As they are fairly well absorbed from the gastro-intestinal tract, they are given orally unless the injection route is necessary.

Chlortetracycline—'Aureomycin'—av. dose 250 mg
Oxytetracycline  —'Clinimycin' — ,,   ,,    ,,    ,,
'Imperacin'  — ,,   ,,    ,,    ,,
'Terramycin' — ,,   ,,    ,,    ,,
Tetracycline   —'Achromycin'— ,,   ,,    ,,    ,,

Side-effects of the tetracyclines are discomforting rather than serious, being occasional nausea and vomiting, and diarrhoea with acute itching of the anus (pruritus ani); the latter has an interesting explanation. Due to not being completely absorbed, part of the tetracycline reaches the bowel and destroys many of the bacteria normally present there; certain other organisms of the yeast type, however, are not sensitive to the drug and are therefore able to multiply profusely, resulting in a superimposed yeast infection. The yeasts excrete irritant toxins, which stimulate the bowel into peristalsis and diarrhoea, and this secondary infection may then spread downwards to the anus, causing the severe irritation referred to. In such cases, one of two antibiotics, nystatin or amphotericin (p. 143), may be prescribed with the tetracycline; these are not absorbed and thus reach the bowel, where they are effective in controlling the growth of the yeast organisms. The mouth may also be affected by the yeast infection, when nystatin or amphotericin is employed as a suspension or lozenge, or natamycin (p. 144) as a cream or suspension.

A further point is that certain of the bacteria in the bowel are beneficial in that they manufacture several of the essential B vitamins, which are then absorbed for utilisation in the body. Hence, during prolonged tetracycline treatment, the patient may be given tablets of Vitamin B Compound to offset deficiency caused by tetracycline action on the bacteria concerned.

One other side-effect of the tetracyclines is that if given during a certain period of pregnancy, or to infant patients, a brownish staining may appear in the teeth of the child. Oxytetracycline is held to have the least effect in this respect.

Further, newer tetracycline derivatives are claimed to have less side-effects and/or to need less frequent dosage. A typical example is **Minocycline** ('Minocin'), two 100 mg tablets of which are taken initially, followed by one twice daily.

The extensive range of activity of the tetracyclines, and other broad-spectrum antibiotics, e.g. ampicillin and subsequent introductions (see later), has led to their wide use, for the following reason in particular. It takes at least 24 hours for the investigation and report to be completed following the sending of a specimen, e.g. pus or urine, to the laboratory. In the meantime, the problem may be one of which antibiotic to commence treatment with, especially if the infection is severe and the laboratory examination does not provide an early clue. Hence the value in such cases of initiating treatment with a broad-spectrum antibiotic which is obviously more likely to cover the organism involved.

## Chloramphenicol

—is another antibiotic with a wide spectrum of activity; it is a white powder, available as capsules, paediatric suspension, intramuscular and intravenous injection, eye ointment and eye drops, etc., and is alone amongst the antibiotics as being entirely synthetically manufactured. Its range of action is similar to that of the tetracyclines, but it is especially effective against the bacterium which causes typhoid.

Chloramphenical is given orally except in severely ill cases, and dosage is usually higher than in the case of the tetracyclines. It is usually employed only when considered essential, for it carries a risk of causing blood abnormalities, which include aplastic anaemia, a serious condition in which there is loss of bone marrow function; the duration of courses is thus also closely controlled.

Chloramphenicol—'Chloromycetin'—av. dose 250–500 mg

It should be appreciated that broad-spectrum activity is not confined to the tetracyclines, ampicillin, and chloromycetin. Certain of the new antibiotics have an even wider range of action, especially against the "difficult" Gram-negative organisms, and these are included in the following section.

### Other Antibiotics

These are numerous, but each has its own range of antibacterial activity, though there is a degree of similarity or overlapping in many cases. Choice is usually controlled, if possible, by the laboratory report, which will indicate the one (or more) most likely to be effective. The following are representative examples.

**Amikacin** is a more recent semi-synthetic antibiotic which is valuable as being effective against certain significant strains of Gram-negative organisms, e.g. proteus and pseudomonas (p. 126), many resistant to gentamicin, as well as against resistant staphylococci—which continue to appear. Amikacin is given twice daily, intramuscularly or intravenously, on body weight basis, an average adult dose being 500 mg; it may also be given intrathecally in Gram-negative meningitis and used as an irrigation solution. A prominent side-effect possible is ototoxicity, and if treatment is likely to be prolonged a hearing test is made before and during the course, and should tinnitus (a constant singing in the ears) or hearing loss occur, then the drug is discontinued.

**Cephaloridin** has a very wide spectrum of activity, covering Gram-positive and Gram-negative organisms and including staphylococci, streptococci, E.coli (against which penicillin is usually ineffective), and proteus, an organism which is sensitive to few antibiotics; it is given only by injection.

**Cephalexin** is a semi-synthetic antibiotic derived from cephaloridin and with a similar range of action. It has the advantage, however, of being effective orally, with a very high rate of absorption. Its toxicity is limited to gastro-intestinal disturbances, as occur with many of the broad-spectrum antibiotics.

Other semi-synthetic cephalosporins (as this cephaloridin-derived group is called) have been introduced as having advantages in one direction or other; examples are **Cephalothin, Cephazolin** and **Cephadrine.**

**Clindamycin**, a further semi-synthetic type, is derived from lincomycin (see later) and is effective orally. It is at least eight times as powerful as lincomycin, and against the same range of organisms, which includes all strains of staphylococci; its action is bactericidal and resistance is rarely encountered.

**Colistin** is one of the few antibiotics which are effective in the treatment of pseudomonas infections; it has to be given by intramuscular injection except in bowel infections, when it is effective orally due to its non-absorption. Carbenicillin has already been referred to for its use in pseudomonas infections (p. 136), and the advantage of having several antibiotics effective against the same organism is that if a particular strain of the organism is resistant to one, it may well be sensitive to another.

**Erythromycin** has a similar range of activity to that of penicillin, but is particularly effective in staphylococcal infections where the possibility of resistance to penicillin is suspected. It is active orally, and is available as capsules and tablets, syrups and suspensions, and intramuscular and intravenous injections.

**Fusidic acid** is also highly active against staphylococci, and produces extremely high bone and tissue levels due to its penetrative effect; it is thus used in conditions such as osteomyelitis, and is taken orally as capsules or syrup. A variety of fusidic acid preparations is also available for external application, these include the 'Fucidin' range of ointment, water-miscible gel, and intertulle gauze square dressings.

**Gentamicin** has an unusually broad range of effectiveness, against both Gram-positive and Gram-negative organisms and including pseudomonas, E.coli and resistant staphylococci. It is not absorbed orally and must be given by intramuscular injection; ototoxicity is a danger if dosage is too high and/or the course too prolonged. Eye drops, ear drops, creams and ointments are also available.

**Kanamycin** is often the antibiotic of choice in the serious infections caused by the proteus organism, against which, as mentioned earlier, few antibiotics are active; it is given by injection, and carries the disadvantage of serious ototoxicity if used too freely.

**Lincomycin** has a similar range of activity to fusidic acid, and is also of particular value in resistant staphylococcal infections.

| | | |
|---|---|---|
| Amikacin —'Amikin' | —av. dose 500 mg | |
| Cephaloridine—'Ceporin' | — ,, ,, | 500 mg–1 g |
| Cephalexin —'Ceporex' | — ,, ,, | 500 mg |
| Cephalothin —'Keflin' | — ,, ,, | 1–4 g |

| Cephazolin | —'Kefzol' | — | ,, | ,, | 500 mg–1 g |
| Cephadrine | —'Velosef' | — | ,, | ,, | 500 mg |
| Clindamycin | —'Dalacin C' | — | ,, | ,, | 150 mg |
| Colistin | —'Colomycin' | — | ,, | ,, | 1 mega unit |
| Erythromycin | —'Erythrocin', 'Ilotycin' | — | ,, | ,, | 250 mg |
| Fusidic Acid | —'Fucidin' | — | ,, | ,, | 500 mg |
| Gentamicin | —'Genticin', 'Cidomycin' | — | ,, | ,, | 40–80 mg |
| Kanamycin | —'Kannasyn' | — | ,, | ,, | 250–500 mg |
| Lincomycin | —'Lincocin' | — | ,, | ,, | 500 mg |

## Mixed infections

Occasionally a mixed infection, i.e. caused by more than one organism, may demand the use of two antibiotics, and the following point is of interest. Some antibiotics are purely bacteriostatic, whereas others are bactericidal, and it is customary to avoid combining a member from each group in treatment, because of the possibility of mutual antagonism of activity. Thus, if two antibiotics are indicated, it is usually preferred that they are both bacteriostatic or both bactericidal.

## Antibiotics used in Fungus/Yeast infections

**Nystatin** and **Amphotericin** have been referred to on page 140 in relation to their specific value in infections of the bowel which may occur during tetracycline therapy; both come from the same commercial source, but amphotericin is the superior antibiotic, for it is active against a wider range of fungus organisms. Common conditions in which amphotericin or nystatin is indicated are the bowel infections already mentioned, which are treated with tablets or suspensions taken orally, both antibiotics being non-absorbed; yeast infections of the mouth and throat which may also accompany tetracycline therapy, and the similar "thrush" infection in young children, when lozenges are sucked or suspensions retained in the mouth; yeast infections of the vagina (due to candida) in which pessaries and creams are used; and skin conditions in which ointments are applied. Fungal infections may also invade the system and become generalised, a severe condition which may occur following tetracycline treatment, and in this event amphotericin is given by intravenous injection and can be life saving; another indication for its use is in "farmer's lung", a condition caused by inhalation of fungal organisms during the handling of hay, etc. Nystatin is not given by injection due to its being too irritant.

**Griseofulvin** is an antibiotic which is excreted via the skin. It has a specific indication in stubborn fungal infections which are resistant to the preparations normally applied externally, examples being "athlete's foot", ringworm, and certain finger and nail conditions. The tablets are taken daily for approximately one month, and after absorption from the gastro-intestinal tract, the antibiotic reaches the skin in high concentration and attacks the fungal infection at a vulnerable point, i.e. where it spreads below the surface.

Nystatin        —'Nystan'  "  —av. dose 500 000 units
Amphotericin—'Fungilin'  —  „    „    100 mg
                'Fungizone'—i/v, dose based on weight of
                                                        patient
Griseofulvin  —'Grisovin', 'Fulcin'—av. dose 500 mg daily

**Natamycin** ('Pimafucin') is particularly active against fungus and yeast infections, but is used essentially for local effect, e.g. as a cream in conditions of the mouth, nail, vagina, etc.; as a 1% suspension for oral thrush; as a 2·5% suspension for inhalation in lung infections; and as vaginal tablets in candida *and* trichomonas infections (p. 146).

**Flucytosine** is not an antibiotic, but is included here as a drug used specifically in a wide range of *systemic* fungus infections; dosage is based on body weight, and the tablets ('Alcobon') are taken in four divided doses daily. Flucytosine acts by interfering with fungal metabolism; possible side-effects include blood abnormalities, hence the drug is carefully monitored in use.

### A further note on the storage and administration of antibiotics

The points already made (p. 134) concerning the deterioration of injections and syrups of penicillin G, once they have been made up, apply also in the case of many of the other antibiotics. Some may be issued by the manufacturing firm in solution form ready for use by injection, or in syrup form ready for taking, but these will always be labelled with the expiry date—after which they should not be used.

A further word of caution concerns injections which are issued as a sterile powder and have to be dissolved for use. If the vial contains one dose, this merely has to be dissolved and administered, but it occasionally happens that a portion only of the contents has to be given, e.g. the vial may contain 1 g, and the dose prescribed may be 250 mg. If the antibiotic is known to remain effective for some time (e.g. 48 hours) after being dissolved, then the vial can be kept in the refrigerator and drawn from for successive doses. However, some antibiotics deteriorate so rapidly after being dissolved that they are directed to be "freshly prepared" for each dose; in such cases the vials must be used for one dose only and then discarded, however much is left unused.

Information covering these points may be available on the label or accompanying leaflet, or instruction may have been given by the pharmacist, but the nurse should always be certain to make herself thoroughly acquainted with the correct routine applicable to the antibiotic being administered.

## Antibiotics mainly employed for external application

Certain antibiotics have a wide range of antibacterial activity but are not used for systemic effect, either because they are not absorbed when taken by mouth (which may then make them suitable as bowel antiseptics, e.g. neomycin) or because they are unsuitable for some other reason, e.g. toxicity; examples are **Bacitracin, Framycetin, Gramicidin, Neomycin** and **Polymixin.** These are reserved mainly for external use as ingredients of eye drops, ear drops, ointments and creams, etc., and in tulle-gras dressings (e.g. 'Neotulle', 'Sofra-Tulle') in which squares of gauze are impregnated with a soft paraffin base containing the antibiotic. Some are included in external steroid applications as a safety measure; neomycin is often used in this connection (see page 192).

This group of antibiotics is contained in a variety of formulae in pressurised sprays (e.g. 'Polybactrin', Framyspray'), which are extensively used in certain procedures, e.g. on the initial incision made during operations, on wounds before dressings are applied, and on bed-sores, etc. The combinations employed are carefully chosen, so that each of the two or three antibiotics used covers any gap in the antibacterial range of the other(s). The spray is held as upright as possible, the nozzle directed at the area concerned and a specified distance away from it (this is important), and the button or cap is pressed. A short burst of spray is then delivered and leaves a film of the antibiotics over the desired site. An important point to note is that caution must be exercised in the disposal of empty containers, which are liable to explode if over-heated or burnt.

## URINARY ANTISEPTICS

Infections of the urinary tract are treated with several types of drugs; apart from irrigation solutions, all are given orally or by injection and are excreted via the urine, where they act as antiseptics against the organism concerned. The treatment may involve the sending of a mid-stream specimen of urine (taken aseptically and transferred to a sterile bottle) to the laboratory for investigation, and the report will then indicate the organism and drug best suited.

Hexamine, once much in favour, is now little used itself, but combined with another urinary antiseptic, mandelic acid, as the tablet **Methenamine Mandelate** ('Mandelamine'), it is employed extensively (av. dose 1 g) as both safe and effective; mandelic acid preparations are more active when the urine is slightly acid, and should it be alkaline ammonium chloride can be used to correct (av. dose 1 or 2 grams).

The use of the systemic **sulphonamides** as urinary antiseptics during their excretion via the urine, and in particular sulphafurazole and sulphamethizole, has been described earlier (p. 129). Cotrimoxazole (p. 129), which is part sulphonamide, has also been referred to in this connection.

The systemic **antibiotics** are similarly effective during their elimination via the urinary tract, choice being usually decided by the laboratory report. Ampicillin (p. 136) is often indicated due to its broad range of activity and the high levels achieved in the urine.

In the event of resistance to the groups of drugs so far mentioned, two further and quite distinct compounds are available.

**Nitrofurantoin** is a yellow compound which is taken in tablet or suspension form, and has a good range of bacterial coverage; high levels are reached in the urinary tract, hence its specific use in urinary infections. It is given at full dosage for relatively short courses only, due to the possibility of toxic side-effects; a harmless one is brown coloration of the urine.

**Nalidixic Acid** is taken as fawn coloured tablets or suspension, and is particularly valuable because it covers almost the whole range of bacteria which commonly cause urinary infections, including those which are resistant to other urinary antiseptics; it is normally free from serious side-effects. As with nitrofurantoin, nalidixic acid concentrates its activity in the urinary system.

> Nitrofurantoin—'Furadantin'—av. dose 100 mg
> Nalidixic Acid—'Negram'    —  „    „   1 g

An infection of the genito-urinary tract met in both sexes (but particularly in women of child-bearing age) is caused by Trichomonas, which is not a bacterium or fungus but a one-celled animal organism; the specific drug used is **Metronidazole** ('Flagyl'), in the form of a tablet which is taken three times daily for one week, and which acts during its excretion via the urine. It is not unusual for both male and female partners to be treated if sexual intercourse is an involvement at the time. The employment of metronidazole in the treatment of anaerobic infections and amoebiasis is described on pages 130 and 152 respectively.

In addition to the use of systemic drugs, infections of the bladder and urethra are also treated with bladder lavage ("washouts"), employing a wide range of antiseptics in weak dilution. Examples are chlorhexidine 1 in 5 000, silver nitrate 1 in 1 000, and phenoxetol

1 in 500. Such irrigation solutions must be sterile, and are usually presented in sealed one litre bottles.

**Noxytiolin** ('Noxyflex') is an antiseptic employed in the control of bladder infections due to both bacteria and fungi. The powder, either with or without amethocaine (the latter for its local anaesthetic effect), is dissolved in sterile water for introducing by catheter; the solution is also used for general cavity irrigation and wet dressings, etc. An advantage claimed for noxytiolin is that being unrelated to the anti-infective drugs commonly used, e.g. the sulphonamides and antibiotics, there is not the danger of its use producing bacterial resistance to these drugs should they need to be used subsequently at any time.

The student nurse will be aware of the strict precautions that need to be observed in order to prevent the ascent of infection via the urethra, as, for example, when introducing a catheter or renewing a bottle or plastic bag into which urine is draining from one of the in-dwelling type of catheter such as the Foley's. Likewise, that if a drainage bag is used for more than one filling, i.e. is emptied and re-used, then it should be of the type fitted with a drain outlet and also a non-return valve to prevent upward creep of infection; a small amount of an antiseptic, such as 1 in 200 chlorhexidine solution, is sometimes added to the bag before each successive use.

# CHAPTER 15

# ANTHELMINTICS
## with an outline of drugs used in tropical diseases

The last Chapter (14) dealt with drugs used in infections mainly caused by micro-organisms of bacterial type. This chapter is concerned with conditions which (with a few exceptions) result from invasion of the body by parasites of *low animal* type, e.g. worms and protozoa. It commences with an account of drugs used in the treatment of worm infestations met in this country, and then proceeds to outline the drugs used in certain tropical diseases. A note on the disease itself is included in each of the latter cases, but this is intended merely as a background to the use of the drug(s) concerned.

## ANTHELMINTICS
—are used to treat intestinal worms; they are sometimes termed vermifuges, or vermicides, indicating that they expel, or kill worms respectively. They are grouped here under the heading of the worms concerned.

### Threadworms
—are found world-wide and are the type most commonly met in this country. They inhabit the large bowel, and infestation is treated by drugs which are given orally. Preparations containing **Piperazine** are much used, and are taken daily for seven days or in one large single dose; commercial examples are 'Antepar', in tablet and elixir form, and 'Pripsen', as flavoured granules which contain piperazine and 'Senokot'—the latter completes the treatment by flushing out the worms by its purgative action. Another efficient single dose drug is **Viprynium** ('Vanquin'), a liquid draught which, incidentally, colours the stools red—the patients are usually warned of this.

Personal hygiene is especially important, not only in the case of the patient but the rest of the family also. Clean and well-shortened finger nails, thorough hand-washing after toilet calls, frequently changed underwear and bed-linen, etc., all such measures are essential in order to avoid re-infestation of the patient and further spread to others.

See also thiabendazole and mebendazole (later).

## Roundworms

—inhabit the small bowel. **Piperazine** is a highly efficient vermifuge to roundworms also, one large dose usually accomplishing the treatment. The worms are paralysed by the drug, and are thus dislodged and passed on to the large bowel by movement of the gut; if the patient is constipated a purge may be necessary to complete the expulsion.

See also thiabendazole and mebendazole (later).

## Hookworms

—occur mainly in tropical and subtropical countries, and may therefore appear in patients who have lived in these areas. The larvae (an immature stage) enter the body through the skin and migrate to the intestine; during the latter process they may cause bleeding, through injury to the tissues, and anaemia may result. A remedy commonly used is **Bephenium** ('Alcopar'), which is given on an empty stomach in the form of granules from a one-dose 5 gram sachet; the instructions are printed in both English and the languages of the areas abroad concerned.

See also thiabendazole and mebendazole (later).

## Whipworms

—are commonly found in the tropics but occasionally also in this country. The parasites inhabit the mid-intestinal tract and appear to have little harmful effect. Their presence is shown when the golden coloured eggs appear in the stools, and a specific anthelmintic in this case is **Dithiazanine Iodide** ('Telmid'), which is given in tablet form three times daily before food for five days; it is used with some caution due to the possibility of severe gastro-intestinal side-effects, and another point to note is that the stools are coloured bluish green.

See also thiabendazole and mebendazole (following).

**Thiabendazole** ('Mintezol') is effective against a wide range of intestinal worms, including threadworm, roundworm, hookworm and whipworm. Dosage is based on body weight, and the tablets may be chewed; two doses are taken the first day, and this is repeated either the next day or several days later, depending on the type of worm involved. Additional purging, etc., is unnecessary, but it is stressed that doses must be taken after a full meal. Side-effects that may occur include gastro-intestinal upset, visual disturbance and skin rash, and the urine may develop a characteristic odour.

**Mebendazole** ('Vermox') is related to thiabendazole, is similarly effective against a wide variety of intestinal worms, including thread-worms, roundworms, hookworms and whipworms, and is claimed to be superior in action in that dosage is lower and success more certain. It is taken orally and no additional measures such as purging are necessary; there is virtually no absorption, and dosage is the same for children as for adults. For threadworms, a single dose of one tablet is taken, and, as is commonly advisable in the case of this worm, any other children in the household should be similarly treated and the dose repeated after a few weeks should a re-infestation appear; for round, hook and whipworms, one tablet is taken morning and evening for three days.

### Tapeworm

This parasite is composed of a head (the scolex) and many segments (body divisions), and is tenacious in its stay in the intestine. The traditional vermifuge used against tapeworm has been **Male Fern** *(filix mas)*; this is taken as capsules or liquid draught, the latter through a duodenal tube as it is highly nauseating in taste. The treatment also includes fasting and purging of the patient, and inspection of the stools for the head of the tapeworm so as to confirm success of the treatment; subsequent fatty meals and oils are avoided as they can foster absorption of the extract which is very toxic.

Treatment with male fern is now little employed, as synthetic alternatives are now available which are both effective and less distressing to the patient.

Two such drugs are **Dichlorophen** ('Anthiphen') and **Niclosamide** ('Yomesan'); both are given in tablet form and normally do not need preceding by fasting and purging, though a requirement in the case of niclosamide is that the tablets must be thoroughly chewed. Likewise, both are vermicidal, i.e. they actually kill the tapeworm; the head is partially disintegrated during the process and is thus not usually identifiable in the stools. A second treatment is used only if further segments are seen in the stools within a period of three months. **Mepacrine,** the drug formerly used in malaria, is also employed in tapeworm infestation, an average dose being 1 gram taken on an empty stomach (preferably as a liquid draught per duodenal tube, as its taste is very bitter and nauseating), a saline purge being given on the previous day and also following the administration of the drug; the head of the parasite is easily recognisable because it is stained yellow.

# DRUGS USED IN TROPICAL DISEASES

## Amoebiasis

Amoebiasis is a condition in which the large intestine is infected with organisms of a parasite type called amoebae. It occurs mainly in warm climates and in areas where sanitation is primitive. The cysts, an intermediate phase of the parasite, are swallowed via contaminated food, and hatch in the large bowel to liberate the amoebae; these then multiply rapidly and invade the intestinal mucosa, causing severe ulceration and diarrhoea with bleeding, hence the common name amoebic dysentery. The organisms frequently penetrate further and reach the liver (causing *hepatic* amoebiasis) and other tissues.

**Emetine** has been the drug mainly used in treatment; it is the active constituent of ipecacuanha, which is employed as an expectorant (p. 84) and emetic (p. 16). Emetine is used by subcutaneous or intramuscular injection to treat acute attacks of tissue amoebiasis; 60 mg are given daily for three to five days or longer, but never exceeding a total of twelve injections, due to its toxic effects, e.g. on the heart muscle. **Dihydroemetine** ('Mebadin') is a derivative of emetine which is less toxic and may thus be used for longer courses. Hepatic amoebiasis may also be treated effectively with the antimalarial drug **Chloroquine** (p. 157); 1 gram is given by mouth daily for one week.

Treatment is also necessary to rid the bowel lumen (channel) completely of the organisms and so avoid systemic re-infection through the bowel wall, and here emetine is given by mouth as 60 mg tablets of **Emetine Bismuth Iodide** (known as E.B.I.) three times daily for ten days; the tablets are coated so as to pass through the stomach into the small bowel before disintegrating, thus forestalling the emetic effect of the drug.

Other drugs may be used for this essential bowel treatment, sometimes in various combinations, and these comprise the arsenical preparation **Carbarsone,** given as 250 mg tablets twice daily; **Diloxanide Furoate** ('Furamide') as 500 mg tablets, and **Phanquone** ('Entobex') as 50 mg tablets, both of which are relatively free of serious side-effects and are given by mouth three times daily for ten days; and **Di-iodohydroxyquinoline** ('Diodoquin'), an iodine containing compound. **Paromomycin** ('Humatin') is an antibiotic which has been used effectively in amoebiasis; it is not absorbed from the intestinal tract, hence its value in the intestinal phase of the disease; the capsules are taken four times daily for five days.

**Metronidazole** ('Flagyl') has been described in relation to its use in anaerobic infections and in Trichomonas infections of the urinary tract (pp. 130 and 146); it is also the drug of greatest importance in the treatment of amoebiasis. Metronidazole treatment is highly successful in all phases of the disease, i.e. both the intestinal and the liver and other tissue forms; it is also efficient in clearing infection from the intestine of carriers, who may themselves be free of symptoms but habitually pass the cyst form of the amoebae in the stools and are thus a potential danger to others. It is given as a short course, either two to four tablets of 200 mg three times daily for five days, or two single doses of twelve tablets each on the same day or consecutive days. Side effects are infrequent and not severe, and its many advantages have made it the drug of choice in amoebiasis and likely to completely supersede emetine and the other drugs previously discussed in this section.

## Bacillary Dysentery

—is also prevalent in areas where sanitation is ineffective, but is most severely experienced in the tropics; the organism concerned is a bacterium which is ingested in faecally contaminated food or drink. The bacteria pass to the large bowel, multiply rapidly, and emit irritant toxins which inflame and damage the intestinal mucosa; diarrhoea with much blood and mucus then occurs. The toxins may be absorbed systemically, and the patient made further seriously ill for this reason.

The drugs used in bacillary dysentery are drawn from the **Sulphonamides** and the **Antibiotics,** but an important reservation is becoming increasingly significant, this is discussed later.

The intestinal sulphonamides, such as succinylsulphathiazole and phthalysulphathiazole (p. 25), may be given in high dosage, as likewise can the systemic sulphonamide, sulphadiazine (p. 128), for its greater effect within the intestinal tissue, measures being taken in the latter case to avoid crystalluria (p. 128). The combination drug, cotrimoxazole (p. 129), which contains a sulphonamide with trimethoprim, is now being used to a noteworthy extent.

Of the antibiotics, chloramphenicol (p. 140) is effective in this condition, and is given in high dosage for short periods of up to five days; or the tetracyclines (p. 139) may be used in place. The non-absorbed antibiotics have a logical place in the treatment of this bowel condition and are also employed, a common example being neomycin.

Drug treatment is continued until bowel movements are reduced to a few times daily, and is often extended for a further short period to ensure complete freedom from the organism.

This disease can be acutely serious, e.g. dehydration may be severe enough to demand urgent fluid replacement intravenously or subcutaneously (p. 47). The patient needs utmost care in nursing, in addition to rigid hygiene and barrier routine in order to prevent the spread of infection.

The reservation mentioned earlier concerns the use of sulphonamides and antibiotics over the years and the resultant problem of increasing development of resistant strains of the bacteria, with subsequent lessening of the effectiveness of these drugs. An added hazard is that such resistance can also be transferred to *other* bacteria, e.g. E.coli, thus producing a resident resistant strain, and this may then endanger the successful treatment of infections due to such organisms should they occur subsequently; this underlines the value of the more newly used components of cotrimoxazole.

## Filariasis

This disease is caused by a type of worm, and occurs in the tropics and subtropics. The immature larvae are injected by mosquitoes when biting, and the worms then develop slowly but in great numbers (appearing in the blood at night and vacating it during the day). The lymph vessels become blocked by the mass of live and dead parasites, and as a result the lymph(fluid) accumulates and causes swelling; eventually the condition known as elephantiasis is reached, in which there is gross extension and thickening of the skin. Thus the scrotum, for example, may be enlarged to an enormous size.

The drug mainly used in treatment is **Diethylcarbamazine** ('Banocide'). A small dose is given orally three times daily for three days; it is doubled for the next two days, then trebled for two further days, and finally quadrupled for the subsequent fifteen days. Side-effects are unpleasant and include inflammation of the eyes, pruritus and oedema.

A form of filariasis which may result in blindness is caused by another species of worm, infestation with which is transmitted by certain small flies or gnats. The worms congregate in nodules which appear on the body, and should the eyes become involved the condition is serious. **Suramin** (p. 161) and diethylcarbamazine are used in this condition.

## Leishmaniasis

—is known as kala-azar when it is generalised throughout the body. It has a wide distribution, e.g. India, China, certain parts of Africa and some countries bordering the Mediterranean, and South America. Hot and moist conditions favour its spread. Kala-azar is caused by a protozoa parasite and is transmitted by sand flies; these bite an infected person, ingest blood containing the parasite, and infect fresh victims by the same biting process. The disease is extremely severe and is characterised by massive enlargement of the liver and spleen (particularly), anaemia, emaciation, and irregular periods of high temperature.

Certain drugs based on antimony are used in kala-azar; non-antimonial drugs, e.g. pentamidine and related compounds, are also employed.

The antimony compound mainly used is **Sodium Stibogluconate** ('Pentostam'), which is given by intramuscular or intravenous injection daily for up to 10 days; several courses given at intervals may be sometimes necessary.

**Pentamidine** is of particular value when infections are resistant to the antimony drugs. It is given daily by intramuscular injection for about two weeks, and the course is repeated after a similar resting period. Another non-antimonial compound used is **Hydroxy-stilbamidine,** which is given by intravenous injection for up to 10 days.

A skin variant of leishmaniasis is caused by a parasite closely similar to that which causes kala-azar; it occurs in many tropical and subtropical countries, but unlike kala-azar its spread is favoured by *dry* climates, as in desert areas. The infection is confined to the skin and is accompanied by ulcer-like sores with protruding walls. Treatment is usually local, the sores being cleaned with eusol (p. 170) and allowed to heal; or they may need to be swabbed with pure liquefied phenol (p. 167), or treated with X-Rays or carbon dioxide snow (p. 222). Injections (e.g. of sodium stibogluconate) may be used if the sores are too numerous and widespread to treat by application.

### Leprosy

Leprosy is a disease caused by a bacterium closely resembling that which causes tuberculosis; it occurs mainly in the tropics and subtropics. Infection is thought to be acquired through the skin by contact; this occurs far more readily in children than in adults. The two main forms of leprosy are tuberculoid leprosy and lepromatous leprosy, and the form taken by the disease depends largely on the degree of response of the defence mechanism of the individual concerned.

In tuberculoid leprosy, there is a vigorous tissue reaction to the bacteria, and this results in extensive skin lesions (tissue damage), but with scanty presence of bacteria; hence, tuberculoid leprosy is relatively safe, or 'closed', in relation to spread of infection. A severe effect of this form of leprosy is damage to the nerve system, in particular the branches leading to the extremities, and resultant muscle wasting may lead to deformity of the hands and feet; there is also local insensitivity to pain, and because of this the patient may suffer severe damage and secondary infection, e.g.

he can be unaware of contact with burning cigarette ends.

In lepromatous leprosy, the reaction of the tissue to the bacteria is weak or absent, hence spread of infection is unimpeded; the bacteria multiply extensively in the mucous membranes (e.g. of the nose and mouth), and the shiny nodules which are a feature of this type of the disease are likewise filled with enormous numbers. Hence, lepromatous leprosy is by far the more infective, or "open", type of the disease.

The drugs chiefly used in the treatment of leprosy are dapsone and clofazimine.

**Dapsone** is given in tablet form by mouth. Typical dosage averages 100 mg twice a week, but commencing in small doses and increasing gradually over several months, this being done to avoid toxic side-effects, which include gastro-intestinal upset and rash. An occasional occurence during dapsone treatment of lepromatous leprosy is a lepra reaction (or leprotic fever); this may follow too high dosage. It would appear that the disintegration in the tissues of the bacteria which have been killed by the drug, and the consequent release of foreign protein substances, causes the body to respond by a rise in temperature and other severe symptoms. Thus, a steroid drug, e.g. cortisone or prednisolone (p. 189), may be given concurrently with dapsone, the anti-inflammatory effect then minimises the possibility of fever being induced.

**Clofazimine** ('Lamprene') is a dye compound which is highly effective against the leprosy bacterium. It has the added advantage of pronounced anti-inflammatory activity, and thus reduces the possibility of lepra reactions occurring; this makes steroid therapy unnecessary. In the long term treatment of leprosy, average dosage is one capsule of 100 mg three times weekly; this is increased in cases where the organisms have proved resistant to dapsone or if lepra reactions (see earlier) need to be treated. Clofazimine has few side-effects, but during prolonged treatment or high dosage, patients often develop a reddish-violet discoloration of the skin, and the skin lesions of the disease may be outlined with a greyish-blue pigmentation; the urine may also be discoloured. The patient is reassured that these effects are of no significance, and the discoloration disappears when the dose is reduced or treatment stopped.

The drugs used in leprosy are given for prolonged periods, e.g. several years, and lower maintenance dosage may then be continued for a long time afterwards. A contributory factor in this connection is that the action of both dapsone and clofazimine is bacteriostatic (p. 127), i.e. they do not directly kill the leprosy bacterium, hence the importance of a drug which has come into use and which is *bactericidal* to the organism concerned; this is **Rifampicin,** the particular importance of which in the treatment of tuberculosis has already been described (p. 139). Even so, treatment of leprosy with rifampicin is still long-term, but is shorter and held to be more certain than in the case of dapsone and clofazimine; also, the period of infectiousness of the patient is less prolonged—an advantage of particular importance. It is unfortunate that rifampicin is a highly expensive drug in the context of prolonged therapy.

It is a matter of concern that development of resistance by the leprosy organism to the drugs hitherto employed is thought likely to become a significant problem.

### Malaria

—is a disease which occurs widely in tropical and subtropical countries, and also in areas of Europe bordering the Mediterranean. There are several different types, caused by distinct parasites belonging to the same family; the transmitting agents are certain species of mosquitoes. The malaria organism is ingested by the mosquito when it bites an infected individual; it then undergoes a change of form, multiplies within the insect, and is injected into further individuals, again during the biting process. Once in the body, the parasite reaches the liver where it undergoes further development and is then released into the blood stream. The erythrocytes (red blood cells) are then invaded, and the organisms multiply rapidly within them until finally the cells burst and discharge a swarm of parasites into the blood stream; many then enter further erythrocytes and the same process is repeated.

The malarial attacks coincide with the rupture of large numbers of cells and the release of the parasites they contain. There is an interval of some 48 hours between each massive discharge in the case of the two main forms of malaria, i.e. the attacks occur every *third* day; hence they are called benign *tertian* malaria and malignant *tertian* malaria. These two malarias differ in several respects.

### Benign Tertian Malaria

The attacks are characterised by rigor (cold shivering with high temperature) followed by sweating; each lasts up to five hours.

Two groups of drugs are employed in the treatment of this type of malaria. The main group is used to overcome the attack by destroying the parasites in the blood; it includes chloroquine (considered the standard drug), amodiaquine and quinine. A complete cure is not effected, because these drugs do not eradicate those parasites which have become established in the tissues of the liver and other organs. Thus, regular dosage with a suitable drug is routinely used to prevent further attacks developing from such parasite sources in the tissues (see "suppressive control", page 158).

The other group of drugs used *does* destroy the parasite forms in the tissues, thus getting rid of the "liver cycle", hence its use when a radical cure (i.e. complete and conclusive) is required, as when the individual is leaving the area finally and permanently. Pamaquine, a drug in this group which has been used, can be the cause of serious blood disorders, hence primaquine, which is related but safer, is now the one almost invariably employed.

### Malignant Tertian Malaria

This is the most dangerous form of malaria. In addition to fever and chills, serious anaemia occurs, and there may be diarrhoea to the point of acute dehydration; the liver and spleen are affected and there is disturbance of respiratory and kidney function. Further severe complications may involve the brain, leading to coma.

In attacks of malignant tertian malaria all the organisms migrate to the blood, and a complete cure may thus be effected in this case with the use of one of the drugs previously mentioned as acting in the blood, i.e. chloroquine, amodiaquine or quinine. Should the serious complications mentioned earlier have set in and the patient be in a condition of shock, chloroquine may be given by intramuscular or intravenous injection; quinine is also used by intravenous injection.

The drugs so far mentioned are now discussed in more detail.

**Chloroquine** ('Avloclor', 'Nivaquine') is available in tablet and injection form; typical dosage is 600 mg of chloroquine (base) to commence with, then 300 mg daily for three days, making a total of 1·5 grams. The *base* is specified because the brand used may contain chloroquine as phosphate or sulphate, and these differ in the amount of actual chloroquine they contain. Resistance to chloroquine is said to be increasingly encountered.

**Amodiaquine** ('Camoquine') is related to chloroquine and may be used in place; it is given orally as tablets of 200 mg, two or three daily for three days.

**Primaquine** is, as stated, effective against the parasites in the liver and other tissues, hence it is used with one of the other main anti-malaria drugs (as mentioned earlier) in the final eradication of the parasite which causes benign tertian malaria; average dosage is 15 mg daily for two weeks. **Quinine,** a drug of natural origin, has long been used to treat and prevent attacks of malaria, and despite the number of newer synthetic alternatives it has resumed an important place in treatment and is resorted to in cases which are resistant to chloroquine and amodiaquine. If used in treatment of an attack, 600 mg is given orally three times daily for 4 days.

## The Use of Drugs in the Suppressive Control of Malaria

There is constant risk of re-infection in countries where malaria occurs. No drug is available which will destroy the parasite in the form injected by the mosquito. The drugs taken to prevent attacks developing are therefore aimed to suppress or destroy the blood forms of the parasites; some may also have variable effect on the liver form.

**Chloroquine** and **Amodiaquine,** already referred to as employed in the treatment of the attack, are also used in suppression routine, one dose being taken weekly. It is often customary for dosage to commence two weeks before entering the malarial area. Two other drugs commonly used are proguanil and pyrimethamine.

**Proguanil** ('Paludrine') destroys the parasites in the blood and also has some effect on the tissue forms. Dosage as a suppressant is one tablet of 100 mg daily, again often commencing 14 days before reaching the area concerned, and continuing for up to one month after leaving. Proguanil is also used occasionally in the treatment of benign tertian malaria.

**Pyrimethamine** ('Daraprim') is widely used for the control of malaria. One tablet of 25 mg is taken weekly, commencing on the day before arrival in the territory and continuing for four weeks after leaving. Resistance of the malaria parasite to both proguanil and pyrimethamine is also not infrequently found.

Combinations of anti-malaria drugs may be used in suppressive treatment, an example being 'Darachlor', which is a combination of pyrimethamine and chloroquine; one tablet is taken weekly.

### "Non-immunes" and "immunes"

The dosage so far mentioned in the treatment and suppression of malaria applies largely to "non-immunes", i.e. those who have come to the territory from non-malarial countries (this includes also those who may have lived there before but have been away for some time). Natives of malarial areas, and others who stay there for long periods, are sometimes termed "immunes", for they gradually acquire a partial degree of immunity so long as they harbour the malarial parasite in their bodies. Total eradication of their parasites would destroy this immunity. Smaller doses of chloroquine are therefore given, just sufficient to control symptoms when they occur.

### Blackwater fever

This condition may follow as a complication of malignant tertian malaria. The prominent symptom is a red to dark brown pigmentation of the urine; this results from haemolysis (disintegration of red blood cells). The urine is kept under regular examination, for a serious possibility is kidney failure.

In treatment, anti-malarial drugs are given in full dosage if the blood is found to be infected, or in suppressive dosage if not.

## Schistosomiasis

—is also known as bilharziasis; it is caused by systemic invasion with certain flukes (parasitic worms, known also as bilharzia or schistosomes) which are found largely throughout Africa and Asia Minor. The organisms concerned have a complicated life cycle; they multiply within snails, which shed the larvae (the immature stage) in the water they inhabit. Infection is acquired by entry through the skin following contact with such water; or, if it is drunk, the larvae penetrate the mucosa of the mouth. In either case the organisms migrate to the liver, where they develop into adult parasites; these eventually reach the bladder and are excreted via the urine. Damage to the urinary tract with resultant haematuria (blood in the urine) occurs. Other types of schistosomes infest the intestine and liver and cause dysentery, i.e. diarrhoea with blood and mucus in the stools.

In the treatment of the various types of schistosomiasis, antimonial compounds are again used. **Antimony Sodium Tartrate** (known as "tartar emetic") is given by slow intravenous injection, commencing with a small dose and increasing three times weekly until the required blood levels are achieved; it produces toxic side effects, e.g. coughing, vomiting, diarrhoea and fainting may occur.

Other antimonial compounds used are **Sodium Antimony Gluconate** ('Triostam'), which is given intravenously for six days, and **Stibophen,** which is given intramuscularly every second day in increasing doses. **Antimony Sodium Dimercaptosuccinate** ('Astiban') is much less toxic, and is given by intramuscular or slow intravenous injection, it being required that the patient then rests for an hour; five injections are given at weekly intervals, and a further requirement is that the total amount of the drug given during a course must not exceed 2·5 g.

The following drugs are being increasingly used in schistosomiasis.

**Niridazole** ('Ambilhar') is much favoured; it is taken daily by mouth for one week, the dosage depending on the weight of the patient. Toxic effects may include mental confusion and epilepsy; also, the urine is coloured brown and may cause alarm, but this is due to the excretion of a harmless breakdown product of the drug and is of no consequence.

**Lucanthone** ('Nilodin') is also given orally, one gram twice a day for three days, but is considered more suitable for mass prophylaxis as it is not as efficient in treatment as niridazole. **Hycanthone** ('Etrenol') is a related drug, but is given by intramuscular injection, a single dose comprising the treatment; this makes it highly suitable for mass programmes of treatment and prophylaxis, frequency being two or three times a year in the latter case.

## Sprue

—is met in widely scattered regions, e.g. India, China, South America and the Philippines; it affects mainly people of middle age. Sprue is associated with malabsorption of fats (particularly) and carbohydrates; errors of diet and consequent deficiency are thought to be the probable cause. Diarrhoea of a watery and frothy nature occurs; later the typical sprue stool is in evidence, this is greasy and offensive. Defective intake of essential factors, e.g. vitamins, leads to severe tongue and mouth conditions, and anaemia develops.

In the acute stage, intravenous fluids are given to reverse the dehydration, and blood to correct the anaemia; a non-absorbed sulphonamide (p. 25) may be used to control the diarrhoea. Subsequently, a diet of high protein and low fat and carbohydrate is routine.

**Folic Acid** (p. 69) is a specific drug in the treatment of sprue. It is given in large doses (e.g. 20 mg) by intramuscular injection daily for a few weeks, followed by similar dosage orally once a week as maintenance. In addition, **Riboflavine** and **Nicotinamide** (page 78) are given to improve the mouth condition.

## Trachoma

—is a virus disease which is common in the tropics and subtropics. The organism causes severe inflammation of the conjunctiva (the inner lining of the eyelid), and the cornea (the outer coat of the eye) may be involved. Secondary infection is the main hazard and may result in permanent blindness.

In trachoma, treatment of secondary infection is the especial need. Systemic **Sulphonamides** (p. 128) or **Antibiotics,** e.g. the tetracyclines (p. 139) or chloramphenicol (p. 140), are given by mouth. These drugs (sulphacetamide in the case of the sulphonamides) are also used as eye drops by day and ointment at night. Such treatment has a high rate of success.

## Trypanosomiasis

—is also called sleeping sickness. It occurs in a wide area of middle Africa, stretching from the East to West coasts, and is caused by a trypanosome parasite which is carried by the tsetse fly. The organism is ingested from infected individuals during the biting process; it then undergoes a change of form within the fly and is transmitted to other individuals via further bites. The infection is accompanied by intermittent high temperature, rash, and swelling of the glands at the back of the neck; finally there is infiltration of the central nervous system, when the lassitude and sleeping phase appear. The eyes may be affected and blindness occur. The disease is extremely serious, but, if treated early, recovery can be expected.

**Pentamidine** and **Suramin** ('Antrypol') are effective in destroying the parasites in the blood. Pentamidine (see also p. 154) is given by intramuscular or intravenous injection daily for up to 10 days, and the course may be repeated after an interval. Suramin is given intravenously once weekly for ten weeks, and as it may cause kidney damage the urine is tested for albumen before each injection to ensure that this is not occurring.

Pentamidine and suramin do not cross the brain barrier and consequently are of no value when the infection has spread into the brain and spinal cord. Hence, treatment is often accompanied by the administration of a compound containing arsenic; **Melarsoprol** (known as Mel B) and **Melarsonyl** (Mel W) are two examples. Melarsoprol is given intravenously twice daily for three days and later repeated, and melarsonyl subcutaneously or intramuscularly daily for three days and likewise repeated. Both drugs cross into the central nervous system and thus ensure that treatment is complete. The arsenical drugs may be extremely toxic, the most serious effect being optic-nerve damage which may result in blindness.

Pentamidine is sometimes given as a prophylactic (preventive) measure against trypanosomiasis, one dose being given every three months. It should be used in this respect, however, only against the West African form of the infection, and not against the East African trypanosome; the reason being that in the latter case the progress of the disease is very rapid, and if infection *has* occurred this can be so masked by the prophylactic dose of pentamidine that the symptoms may not become apparent until dangerously late.

## Yaws

This disease occurs throughout the tropical countries. It is caused by a bacterial organism and is spread by contact via skin injury, e.g. cuts and sores. Hence yaws occurs mainly in territories where the inhabitants, particularly children, wear few clothes and are thus more unprotected. The disease commences with skin eruptions and scabs on the face and body; severe bone changes are subsequently involved, e.g. the bridge of the nose may be thickened to a grotesque degree.

For treatment, **Penicillin** is given by injection or one of the **Tetracyclines** by mouth. Courses are short (e.g. two large doses of procaine penicillin) and are remarkably effective.

# CHAPTER 16

# SERA AND VACCINES

Before reading this section, the student should refresh his or her understanding of the terms "prophylactic" and "therapeutic"; the former applies to treatment intended to prevent a disease occurring, the latter to treatment of a disease already established.

## SERA

The serum is the thin, clear liquid part of the blood, and the sera (plural) used in medicine are usually obtained from cattle or horses. Sera are given by injection for either prophylactic or therapeutic effect, i.e. in the prevention or treatment of certain diseases caused by infection. But firstly, how a serum is prepared, with anti-tetanus serum as an example. The tetanus bacteria produce the poisonous tetanus toxin, and this is collected and injected into horses in gradually increasing doses; during this process, and *in response to the toxin*, the animal produces antibodies in the blood. Finally, the blood is withdrawn from the horse and the serum separated, tested and adjusted for potency, and finally sterilised ready for injection. It will now be clear that the serum contains antibodies, or antitoxins as they are also termed, which can destroy the tetanus organisms and so prevent them multiplying.

**Anti-tetanus** serum is given both prophylactically and therapeutically. Thus, in injury involving tissue damage and risk of tetanus, with patient known or presumed to need protective coverage, a subcutaneous or intramuscular injection of the serum is given in moderate dosage of 1 500 units, and this confers immediate but short-term immunity (i.e. for the following few weeks) against the disease. If, however, tetanus *has* developed, the patient will be given one or two intravenous injections of 50 000 units of anti-tetanus serum, this being therapeutic treatment, where the much larger amount of antibody will be needed to overcome the already established tetanus infection. Another example of the use of a serum both prophylactically and therapeutically is in diphtheria; if a patient has been exposed to the disease and is therefore at risk, a small dose of **anti-diphtheria** serum is given for short-term protection, whereas if the disease is established, large doses are required for actual treatment. The short-term protection described provides what is termed *passive* immunity, because the patient is given the antibodies (i.e. antitoxins) "ready made", as it were, and does not have to produce them himself.

With further reference to anti-tetanus serum, a preparation of *human* antitoxin is now available. Serum is collected from healthy human donors who have had active immunisation with tetanus vaccine (see later) and are known to have a high serum level of the antitoxin; the antitoxin is separated and made available as a solution for injection in 1 ml ampoules ("Humotet"). **"Humotet"** is employed similarly to the anti-tetanus serum already discussed, but its advantage is that severe reaction, e.g. anaphylactic shock, as may occur due to sensitivity to a foreign protein in products of animal source, is far less of a possibility.

## VACCINES

Vaccines are used almost entirely for their prophylactic effect in stimulating the development of antibodies, and the immunity they produce is long-term and is called *active* immunity, because in this case the patient *himself* produces the antibodies concerned. In general, such immunity does not become effective immediately, some weeks elapsing before a sufficient level of antibodies has been developed. There are several classes of vaccines; each is discussed separately.

Firstly, the toxoids, of which **tetanus toxoid** is a good example. The poison, or toxin, produced by the tetanus organism is rendered relatively harmless by treatment with formalin; after standardising the strength of the preparation, it becomes tetanus toxoid, which is used by injection (repeated twice at prescribed periods) to produce active, long-term immunity against tetanus. A newer, more active form of tetanus toxoid, called the *adsorbed*, is now widely used, and because of its improved effect it is favoured both to initiate the course of injections given for active immunisation and as a booster dose when the need arises.

Certain vaccines are in the form of dead bacteria suspended in normal saline, e.g. **T.A.B.,** which is given to produce active immunity against typhoid and paratyphoid, particularly before travelling abroad. In this type of vaccine, the presence of the dead typhoid and paratyphoid bacteria stimulates the production of antibodies in the blood against these two organisms. This vaccine, being a suspension, needs shaking gently before use.

Live bacteria can also be used as vaccines, an example being **B.C.G.** vaccine, which is used for protection against tuberculosis. It may appear puzzling that live bacteria are introduced into the body to produce immunity against the same organisms, but the T.B.

bacteria used in B.C.G. vaccine are from a deliberately weakened strain, and this ensures freedom from the possibility of a dangerously active infection developing.

Decision to inoculate with B.C.G. vaccine is dependent upon the Mantoux skin-test with solutions of tuberculin, except in very young children. Tuberculin is produced by the T.B. bacterium, and is collected from the liquid medium in which the organisms have been grown; it is available in solutions of 1 in 100, 1 in 1 000, and 1 in 10 000, and the patient is skin-tested by intradermal injection, using the weakest first, and following with increasing concentrations if necessary. A positive reaction—shown by a raised area encircled by a reddening of the skin (erythema)—indicates that immunity has already been acquired by previous contact with the infection. A negative reaction (absence of this response) indicates that immunity is not present, and it is then advisable for the patient to be given B.C.G. vaccine to provide the necessary protection. The "Heaf" multiple-puncture apparatus is also used for testing, but with a special tuberculin solution; and the 'Tine Test' sterile, disposable, plastic unit, with four "tines", or needles, ready coated with tuberculin, is pressed on the forearm to give four punctures, the reaction being read after the appropriate interval.

The vaccines discussed so far have been those used for protection against diseases caused by bacteria, but infections are also caused by viruses. These are minute organisms, much smaller than bacteria, which can multiply only in living cells. Vaccines for protection against virus infections actually contain the live virus concerned, but, as with B.C.G. vaccine, it is of a safe, weakened or inactivated type (sometimes termed attenuated). Three well known examples are **poliomyelitis** vaccine, which is taken by mouth on a lump of sugar; **influenza** vaccine, which is given by deep subcutaneous injection; and **calf lymph,** which contains the virus of cow-pox and produces immunity to smallpox, and is applied to the upper arm after scarifying the skin.

**Rubella** vaccine ('Cendevax') is a vaccine of particular importance, as it produces active immunity against rubella (German measles). If this disease is contracted during early pregnancy, there is a risk of damage to the foetus, hence the value of immunising women of child-bearing age. The vaccine contains the live virus of rubella, but, as in the case of other vaccines already referred to, from an appropriately attenuated and thus safe strain. It should be noted that it must not be given to women who are already pregnant.

## Autogenous vaccines

It occasionally happens that the organism responsible for an infection persists in reappearing, despite the use of a drug to which it is sensitive, e.g. in the case of recurrent boils. In such an event an autogenous vaccine may be used. This is prepared from the organisms which have been isolated from a specimen obtained from the patient, e.g. pus in the case of boils, and is then injected back into the patient.

## Vaccines used in allergies

The term allergy has been explained on pages 101 and 102, together with the use of the antihistamine group of drugs in the treatment of this condition, which is characterised by extreme sensitivity. Another approach to the problem of recurring or persistent allergy is the administration of a course of the appropriate vaccine. Thus, if the symptoms of hay fever or a similarly allergic condition are severe and distressing, or in the allergic type of asthma which is usually unresponsive to antihistamine treatment, a course of vaccine to produce immunity (by desensitisation) is often preferred—as a case of "prevention being better than cure". The patient is "prick-tested" for sensitivity, in the forearm or thigh, using a wide range of solutions of possible allergens (the substances which cause allergy); the *group* is sought first, e.g. "cereals", and then the *individual member*— which might be wheat, rye or oats, etc. Sensitivity is indicated by a circular area of reddened skin (erythema). When the allergen responsible has been found (there may be several), a vaccine is prepared from a concentrated extract of the substance(s) concerned, and is then administered by subcutaneous injection, commencing with a very weak concentration and gradually increasing this until the course has been completed; the production of antibodies which has been stimulated will (or may) enable the patient subsequently to withstand the effect of the allergen(s) concerned.

In hay fever, vaccines are prepared from the pollen of mixed grasses and are often reasonably successful; an example is 'Pollinex', three injections of which are given subcutaneously at intervals of seven to fourteen days, the course being completed before mid-May.

House-dust mites are established as a frequent cause of asthma and persistent rhinitis (p. 216), and short courses of vaccines containing house-dust mite extract ('Allpyral Mite Fortified house dust', 'Migen') are widely employed.

## The use of vaccines in malignant disease

Reference to this approach in the treatment of appropriate conditions of this nature is contained in chapter 19 (see page 209).

# CHAPTER 17

# ANTISEPTICS AND DISINFECTANTS

These terms have very much the same broad meaning, in that both groups of preparations kill or inactivate pathogenic (disease producing) organisms, such as bacteria, etc., and are employed to prevent or check infection; thus antiseptics may be held to function as disinfectants, and vice-versa. A general and helpful distinction is that antiseptics may be said to be used for application to human skin and tissue, as well as for other purposes, whereas disinfectants are usually employed in a "domestic routine" sense, i.e. for removing sources of infection from, e.g., ward furniture, equipment, baths, floors, sluices and toilets, etc. This distinction is not clear cut, however; for instance, the application of an antiseptic to the skin before operations or injections is actually a disinfecting process. In addition to physical advantages, such as being easy to recognise, i.e. by colour and/or smell, and convenient in use, the attributes desirable in an antiseptic or disinfectant include:—

1. activity against a wide range of organisms at high dilution,
2. speed of activity,
3. activity not only under laboratory conditions but also in the presence of organic matter such as pus or serum, and
4. safety in use.

Few, if any, of the antiseptics and disinfectants available fulfil all these requirements completely. Thus, some preparations may have a wide range of "kill" (i.e. effectiveness against organisms) but may need care, or be unpleasant, in use. Or they may be less effective in actual conditions of use than when tested in the laboratory. In particular, many are *selective* in action, i.e. they are not effective against certain organisms, and this is sometimes an important factor to be borne in mind. Hence the perfect preparation is probably not yet to hand. However, the range available offers a wide choice, and, used appropriately and with common sense, provides a valuable measure of protection against commencement or spread of infection. The need to use at the correct dilution specified cannot be too strongly emphasised; the adding of "some" of the antiseptic or disinfectant to "some" water is bad practice.

## Carbolic acid

—also known as **phenol**, is basically a white crystalline substance obtained from coal tar, which has a not unpleasant "antiseptic" smell and a wide range of activity, or "kill"; it is also available as a concentrated liquid known as liquefied phenol. In these pure or concentrated forms, phenol is extremely caustic and must be handled with care. The 1 in 20, or 5%, solution in water is also caustic and is now only occasionally used in the hospital ward, e.g. for disinfecting certain items of equipment.

## Cresol-type preparations

Cresol is an antiseptic related chemically to carbolic acid, and has long been used as **Lysol,** a 50% solution in a soap base. Neat lysol, a thick, brown clear liquid, is highly corrosive to the skin, and an average dilution for general use is 5 ml made up to 600 ml, or 1 in 120; the soap base provides additional valuable cleansing properties. Lysol is losing favour due to the danger associated with its use, and several preparations are now available which are similar to it in type, appearance and germicidal (i.e. germ-killing) power, but with minimal caustic effect; examples are 'Sudol', 'Clearsol' and 'Stericol'; the latter also incorporates a detergent ingredient, and is used at strengths of from 1 in 50 to 1 in 100. For general ward purposes (except for application to the patient) there is much to be said for this type of preparation, which is relatively safe in use and has a good range of "kill".

## 'Jeyes Fluid' and 'Izal'

—are sometimes called "black" and "white" disinfectants, respectively, and are also obtained from coal tar. These are cruder preparations intended for ordinary common use, such as on floors, toilets and sluices, etc.; they have a wide range of "kill". A disadvantage is the pronounced odour, which, though evidence of their disinfecting presence, may not be acceptable in certain areas of the hospital field. Both are employed at high dilution, e.g. 1 in 300, forming a milky type of emulsion, and points in their favour are cheapness and their relatively non-corrosive nature, even in the neat state.

## The Chlorinated Xylols

—again derive from coal tar. The antiseptics prepared from them have additional soap-based cleansing qualities, and are entirely without corrosive effect; 'Dettol' was the first of this series. These preparations can be used in concentrated solution, such as 1 in 3, or even neat, in conditions where antiseptic effect is vital, as in obstetrics (midwifery); an advantage is their highly effective action against the streptococcus organism (p. 126) which can be responsible for serious sepsis in childbirth. 'Dettol' and other brands continue to be used, usually at a 5%, or 1 in 20, dilution for ordinary purposes, but it should be appreciated that they are *selective* in action and are relatively ineffective against certain organisms commonly encountered, e.g. the staphylococcus (p. 126). Hence, they are being progressively replaced in hospital wards, Maternity Units and Operating Theatres with antiseptics of superior performance, such as chlorhexidine (see below).

## Cetrimide

—also known as C.T.A.B. and 'Cetavlon', is an antiseptic of medium effect and moderate range of activity; however, it is neither toxic nor irritant and has the especial advantage of a highly detergent action, which makes it an excellent preparation for cleansing wounds, etc., in the initial stages of treatment. The strengths used vary from 1 in 100 to 1 in 1 000. A point that should be noted is that although it has a frothy, soap-like appearance and "feel", solutions of cetrimide are not compatible (i.e. they do not "mix") with ordinary soap, and thus should not be used together.

**Benzalkonium** ('Roccal') is a related compound; it is usually coloured blue, and is mainly used at strengths of 1 in 1 000 or 1 in 2 000.

## Chlorhexidine and 'Savlon'

Chlorhexidine ('Hibitane') is a much favoured antiseptic in hospital routine; solutions are light to reddish pink in colour, according to the strength. It is active in high dilution against an extensive range of organisms, is non-irritant, and is effective in the presence of pus and serum. Chlorhexidine is used for many purposes, e.g. as a 1 in 200 solution in 70% spirit (sometimes with added colour as visual aid) for pre-operative and pre-injection skin sterilisation; at the same strength in spirit for speedy (2 mins.) emergency sterilisation of instruments; as a 1 in 5 000 solution in spirit for the storage of pre-sterilised surgical instruments; as a 1 in 5 000 sterilised solution in water for bladder wash-out; and as creams for obstetric use and for application to wounds. It should be noted that chlorhexidine is also selective in action, i.e. it is not effective against *all* micro-organisms, but its range is a practical one, and for general medical and surgical purposes it is justifiably popular.

Certain solutions of chlorhexidine will be found labelled as containing also sodium nitrite, this is to prevent the corrosion of instruments, etc., which may occur in certain cases.

Chlorhexidine, like cetrimide, is not compatible with soap-based cleansers, hence the value of the preparation 'Savlon', which combines the detergent and antiseptic effect of cetrimide with the more specific and powerful action of chlorhexidine. 'Savlon' is a clear, amber coloured liquid of smooth "soapy" feel, is miscible with water and spirit, and has a fresh, pleasing smell; it is non-toxic and non-irritant to the skin. The dilutions used vary from 1 in 100 and 1 in 200 to even weaker strengths for various purposes.

### Hexachlorophane

—is an antiseptic used mainly for its highly effective action against organisms commonly present on the skin. Thus, it is much employed in a range of preparations (e.g. 'Ster-Zac')—soap, tablet and liquid, bath concentrate and dusting powder, for disinfection of the hands and skin, e.g. in Children's and Maternity Wards; also as the 'pHiso-MED' hand cream for the customary scrubbing-up routine before surgical procedures.

Hexachlorophane has been incriminated as dangerous in use if various preparations are used too lavishly and frequently; in such an event, absorption of the antiseptic can take place and may lead to brain damage. Hence, whilst such preparations are held to be safe *if used sensibly*, an Order now requires that any medicinal product containing hexachlorophane may be used on children under 2 years of age only on medical direction.

### Iodine

—in the pure form is a dark blueish-brown crystalline substance with a characteristic odour; it is used as a solution in spirit, either at the "weak" strength, 2·5%, or the "strong", 10%. Its range of activity is very wide, and few organisms are resistant to its action.

An application of the weak solution of iodine to cuts or wounds will do much to ensure freedom from infection; it is also highly effective for pre-operative skin sterilisation, for it evaporates quickly (being spirit based) and leaves a penetrating and protective film of iodine, which has the additional advantage of being easily visible. The use of iodine has certain drawbacks—it stings on application to cuts and wounds, its stain is difficult to remove and takes time to disappear, and, lastly, it is a substance to which the patient can have an idiosyncrasy, i.e. a sensitivity or allergy. Thus "iodine rash" is occasionally met, and patients on whom it is to be applied extensively before operations are often routinely tested on a small area first, so as to confirm non-sensitivity.

The 10% solution of iodine is rarely used. It produces a very deep layer of stain on the skin, and is of value in certain fungus infections.

### Iodophors

The value of iodine as a germicidal agent has led to the evolution of iodophors, compounds of iodine which do not leave a persistent stain. The best known is **Povidone-Iodine** ('Betadine'), which is available as a solution for pre-operative skin disinfection, as other applications of various kinds, and as a "Surgical Scrub". The latter is a thick liquid cream with a detergent action; it lathers easily, and washes off readily with water. This non-staining iodine scrub is often used in place of the hexachlorophane preparations in surgical and medical procedures, as considered more efficient, i.e. with a wider and more certain range of antibacterial action.

## Iodoform

—is a yellow powder with a persistent antiseptic smell, and is chiefly used with bismuth subnitrate and liquid paraffin as "B.I.P.P." (bismuth, iodoform and paraffin paste). B.I.P.P. is used as an application to ulcers, etc., and on gauze for packing wounds and cavities; the iodoform acts as an antiseptic by slow release of the iodine it contains. A liquid preparation is the compound paint of iodoform known as Whitehead's Varnish, which evaporates and leaves a protective coating impregnated with iodoform, thus making it a suitable dressing following minor sutures in Casualty Departments, etc.

## The Chlorine Antiseptics

Chlorine is a gas with a pungent smell and powerful antiseptic action; it is contained in several preparations which act by releasing it in solution. The best known is **Eusol,** a clear white liquid with a typical odour, which is used neat in the treatment of leg ulcers, etc.; its effectiveness as a deodorant, i.e. in removing offensive smell, is an added advantage, and is typical of chlorine antiseptics. A mixture of equal parts of eusol and liquid paraffin is also commonly used, but as there is separation on standing, the oil above the eusol, the bottle should be shaken vigorously before application.

Solutions of sodium hypochlorite also yield chlorine, and a well known commercial preparation is **'Milton',** which has a wide range of uses, an interesting one being the cold sterilisation of infants' feeding bottles and teats, a routine employed in many Paediatric Units. 'Milton Crystals', in separate sachets, can be used in place of the liquid form and represent an advance in convenience and claimed performance.

**Chlorinated Lime** is a chlorine-releasing compound of crude type; it is also known as "bleaching powder", and is used for disinfecting swimming pools and toilets, etc., and also for purifying drinking water in certain circumstances.

## The Mercurial Antiseptics

**Mercurochrome** is a complex derivative of mercury which is in common use; its solutions are deep red in colour and stain the skin. It has a useful antiseptic action, and is safe in use and non-irritant to the skin, hence its value in pre-operative skin disinfection, where, as referred to earlier, the staining effect itself provides a safe indication that the area to be prepared has been fully covered. 'Merthiolate' is another complex mercurial preparation; it is also used, as an alcoholic solution (the 'Tincture'), for preparing the skin before operations.

## The Dye Antiseptics

—comprise certain chemical dyes of pronounced colour and staining properties; they are employed as solutions in spirit or water in a variety of conditions and against several types of infection. The **Flavines** (acriflavine and proflavine) stain the skin yellow, and are used at a strength of 1 in 1 000 for pre-operative skin sterilisation, etc., and as creams for wounds and burns. **Gentian Violet** is a powerfully staining dye, of colour as its name, and is extremely persistent; it is used mainly in aqueous (watery) solution, at strengths of from 1 in 200 to 1 in 1 000, for application to the mouth, nose, ears, vagina and skin, etc., and it is especially effective in infections of the yeast or fungus type. **Brilliant Green** is another dye similar in effect and use to gentian violet; a 1 in 1 000 solution is occasionally inhaled as a fine spray in lung infections of the yeast type.

## The Oxidising Antiseptics

These comprise two distinct preparations, which, by virtue of their release of oxygen, have both antiseptic and deodorising properties; they are potassium permanganate and hydrogen peroxide.

**Potassium Permanganate** is in the form of tiny free-running crystals of a metallic blueish-red colour, which dissolve in water to make solutions varying in tone from pale pink to purple depending on the degree of dilution. It is used in strengths of from 1 in 1 000 to 1 in 5 000 for several purposes, e.g. swabbing ulcers, irrigation of various parts of the body, and as soaks in conditions such as athlete's foot.

**Hydrogen peroxide** has the appearance of water, and indeed only differs by the addition of an extra atom of oxygen, i.e. it is $H_2O_2$ instead of $H_2O$; it releases this oxygen, which then acts as a mild antiseptic and powerful deodorant. Hydrogen peroxide is usually labelled in strength as "10 volume" or "20 volume", and this means that it is capable of releasing, respectively, 10 or 20 times its own volume of oxygen. The strength mainly used is "10 volume", a useful and safe antiseptic in the treatment of leg ulcers, etc.

## Formaldehyde

Formaldehyde is a gas with a pronounced, irritant odour, and is an extremely powerful disinfectant; it is penetrating in effect and rapidly kills all forms of bacteria and other sources of infection. Formaldehyde is available as **Formalin,** a clear white solution containing approximately 40% of the gas, but its employment as an antiseptic in treatment is handicapped by its irritant vapour and its injurious and hardening effect on the skin. It is used as a 3% solution for application in certain conditions of the feet, including plantar warts, i.e. on the sole.

The efficient disinfectant action of formaldehyde is made use of in the fumigation of rooms and mattresses, etc., when the gas is liberated from commercial unit packs, the room being kept sealed for several hours afterwards.

Formaldehyde gas is also liberated from formalin tablets, which contain paraformaldehyde, a solid form of formaldehyde, and these are used by placing under a bottom layer of lint in a closed container holding instruments which cannot be boiled; the gas then penetrates and sterilises the entire contents. These tablets are clearly labelled *"for disinfection"* and are usually distinctively coloured, lest they be mistaken for the very much weaker white formalin *lozenges* which are sometimes sucked for sore throat.

A valuable property of formaldehyde is its sporicidal (spore killing) effect, which is possessed by few antiseptics, hence the use of solutions containing formaldehyde (e.g. 'Ethicon Fluid') in the storage of sutures, etc., in the Operating Theatre. Formaldehyde is used as a 4% solution in the preservation of pathological specimens.

**Glutaraldehyde** is related chemically to formaldehyde and has a similar sterilising action, but is relatively free from unpleasant vapour or effect on the skin and is thus more acceptable in use. A commercial preparation, 'Cidex', is mainly employed for the immersion sterilisation of delicate instruments, etc., especially endoscopic instruments used for internal examination (e.g. bronchoscopes and cystoscopes), the lens and bulb systems of which may be damaged by other sterilisation methods.

## Spirit

—refers to industrial methylated spirit, which is fully discussed in Chapter 22. It has but moderate antiseptic value, and if intended for antibacterial effect it should be diluted to contain 30% of water, making it "spirit 70%", for this is the strength at which it has maximum germicidal quality. Hence the use of 70% spirit in the preparation of spirit-based solutions of chlorhexidine and other antiseptics, and in the pressurised sprays which are used for cleansing the skin prior to injection and for spraying trolley tops, etc., before laying out for dressing procedures.

## Storage of antiseptic solutions—a word of caution

It may easily be thought that because an antiseptic solution is antibacterial in effect, it will retain its action indefinitely and thus presents no "keeping" problems. This is not so in many cases; for example, solutions of chlorhexidine or 'Savlon' in water may quickly develop contamination with certain common organisms which are resistant to them. Thus, before being refilled, the containers are always thoroughly cleansed, or even sterilised, and the solutions should be used as freshly made as possible, within a week of preparation being reasonable; a dated label is a customary and excellent safeguard. In the ward, the use of sterile "Non-injectable Water" (p. 238) is advisable for diluting antiseptics should this need to be done before use.

The chlorine antiseptics should also be dated, e.g. eusol and dilutions of 'Milton', a fortnight being a reasonable "life"; loss of effective chlorine concentration is thus avoided. A similar example is hydrogen peroxide, which can lose its available oxygen content gradually during keeping and exposure to air when used.

The phenolic/cresylic antiseptics, e.g. lysol, etc., which have been relatively non-suspect hitherto, are now also incriminated in respect of the possibility of development of bacterial growth in dilutions on keeping. Thus it is wise to presume the possibility of deterioration and/or contamination in dilutions of *all* antiseptics and disinfectants, and to use them as freshly prepared as possible (and certainly within the stated period if specified on the label), so as to ensure maximum effect and avoidance of risk of initiating infection.

## Pre-packed sachets

Antiseptics are now available, e.g. chlorhexidine with cetrimide ('Savlon'), in sealed plastic sachets containing a measured amount which, when added to a stated volume of sterile water, makes a solution of appropriate strength for use. The sachets are easy to open and there is much to commend their use, *as long as prepared solutions are used up speedily and not allowed to "stay-around".* A further development is plastic sachets containing solutions *ready diluted* and in convenient amounts for "one use"—in the gallipot or as irrigation, etc., an example being 'Savlodil' (i.e. diluted 'Savlon').

Also widely employed are sealed plastic sachets in strip form, each containing a pad saturated in a 70% alcohol. Two sizes are

available, the smaller (e.g. 'Medi-Swab') for cleansing the skin
before giving injections, and the larger (e.g. 'Alco-Wipe') for disinfectant wiping of trolley surfaces, bowls, thermometers, etc. Disinfectants proper are also available in convenient form, e.g. the tube-
sachet of "Clearsol" which is diluted to 10 litres with water for use.

# CHAPTER 18

# DRUGS USED IN ENDOCRINE THERAPY

*—the functions of the glands*
*—the hormones—deficiency—excess*
*—preparations used in treatment*

The *endocrine* glands, also known as the ductless glands, are the glands of *internal* secretion, for the substances they secrete (i.e. produce), known as *hormones*, are released directly into the blood as it passes through them. In contrast, *ex*ocrine glands (i.e. glands of *ex*ternal secretion) supply their products in liquid form through ducts or channels, as, for example, the salivary glands in the mouth. The pancreas is a gland which combines both functions, for the liquid substance it produces, the pancreatic juice, is conveyed through a duct into the small intestine, and, in addition, it contains small groups of cells (the islets) which release the hormone insulin into the blood stream (as will be referred to later).

The endocrine glands—the pituitary, thyroid, parathyroids, adrenals, pancreatic islets and the ovaries and testes, are sometimes termed the endocrine "orchestra", for they function as a team in health, and their hormonal output is interdependent in many cases. The anterior lobe of the pituitary gland is often referred to as the "leader", for its secretions control the activity of almost all the other endocrine glands. The hormones are complex substances which play an important part in bodily function, and the level of their secretion by the various endocrine glands is carefully controlled by a "feedback" mechanism, involving the anterior pituitary, the "leader". Broadly, what happens is that changes in the blood level of a hormone act as signals which are conveyed (i.e. "fed-back") in the blood and activate the anterior pituitary into re-adjusting the level to normal requirement; *this is the basic point to grasp.* As an actual example let us take the thyroid gland (p. 179), which produces the hormone thyroxine under stimulation by the thyrotrophic hormone (also known as thyrotrophine or T.S.H., p. 178) secreted by the anterior pituitary. Thus, as the thyroxine level rises, this has a restraining, or braking, effect on the anterior pituitary, which then reduces its output of thyrotrophin to correspond; production of thyroxine is then slowed in turn. Similarly, as thyroxine is being used up in the body's metabolic processes, its falling level in the blood "feeds back" and the anterior pituitary is activated into raising its production of thyrotrophin accordingly; this, in turn, stimulates the thyroid to increase its production of thyroxine. The process can be likened to a delicate "rise and fall", so instantly reacted to on each side as to maintain the output of the hormones at levels correctly adjusted to body requirements. However, in the case of gross malfunction of an endocrine gland, this mechanism is disturbed, imbalance of hormone production results, and clinical disease will become apparent and need treatment; this may entail either replacement therapy if there is deficient production of a hormone, or regulation of hormone activity if it is excessive.

A reference is needed at this point to the important role played in the feed-back process by the *hypothalamus*, that part of the brain to which the pituitary gland is attached. Thus, the hypothalamus is involved in "picking up" the variations in hormone blood levels which signal the need for adjustment by an increase or decrease in the output of the hormones of the anterior pituitary (as just described in the case of thyrotrophin and thyroxine); in addition, the output itself of the anterior pituitary hormones is controlled by factors which are released by the hypothalamus. Hence, the hypothalamus can be said to *mastermind* the feed-back process. However, the explanation of this process already given has been intentionally confined to the relationship between the anterior pituitary and the endocrine glands, so as to enable an easier understanding of a mechanism which has an important bearing on so many aspects of this Chapter.

Two of the hypothalamus factors referred to above are now available as synthetic preparations, and their use is discussed on pages 225 and 227.

In order to fully appreciate the actions and uses of the endocrine gland preparations, it is helpful to have an acquaintance with the functions of the glands themselves, and also with the conditions being treated; this will be covered in each case. Likewise, it should be explained that the endocrine, or related, preparations used in treatment are generally based on the hormone substances themselves. They may be of *natural* origin, i.e. extracted from an animal source, e.g. insulin (p. 181), or from a human source in a few cases, e.g. chorionic gonadotrophin (p. 195). Or they may be *synthetic* i.e. artificially prepared, examples being salcatonin (p. 181) and the corticosteroids (p. 188).

## THE PITUITARY GLAND

This is a small organ suited at the base of the skull, and consists of two lobes, the anterior and posterior.

## The Posterior Lobe

—secretes two hormones, oxytocin and vasopressin. **Oxytocin** stimulates contraction of the uterus, especially in the late stage of pregnancy, and the use of preparations of this hormone in obstetrics (midwifery), and in facilitating lactation, has been described on page 109.

**Vasopressin** is the more versatile and interesting of these two hormones. Firstly, its chief function in the body (termed the antidiuretic effect) is to ensure the reabsorption of water into the blood stream following filtration of blood through the glomeruli (p. 27); lack of its secretion leads to diabetes insipidus, and this is treated by replacement with commercial preparations containing vasopressin, or an equivalent, see page 37. Secondly, vasopressin is also used in the diagnosis of diabetes insipidus (p. 228). Lastly, vasopressin is employed in the halting of bleeding from oesophageal varices (swollen and congested, i.e. *varicose,* veins in the oesophagus), the effect of the drug being to constrict the vessels concerned.

Oxytocin and vasopressin preparations are labelled in terms of units; both hormones are destroyed in the stomach and hence must be given by injection, except in the case of the buccal tablets of oxytocin (p. 109) and the nasal preparations containing vasopressin or its equivalents (p. 37).

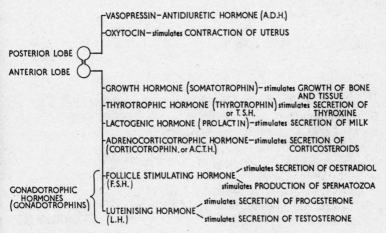

Fig. 7. Hormones secreted by the pituitary gland.

## The Anterior Lobe

—is, as already stated, the leader of the endocrine orchestra, and the hormones it produces stimulate the activity of other endocrine glands. The terms "trophic" or "trophin" are used to denote this effect, as, for example, the *thyrotrophic* hormone, or *thyrotrophin*, which stimulates the production of the hormone thyroxine by the thyroid gland. Of the many hormones produced by the anterior lobe, the following have been isolated and are of significant interest.

**The Growth Hormone** (or somatotrophin—from "somatic" which means "pertaining to the body") governs the development of bone and soft tissue during the growing period. If it is lacking in a child, growth is stunted, resulting in dwarfism. If it is excessive *during the growing period*, there is elongation of the long bones of the legs and arms, so that persons are abnormally tall. If, however, excessive secretion of the growth hormone occurs *after growth is complete* (possibly due to a tumour in the anterior pituitary lobe), the bones, being now set and unable to lengthen, respond by widening; this condition is known as acromegaly, symptoms being spade-like hands, enlarged feet and jaw, and humped spine. Surgery and radiotherapy are employed in cases of acromegaly, but a new medical supportive measure is the administration of bromocriptine tablets ("Parlodel", p. 198), commencing with moderate dosage and increasing gradually to a high level; the action is one of reducing the output of growth hormone by the anterior pituitary. Growth hormone is used occasionally by injection to stimulate growth in dwarfed children, but is effective only in the rare case of true deficiency of the hormone.

**The Thyrotrophic Hormone** (T.S.H., or thyrotrophin) stimulates the secretion of thyroxine by the thyroid gland. It is not used to treat deficiency of thyroxine production, for this is easily corrected by the administration of tablets of thyroid or, most usually, thyroxine (see later). However, thyrotrophin has a use by injection in the differential diagnosis of the cause of thyroxine deficiency; this is described on page 227. The use of a synthetic compound 'T.R.H.' in the further investigation of thyroid disease is described on p. 227.

It should be noted that 'T.S.H.' stands for "Thyroid Stimulating Hormone", and 'T.R.H.' for "Thyrotrophin Releasing Hormone".

**The Lactogenic Hormone** (or prolactin) is concerned with the growth of the mammary (or breast) glands and the production of milk following childbirth, and has been thought to be a factor in the nourishment of the corpus luteum (see page 195) during pregnancy; it is not used therapeutically.

**The Adrenocorticotrophic Hormone** (A.C.T.H., or corticotrophin) controls the production of the steroid hormones by the cortex of the adrenal glands, and is thus often used in place of cortico-steroid drugs (e.g. cortisone, prednisolone, etc.) in order to stimulate the patient's adrenal cortex to produce more steroid hormones itself. Hence, discussion of the various preparations of A.C.T.H., and their use in treatment, will be more appropriate in the section dealing with the corticosteroids (p. 193).

**The two Gonadotrophic Hormones** (or gonadotrophins) produced by the anterior pituitary are the follicle stimulating hormone (F.S.H.) and the luteinising hormone (L.H.); these govern the development and function of the organs of generation (the gonads) in both sexes. Secretion of F.S.H. and L.H., commences at puberty, i.e. at the onset of sexual maturity. F.S.H. and L.H. are not available *separately* for use in treatment, but two other hormones of equivalent effect and derived from certain natural sources are employed in place (p. 195). F.S.H. and L.H. are available *together* in a preparation of human source which is used in infertility; this is described on page 200.

Secretion of F.S.H. and L.H. can be stimulated by the synthetic compound gonadorelin, and the use of this in diagnosis is explained on page 225.

## THE THYROID GLAND

—secretes the hormone, thyroxine, which controls body activity in general, and metabolic function in particular.

Deficiency of thyroxine secretion is termed *hypo*thyroidism. If extreme insufficiency is present before, and from birth, this results in cretinism, a condition in which the child's growth is stunted and mental development retarded. In middle age, women (usually) may be affected by thyroxine deficiency, when the outcome is a slowing down of body metabolism accompanied by lethargy, mental sluggishness, dry and lank hair, and a typical coarsening of the skin; this condition is known as myxoedema. In the treatment of both cretinism and myxoedema, tablets of synthetic **Thyroxine** ('Eltroxin', 50 and 100 micrograms) are taken daily in carefully assessed dosage; tablets of dried animal thyroid gland have been much used in the past, but thyroxine is now routinely prescribed, as being far more dependable in action. The use of thyroxine is a typical example of *replacement* therapy in endocrine disorders.

Treatment with thyroxine needs to be carefully adjusted, for overdosage results in significant side-effects. Thus the stimulation of excessive activity can cause persistent tremor of the hands, rapid heart beat (tachycardia), insomnia, loss of weight and sweating. Stopping of treatment, and resuming later with a lower dosage, is then indicated.

Over-activity of the thyroid gland is known as *hyper*thyroidism, or thyrotoxicosis. As in the case of overdosage, excessive secretion of thyroxine results in extreme activity, restlessness and insomnia; loss of weight is marked despite a keen appetite, this being due to the very high rate of metabolism. Another typical symptom is the prominent eyeballs (termed exophthalmos), and there may also be goitre, or visible enlargement of the gland. Treatment may be either medical or surgical, and in both cases interesting drugs are concerned. Medical treatment is based on drugs which act by reducing the output of thyroxine. Thiouracil was formerly used but has now been superseded in this country by **Carbimazole** ('Neo-Mercazole'), tablets of which (5 mg) may be given up to several times daily, the dosage being adjusted to control thyroid function at a normal level. Carbimazole may also be given as a course before the operation for removal of part of the gland (partial thyroidectomy).

An aqueous solution of iodine, known as **Lugol's** solution, is also used before thyroidectomy, 0·6 ml being given three times daily in milk for approximately two weeks. Iodine is essential to the thyroid gland for the manufacture of thyroxine, and its administration sedates the gland, which then reduces in size and becomes firmer, with consequent less risk of excessive haemorrhage during the operation.

A point of interest is that iodine is deficient in the soil in certain areas, and vegetables and dairy produce (from grass-eating stock) are therefore likewise deficient in this element. The consequent lack of iodine in the diet leads to the swelling of the neck previously referred to as goitre, but resulting, in this case, from the gland's effort to produce thyroxine on an insufficient supply of iodine. Examples of areas affected are Derbyshire and certain parts of Switzerland and Canada, where the problem is overcome by the use of "iodised" table salt (i.e. containing iodide of sodium or potassium).

It needs to be mentioned that the hormone **Liothyronine,** of similar function, is also associated with thyroxine in the output of the thyroid gland; however, thyroxine is almost invariably used in treatment, as being more gradual in effect and hence safer and more controllable. The very quick and short action of liothyronine is used when immediate response is needed, as in the coma which may occur in myxoedema; it is issued as the synthetic 20 microgram tablet 'Tertroxin'.

## THE PARATHYROID GLANDS

—produce a hormone which controls the levels of calcium and phosphate in the blood; the source from which it obtains calcium is the bones. Deficiency of parathyroid hormone secretion (*hypo-parathyroidism*) results in raised phosphate and lowered calcium levels. Calcium is essential to the control of muscle and nerve tissue, and a low blood level leads to nerve irritability and tremor; this may result in tetany, a condition which is occasionally met in young children and is characterised by severe muscle spasms. Treatment consists of raising the calcium level by giving calcium gluconate by intravenous injection, and vitamin D, or one of its derivatives such as 'A.T.10' (p. 77), by mouth so as to increase the absorption of calcium from the intestinal tract. **'Para-Thor-Mone'** is an extract of animal parathyroid which contains parathyroid hormone; it is given by injection and is occasionally combined in the treatment of tetany.

**Calcitonin** is a hormone produced by certain thyroid (and possibly parathyroid) tissue. It has an effect opposite to that of the parathyroid hormone, for it *reduces* the amount of calcium taken from the bones and thus lowers its level in the blood; hence it assists in regulating calcium balance when necessary, i.e. if levels are high. Calcitonin is available as 'Calcitare', and is given by intramuscular or intravenous injection in the treatment of serious hypercalcaemia (excessive calcium level), as occurs in hyper-activity of the parathyroid glands (*hyper*parathyroidism). In Paget's disease, where the bones lose calcium to the blood and become soft and then deformed, calcitonin is employed for its action in correcting further loss and so maintaining the soundness (termed the integrity) of the bones; the pain which may accompany the condition is also relieved.

The calcitonin in 'Calcitare' is natural, as it is obtained from porcine (pig) tissue; **Salcatonin** ('Calcynar') is a synthetic compound which is identical with the calcitonin present in salmon. Unlike 'Calcitare', which needs dissolving before use, 'Calcynar' is a ready dissolved injection; also, whilst the place of both in treatment is the same, the chemical purity of 'Calcynar' ensures minimal risk of reaction compared with a product of animal origin like 'Calcitare'.

## INSULIN

### —and other Antidiabetic Drugs

[**To note**—"blood sugar" is a term frequently used when discussing aspects of diabetes mellitus, etc., but whilst other sugars may be present (in small amount) in the blood, *glucose* is the one normally implied, hence *"blood glucose"* is more accurate and will be used whenever applicable in the text.]

Insulin is the hormone produced by the *beta* cells of small areas of tissue in the pancreas called the islets of Langerhans; its function is to control the level of the blood glucose which is formed from the carbohydrates, i.e. the sugars and starches, etc., contained in the diet. Under its influence the glucose is stored as glycogen in the liver and the muscles; it is then called upon as required, and insulin facilitates its entry into the cells for immediate production of energy. If insulin production is deficient, there is an inevitable rise in the blood glucose level, termed *hyper*glycaemia, which leads to excretion of excess glucose in the urine, termed glycosuria; the output of urine is greatly increased by the larger volume of water taken out with the sugar through osmotic effect (p. 28). Due to its inability to utilise glucose, the body falls back on metabolising fats and protein for energy; some fat metabolism is incomplete, and resultant ketone substances are excreted in the urine (see under 'Acetest', p. 230). The condition is then one of diabetes mellitus, in which large volumes of urine are passed, severe thirst results, and weakness and loss of weight are striking. When this occurs at a young age, failure to secrete insulin is usually complete, or relatively so, and replacement treatment is essential for maintenance of life and health; commercial insulin is used, obtained from the pancreas of cattle or pigs. The additional importance to all diabetic patients of a carefully regulated diet, especially in respect of carbohydrate intake, is referred to on page 186.

**Insulin** is effective only by injection, and is given subcutaneously; several forms are available. **Soluble** insulin acts very quickly, but two or more injections daily are required due to its short action of 6 to 8 hours. A reduction of injections to once daily is an obvious boon to the diabetic patient, and this has led to the wide use of the longer-acting insulins. The first of these was **Protamine Zinc,** or P.Z., insulin, a combination of insulin with zinc and a protein substance, one dose of which given early in the day is sufficient; as it is insoluble the vial must be shaken gently but thoroughly before use. P.Z. insulin takes some hours to exert effect, and patients may need soluble insulin in addition in order to deal with the carbohydrates taken at breakfast. If this combination is used in one injection, the soluble insulin should be drawn into the syringe first, and then the P.Z., for if the order be reversed there is a risk of traces of P.Z. contaminating the soluble insulin vial and reducing its efficiency; incidentally, it is thought that mixing P.Z. and soluble insulins in one injection may reduce the overall effect. Two other protein/zinc insulins of prolonged action are **Globin** and **Isophane,** but the use of these appears confined to certain special cases.

The **Lente** insulins are insoluble combinations of insulin and zinc, and have the advantage of not containing protein, which is a possible source of allergic reaction (p. 101). There are three in all, each differing in physical properties and hence in duration of action. The quickest acting is the **Semi-Lente** suspension, which is in the form of an extremely fine powder, termed amorphous; its duration of action is approximately 12 hours. The longest acting is the **Ultra-Lente** suspension, which is in crystalline form and is thus slowly absorbed; its duration of action may be as long as 36 hours. The middle member, and the most widely used of this group, is **Lente** insulin, a mixture of three parts semi-lente and seven parts ultra-lente; the fine particles of the semi-lente ensure rapid initial action following the early morning injection, and the crystalline ultra-lente maintains its effect throughout the 24 hours, so achieving a perfect one-dose-daily regime. As with all insoluble insulins, the vials need shaking before use.

Two other insulins are 'Actrapid' and 'Rapitard'. 'Actrapid' is a soluble pork (i.e. pig) insulin which is used in certain especially sensitive patients, and 'Rapitard' is a mixture of 'Actrapid' and a long-acting crystalline beef (i.e. cattle) insulin. Both are used in patients who for some reason find the other types of insulin unsuitable.

The insulins discussed have long been established in use; several of them, however, have recently been subject to certain significant changes and improvements, and the following relevant points should be noted.

(1) As mentioned earlier, the animal origin of the pancreas from which insulin is obtained may be either cattle (hence the description *"beef"* or *"bovine"*) or pig (i.e. *"pork"* or *"porcine"*), and certain patients may be sensitive (i.e. get a reaction) to insulin from one or other of these two sources. This can be a factor in the prescriber's choice, and it is now required that the label *must clearly state* whether "beef" or "pork".

(2) The conventional soluble insulin is *acidic* in reaction, i.e. it has a pH (p. 231) of between 3 and 4; so also has globin insulin. All other insulins are *neutral* in reaction (i.e. a pH of about 7) and so carry less risk of pain and local reaction. Soluble insulin is available in both acidic *and* neutral forms, but the neutral is employed *only if so specified by the prescriber*.

(3) Preparations are now also available in which the insulin is in one of the following three more highly purified forms.

   (a) If labelled **"Proinsulin-freed"**, the insulin does not contain any proinsulin, a related substance which is normally associated with insulin and which can reduce its effectiveness.

   (b) If labelled **"Monocomponent"** (or "MC"), the insulin has been largely freed from undesirable related substances also normally present with it.

   (c) If labelled **"Rarely Immunogenic"** (or "RI"), again the insulin has been highly freed of undesirable constituents capable of provoking resistance to the insulin itself.

It will be clear that the advantages associated with these purer forms of insulin include the possibility of *reduced dosage need* and *less likelihood of reaction*.

Further developments, or maybe a simplification of the position, are yet possible, but it is emphasised that the nurse administering insulin, or advising the patient regarding it, should always observe the absolute rule that only the insulin *clearly prescribed* should be employed; and in view of the number of factors and combinations now involved, e.g. source, pH, types ("MC", etc.), it will be good practice to read carefully *the full wording* of the insulin description on the label and not rely on any abbreviations or trade captions, e.g. "Nuso", etc. Indeed, and again stressing this point, official advice is that the same brand (or "make") should be adhered to, as a further precaution against variation in therapeutic effect.

It should be noted that soluble insulin is always the one used in an emergency, e.g. in *diabetic* coma, where insufficient insulin dosage and/or possibly too high a carbohydrate intake has led to seriously excessive blood glucose levels. Treatment consists of giving soluble insulin (intravenously if need be), together with an intravenous injection of glucose solution to "buffer" the possible shock effect of too extreme a fall in blood glucose due to the insulin. In addition, the dehydration, and metabolic acidosis and disturbance of electrolyte levels, which are features of this condition, are treated with appropriate intravenous solutions (p. 42).

*Insulin* coma may also occur in diabetics. This is caused by too high a dosage of insulin and/or too low a carbohydrate intake, resulting in a severely reduced glucose level in the blood, termed *hypo*glycaemia; treatment consists of giving 'Glucagon' (p. 187), or a 50% glucose solution by intravenous injection (up to 50 ml). It is useful to note that insulin coma can be reversed by giving 0·5 to 1 ml of injection of adrenaline subcutaneously; this releases glycogen from the liver, and the glycogen is then converted to glucose, which raises the blood glucose level sufficiently to arouse the patient and enable him to take glucose or some other form of sugar by mouth. Diabetics often make a point of carrying lumps of sugar, which can be taken should the onset of such symptoms as a sinking feeling be a timely warning of too reduced a blood glucose level.

The symptoms of diabetic coma are, of course, directly opposite to those of insulin coma. In *diabetic coma,* the skin is flushed, the breath smells of acetone, breathing is deep and laboured, and urinary and blood glucose levels are very high. In *insulin coma,* the skin is pale, the breath acetone-free, breathing shallow, and urine usually glucose-free and blood glucose levels very low.

Strict regulations apply to the packaging of insulin by the various manufacturers and are essential for safety, because the treatment of the diabetic patient is finely balanced and accurate dosage is vital. Thus, all insulins are labelled and packaged with a distinctive colour, or colours, to denote both the type and its strength. The strengths employed are 20, 40 and 80 units per ml in the case of soluble insulin, and 40 and 80 units per ml in the case of the longer acting types; the figures are printed boldly.

It is likewise important that only "Insulin Syringes" be used for giving insulin; several are available, in 1 ml and 2 ml sizes. They may be all-glass, glass and metal, or the disposable single-use plastic type, but the important point is that *all* conform to the essential requirement—that they are graduated in *20 divisions per ml* and bear *no other division markings*—such as fifths of a ml; this ensures that the nurse or patient can give his or her undivided attention to the insulin divisions, with nothing else to confuse.

Estimation of the dose is greatly simplified by this standard set of 20 divisions; thus—

1. If using insulin of 20 units per ml, the dose will be exactly the *same* number of division markings as units needed—e.g. if 16 units needed, 16 division markings are used.
2. If using insulin of 40 units per ml, the dose will be exactly *half* the number of division markings as of units needed—e.g. if 30 units needed, 15 division markings are used.
3. If using insulin of 80 units per ml, the dose will be a *quarter* the number of division markings as of units needed—e.g. if 48 units needed, 12 division markings are used.

A point to note is that for convenience of injection the volume of the dose is best kept below 1 ml by the use of the appropriate strength insulin. Also, as in the case of all injections, aseptic technique is essential; this includes absolute need for sterile equipment (e.g. syringe and needle), plus the customary attention to the vial cap and the skin site itself.

Insulin is also used to ascertain if the operation known as vagotomy, in which the stomach branch of the vagus nerve is removed, has been successfully completed (see page 226).

## The Oral Hypoglycaemics

If diabetes mellitus appears in older patients, broadly from middle-age onwards (sometimes termed "maturity onset" diabetes), inability to produce insulin is often only partial, and the symptoms can be controlled by a comparatively small amount of insulin, perhaps less than 30 or so units per day; this is an indication that the patient is producing *some* insulin, *but not enough.* In such cases insulin therapy is often unnecessary, and oral hypoglycaemic drugs are used (note *hypo*glycaemic—to lower the blood glucose level and so prevent *hyper*glycaemia). The drugs concerned are in tablet form, and fall into two general groups according to their mode of action.

The first group, composed of certain sulphonamide derivatives, acts by stimulating the beta cells of the islets (i.e. those which are still functioning) to produce more insulin. The drugs mainly used are **Tolbutamide,** which has short action and is thus taken three times daily, and **Chlorpropamide,** which has more prolonged effect and is taken only once daily, at breakfast time. Tolbutamide is also used by injection in the diagnosis of diabetes mellitus (p. 228).

Other drugs related to tolbutamide and chlorpropamide are also used as hypoglycaemic agents, e.g. **Glibenclamide, Glypizide** and **Glibornuride,** for which are claimed the advantages of smaller dosage and less risk of side-effects, etc.

Tolbutamide     —'Rastinon'            —av. dose 500 mg
Chlorpropamide—'Diabinese'            — „    „    250 mg
Glibenclamide  —'Euglucon', 'Daonil'— „    „    5 mg
Glypizide       —'Glibenese'           — „    „    5 mg
Glibornuride   —'Glutril'              — „    „    25 mg

The second group of oral hypoglycaemics acts by increasing the utilisation of dextrose by the body, thus lowering the blood glucose level; **Phenformin** and **Metformin** are two examples. Long-acting capsules of the former are available which ensure slow release of the drug and thus allow once-daily dosage.

Phenformin therapy may involve risk of development of a metabolic acidosis which can be serious, especially in patients with certain heart, kidney or liver conditions; hence it is now employed with caution and due choice of case.

Phenformin—'Dibotin'     —tablets 25 mg, capsules ('SR')
                                              25 & 50 mg
Metformin —'Glucophage'—   „    500 & 850 mg.

In oral therapy, combinations of these drugs are occasionally used, and they may also be employed in certain cases to supplement insulin therapy.

As a final note on antidiabetic drugs, it must be emphasised that wisdom in restriction of carbohydrate intake is essential in the treatment of diabetes mellitus; reduction of weight to normal in respect of height, age, sex and build can effect profound improvement in many cases. Another important point is that the distribution of the carbohydrate content of the diet may have to be varied during the day to correspond with the type of insulin being used (i.e. quick acting or long acting). It is also held that diabetes mellitus may be prevented in many potential patients by a rational approach to diet *from infancy*, i.e. by limiting the intake of refined carbohydrates *in concentrated form*. Thus, if a diet is so adapted, for example by eating bread which is brown wholemeal only, and by a sparing intake of sugar in any concentrated form, then it is probable that many who inherit, not actual diabetes mellitus, but merely an inability to deal with the high level of processed carbohydrates in the modern diet *which may lead to the condition,* will remain healthy in this respect all their lives.

## Drugs used for their hyperglycaemic effect

### Glucagon

It will be recalled that insulin is secreted by the *beta* cells of the islets of Langerhans. The islet tissue also contains *alpha* cells, and these produce a substance called glucagon. The function of glucagon is to stimulate conversion of glycogen (which has been stored in the liver under the influence of insulin) back to glucose when it is required for utilisation; thus it is a *hyper*glycaemic agent and acts in reverse to insulin, another example of the comprehensive mechanism of the body.

Glucagon is available as an injection, which may be used in the treatment of insulin coma (together with intravenous glucose if necessary). It may also be given to, or self-administered by, the patient subcutaneously at home if symptoms of impending coma do not respond to the taking of sugar, etc. An important point regarding the use of glucagon is that as soon as the patient has recovered he should take food (carbohydrate) immediately, lest a relapse occur.

### Diazoxide

In contrast to the *hyper*glycaemia of diabetes mellitus, a condition of *hypo*glycaemia may also occur, in which insulin continues to be produced excessively and the blood glucose is maintained at an abnormally low level in consequence; the cause may be one of several factors, e.g. stimulation of the pancreatic islets by a tumour (i.e. a growth). Diazoxide ('Eudemine') may be used in this condition as tablets of 50 mg; it is thought to act by suppressing the activity of the insulin-producing beta cells, thus allowing blood-glucose levels to rise. The other use of diazoxide, in hypertensive emergency, is referred to on page 57.

## THE ADRENAL GLAND PREPARATIONS

There are two adrenal, or suprarenal, glands, one lying above each kidney. They consist of two parts, the inner, called the medulla, and the outer, the cortex; both secrete hormones essential to bodily function.

### The Medullary Hormones

The adrenal medulla secretes two hormones, adrenaline and nor-adrenaline, which reinforce and maintain bodily function during activity or stress; thus they increase blood pressure and stimulate the heart, raise blood glucose by release of glycogen (p. 181) from the liver, and improve the action and vital capacity of the lungs. The actions of these two hormones are similar in some respects but differ in others; this will be clarified later.

**Adrenaline** is prepared synthetically, and is used mainly as a 1 in 1 000 injection and as a solution for application. When applied to a bleeding point, solutions of adrenaline immediately constrict the vessel concerned, thus acting as a prompt haemostatic (p. 69). Adrenaline is also included in solutions of local anaesthetics such as lignocaine, at very dilute strengths, e.g. 1 in 200 000, or even weaker, the effect being to constrict the tissue locally at the site of injection and thus prolong the action of the local anaesthetic by slowing down the rate at which it diffuses away (p. 125).

Adrenaline has a powerful dilating effect on the bronchi, and its use by injection and inhalation in severe asthmatic attacks is described on pages 85 and 86. It is also a powerful heart stimulant, and in cardiac arrest it may be given by injection through a long "cardiac" needle directly into the heart muscle; it is more usually given intravenously in this condition as a 1 in 10 000 solution (p. 63).

Adrenaline is inactive by mouth as it is destroyed in the stomach, but two derivatives that are employed orally are isoprenaline and orciprenaline, their use as bronchodilators is discussed on pp. 85 and 86.

**Noradrenaline** differs from adrenaline in that it constricts the peripheral blood vessels, thereby raising the blood pressure, and has no direct effect on heart action; whereas adrenaline has an overall dilating effect on blood vessels and is a direct heart stimulant. Noradrenaline is available in 2 ml and 4 ml ampoules of a 1 in 1 000 solution ('Levophed'), which are diluted to $\frac{1}{2}$ litre and 1 litre respectively for use by intravenous drip to counteract shock; it is now seldom used in this connection.

### The Corticoid Hormones

—are produced by the cortex of the adrenal glands. They are often called the **corticosteroid,** or just **"steroid"**, hormones; the term "steroid" refers to a particular chemical structure which is common to these compounds. The corticosteroid compounds in use are all synthetic, and **Cortisone** is perhaps the best known.

The corticoid hormones exert several essential functions in the body. They take part in regulating carbohydrate, fat, and protein metabolism; this is termed the *glucocorticoid* effect, glucose being the prominent carbohydrate. They are also concerned with maintaining the salt and water balance of the body; this is termed the *mineralocorticoid* effect, salt (sodium chloride) being a mineral substance. All these mechanisms are vital to health, and play an essential role in conditioning the body to withstand stress, strain and shock, physical or mental, at which times it is known that secretion of the corticoid hormones is greatly increased.

Since the synthesis of cortisone, a number of derivatives have been introduced; the aim has been to increase effectiveness in one or other direction and reduce dosage and incidence of side-effects (the latter does not always follow), which can be a problem in corticosteroid therapy. Of the examples listed below, **Hydrocortisone** is identical with cortisol, the main hormone secreted by the adrenal cortex; **Prednisolone** and **Prednisone** are largely identical in action and interchangeable; and **Fludrocortisone** contains fluorine, which appears to greatly enhance the action. All these steroid drugs are effective orally; most of them may also be given by injection.

| | | | | |
|---|---|---|---|---|
| Cortisone | —'Cortelan' | —av. dose | | 25 mg |
| Hydrocortisone | —'Hydrocortone' | — „ | „ | 20 mg |
| Prednisolone | —'Precortisyl' | — „ | „ | 5 mg |
| Prednisone | —'Decortisyl' | — „ | „ | 5 mg |
| Triamcinolone | —'Ledercort' | — „ | „ | 4 mg |
| Dexamethasone | —'Decadron' | — „ | „ | 0·5 mg |
| Betamethasone | —'Betnelan' | — „ | „ | 0·5 mg |
| Fludrocortisone | —'Florinef' | — „ | „ | 0·1 mg |

The actions of this main group of corticosteroid drugs follow a pattern broadly similar to that of the functions of the natural body corticosteroid hormones as referred to earlier. Thus there is a glucocorticoid effect concerned with vital metabolic processes; a mineralocorticoid effect which influences electrolyte levels, and also the fluid balance of the body—due to the osmotic power of sodium; and a general protective effect in stress and shock. In addition, they have a striking anti-inflammatory action, which is not clearly understood but makes them extremely valuable in diseases characterised by allergic and inflammatory response. It should be noted, however, that the glucocorticoid/mineralocorticoid ratio varies from drug to drug, some being more active in the former respect and some in the latter, and this may influence the decision re which to use. Two other steroid hormones which are entirely mineralocorticoid in effect are discussed on page 193.

Now to outline the wide range of applications in which the steroid hormones are employed.

Firstly, they are used for their anti-inflammatory effect in rheumatoid arthritis (p. 117), where inflammation of the connective tissue in the joints is involved. Cortisone and prednisolone (or prednisone) are taken in tablet form for their systemic effect via the circulation, and hydrocortisone or prednisolone can be given by intra-articular injection (p. 118) to relieve pain in a particular area, e.g. knee, elbow or hip joints; a long acting "depot" form is often used for this purpose. Corticosteroids may also be used in high dosage in rheumatic fever (p. 119).

The inflammatory reactions associated with allergies and eye and skin diseases are special fields for corticosteroid therapy; in addition to systemic administration, powerful derivatives are used as external applications in cream, ointment, lotion and spray, etc., form, e.g. **Betamethasone** in the 'Betnovate' preparations and **Clobetasol** in the 'Dermovate' range. The inclusion of fluorine in the chemical structure again appears to greatly increase the potency of certain steroid drugs used externally, e.g. the "Synalar" range of preparations containing **Fluocinolone,** the "Topilar" range (**Fluclorolone**) and the "Metosyn" range (**Fluocinonide**). A point to note is that the steroids can be *absorbed* through the skin, and too lavish or prolonged use may induce systemic side-effects, particularly in infants, in whom there is also the danger of brown areas of atrophied skin (striae) developing where the folds have held substantial amounts of the application. These powerful preparations are frequently prescribed by the dermatologist in diluted form.

Some asthmas may improve on daily prophylactic dosage with prednisolone, for example, or an intensive course may be employed at intervals, commencing with a large dose and tapering off over seven days or so. Severe hay-fever, also, may be prevented in certain cases by a single long-acting injection given at the appropriate time.

Corticosteroids are of specific value for their anti-inflammatory effect in ulcerative colitis (a condition referred to on page 130). In certain cases prednisolone is given orally and reaches the affected tissue of the colon via the circulation. However, it is more often used as a retention enema solution ('Predsol'); this is contained in a disposable plastic bag and is administered daily as described on page 22.

It needs mentioning that in many of their uses the steroid hormones do not *cure* the condition but merely act as *palliatives*—e.g. in rheumatoid arthritis. Likewise, their use as creams and ointments, etc., is of benefit mainly in allaying the inflammation involved whilst the curative processes continue.

The corticosteroid drugs are often used specifically in treating or preventing shock, where the circulation is unable to provide an adequate blood flow to vital organs and tissues such as the brain and kidneys. Causes of shock include severe trauma (injury), blood loss, fall in cardiac output (as in coronary thrombosis), acute bronchial asthma, and overwhelming infection. In such conditions hydrocortisone or dexamethasone may be given by intravenous injection, sometimes in "heroic" (i.e. very high) dosage, as much as two grams or 80 mg, respectively, over 24 hours being not uncommon. The mechanism of action is not completely understood, but the vital function of the natural corticosteroids in conditions of stress has been referred to (p. 189).

The corticosteroids are given as specific replacement treatment when the adrenal cortex is unable to produce its hormones, as in Addison's disease in which the cortex is atrophied (often due to tuberculous infection), or following surgical removal of the adrenal glands (adrenalectomy) in advanced breast cancer. Maintenance therapy, e.g. with prednisolone (and fludrocortisone, p. 193) must then be continued with, because of the essential position of the corticoid hormones in the metabolic and electrolyte-regulating processes of the body.

The frequent use of the corticosteroids in the treatment of malignant conditions is referred to in Chapter 19.

### Side-Effects of Corticosteroid Therapy

These are numerous and can be serious, particularly if treatment is long-term. Oedema may occur due to retention of sodium (and hence also water—p. 28), and this may lead to hypertension, i.e. raised blood pressure. In contrast, the excretion of potassium is increased, and in view of the importance of an adequate level of this electrolyte (p. 31) it may be given as slow-release tablets (p. 33) during steroid treatment, in order to make up the deficiency.

The corticosteroids are also diabetogenic, i.e. they may cause a rise in blood glucose, probably due to antagonism of the action of insulin; a form of diabetes mellitus results and may be "insulin-resistant".

Long-term corticosteroid therapy may cause distressing facial effects; hirsutism (growth of hair) may result, and also acne and the condition known as "moon face", caused by deposition of fat about the cheeks and under the eyes. Mental balance may be disturbed, resulting in either elation or depression. Bone substance may be affected due to protein loss, and osteoporosis result, a brittle condition of the bone which is difficult to treat, though the anabolic drugs are claimed to be of some value (p. 201). The side-effects so far described are collectively known as "Cushingoid" features, for they are similar to the symptoms known as "Cushing's syndrome", which are caused by excessive activity of the adrenal cortex in certain diseases.

A hazard of long-term corticosteroid therapy is peptic ulceration of the stomach and/or duodenum. This has been ascribed to an increase in gastric acid secretion, but it is also thought possible that during prolonged therapy the mucosal tissue itself is rendered less resistant to the effect of gastric acid and/or digestive processes, and that repair is likewise delayed.

Two final points regarding corticosteroid therapy are especially important.

Firstly, when treatment is to be discontinued (and particularly if it has been long-term) abrupt cessation is invariably avoided, because the prolonged high blood level produced by the *administered* steroid will have suppressed the output of A.C.T.H. (p. 178) from the anterior pituitary (see page 175 re the "feed-back" mechanism), and the lack of this cortex-stimulating factor will have resulted in a very low output of the *natural* steroid hormones from the adrenal cortex. Hence, steroid dosage is tapered off gradually over a period of two or three weeks, which allows time for the production of A.C.T.H. to pick up *in response to the falling steroid blood levels;* the adrenal cortex, in turn, increases its output to normal by the time dosage ceases entirely. An injection of A.C.T.H. is sometimes given during the tapering-off process, because its additional stimulating effect on the adrenal cortex hastens the return to normal of the output of corticosteroid hormones.

It is customary for patients to carry a card recording that they are on corticosteroid therapy. Then, in an emergency, such as an accident or operation, the doctor will be aware that the patient's own production of corticosteroids is low, and that he will need additional steroids (e.g. hydrocortisone intravenously, p. 190) for protection against shock, etc.

Secondly, the anti-inflammatory action of the corticosteroids may actually facilitate the spread of infection, for inflammation is the body's protective response, or barrier, to infection. Thus, eye-drops containing a corticosteroid often incorporate an antibiotic such as neomycin; otherwise, although inflammation of the eye may resolve and all appear well, it is possible for infection, if present, to spread more easily in consequence, with possible serious results. Similarly, tubercular disease which is under control may become active once more when steroids are given for some other condition.

The decision as to which steroid drug to use may largely depend on the extent of its glucocorticoid or mineralocorticoid effect. Thus, when a predominantly glucocorticoid drug is required, prednisolone appears to be most commonly used. An example of the utilisation of mineralocorticoid effect is the use of fludrocortisone in Addison's disease (see next section).

## The Mineralocorticoid Drugs

The corticosteroids so far discussed have both glucocorticoid and mineralocorticoid action, though in varying proportions. Deoxycortone and aldosterone are two further corticoid hormones which have mineralocorticoid effect only.

**Deoxycortone** has been used in Addison's disease for its action in retaining sodium and chloride and thus regulating water balance; it is now seldom employed; brand name 'Percorten M'.

**Aldosterone** is the major natural mineralocorticoid produced by the adrenal gland; its function is to promote the reabsorption of sodium and chloride in the distal tubule of the nephron (p. 32); it is available in injection form as the synthetic 'Aldocorten', and is more powerful and specific than deoxycortone.

Deoxycortone and aldosterone are effective by injection only, and when mineralocorticoid action is needed, fludrocortisone is usually the drug of preference, for it has very powerful sodium retaining properties, approaching aldosterone in this respect. Thus, in the treatment of Addison's disease (p. 191), cortisone or prednisolone may be used as replacement for their pronounced glucocorticoid action, together with fludrocortisone in small doses to ensure maintenance of sodium levels and fluid balance; both drugs being taken orally.

### A.C.T.H. (Corticotrophin)

—has been referred to (page 178) as controlling the secretion of steroid hormones by the adrenal cortex. It has also been mentioned that it is used in place of steroid drugs in many conditions; these include rheumatic diseases, acute asthma, severe allergies and serious skin conditions. It will be clear that treatment with A.C.T.H. is effective only if the adrenal cortex is functioning and is able to respond to stimulation. In cases of cortex failure, as in Addison's disease, A.C.T.H. is of no value, and therefore steroid drugs must be given.

A.C.T.H. is obtained from the pituitary gland of pigs, though an almost identical synthetic equivalent is also available (see later); it is effective only by injection. It is issued as a white powder, labelled in units of strength, which is dissolved in water immediately prior to injection as it does not keep in solution; its effect is short and several injections a day are needed. A 'Gel' solution thickened with gelatine is available, this is stable, and one injection lasts for 24 hours; a zinc suspension with similar prolonged action is also employed, this needs to be well shaken before use. The injections are normally intramuscular, but in acute conditions the pure powder form is dissolved and given intravenously.

The side-effects of A.C.T.H. are naturally similar to those which occur during steroid treatment, due to the fact that it acts by stimulating increased production of steroid hormones. However, it has two important advantages over the steroid drugs. Firstly, it does not suppress the adrenal glands and reduce their output of steroids, as happens during treatment with steriod drugs (p. 192). Secondly, although the high level of corticosteroids produced by A.C.T.H. injections depresses the *natural* secretion of A.C.T.H. by the anterior pituitary lobe (see "feed-back" mechanism, p. 175), this natural production rapidly increases again when the injections are stopped. Hence the danger associated with interruption or cessation of therapy (p. 192) is far less when A.C.T.H. is used.

The A.C.T.H. preparations which contain the natural hormone, i.e. the powder form, the "Gel", and the zinc suspension, all carry the disadvantage that being derived from animal (pig) sources, traces of foreign protein may be present and cause reactions. Synthetic A.C.T.H., known as **Tetracosactrin,** is now available and is free of the risk of sensitivity due to impurity. In addition, the effect of one injection may last for 2 or 3 days or even longer. Because of its complete purity, doses of tetracosactrin may be weighed accurately and are thus expressed not in terms of units, as in the case of natural A.C.T.H. preparations, but as milligrams (see "Units", p. xiv).

Both A.C.T.H. and tetracosactrin are used in testing the function of the adrenal cortex (see page 224).

| | | | | |
|---|---|---|---|---|
| A.C.T.H. powder | —'Acthar' | —av. dose | | 25–40 units |
| gelatine solution | —'Acthar Gel' | — „ | „ | 20–80 „ |
| zinc suspension | —'Cortrophin ZN' | — „ | „ | 40–120 „ |
| Tetracosactrin-diag-<br>nostic & therapeutic } | —'Synacthen' | — „ | „ | 0·25 mg |
| -therapeutic | —'Cortrosyn Depot' | — „ | „ | 1 mg |
| | —'Synacthen Depot' | — „ | „ | „ „ |

## THE SEX HORMONES

—are the complex chemicals which stimulate the growth, and control the function, of the organs of generation.

The actions of the female sex hormones are by far the more complicated, and in order to clarify the explanation of their use in treatment it will be helpful to outline the pattern of events involved in the menstrual cycle. The uterus, or womb, is connected to the ovaries by two ducts (the fallopian tubes), and at its lower end it narrows to form the cervix, which terminates within the vagina; the inner lining of the uterus is called the endometrium. Both ovaries contain a number of minute sacs, or chambers, called follicles, each of which contains an unfertilised ovum, or egg, i.e. female reproductive cell. The menstrual cycles commence at puberty, and each cycle lasts about 28 days, during the first three or four of which menstruation occurs, involving the breakdown and shedding of the endometrium together with blood. Following menstruation, the follicle stimulating hormone (F.S.H.) from the anterior pituitary lobe (p. 179) stimulates growth of the follicles; these in turn secrete the sex-hormone, oestradiol. This process continues for approximately half the menstrual cycle, i.e. to about the fourteenth day, by which time one (usually) of the follicles has matured in size together with the ovum inside. At this stage the follicle bursts and releases its ovum (this is termed ovulation); the ovum then travels down the fallopian tube towards the uterus, and, if it is not fertilised, is ejected during the next menstruation. The ruptured follicle, under the influence of the luteinising hormone, L.H. (p. 179) which is now involved, develops into the corpus luteum, a yellow body. The corpus luteum then proceeds to secrete the other ovarian sex-hormone, progesterone, for the remaining 12 or 14 days (still under stimulation from L.H.), when production of progesterone and oestradiol falls sharply and menstruation again commences.

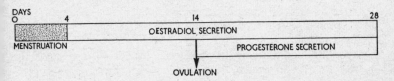

Fig. 8. Illustrating the menstrual cycle.

The above has been the accepted explanation of the part played by F.S.H. and L.H., but it is now thought possible that L.H. may be concerned to a greater degree.

We can now proceed to discuss the uses of the sex hormones and their synthetic equivalents and derivatives.

The gonadotrophic hormones, F.S.H. and L.H., are difficult to extract separately from animal sources for therapeutic use, but two other hormones, similar chemically and in certain therapeutic effects, are freely available.

**Serum Gonadotrophin** is obtained from the blood of pregnant mares, and its action resembles that of the follicle stimulating hormone, F.S.H. Thus, it is used by injection in disturbances of the menstrual cycle, e.g. certain types of amenorrhoea (absence of menstruation), where it may assist in the resumption of regular monthly periods; brand name is 'Gonadotraphon F.S.H.'.

**Chorionic Gonadotrophin** ('Pregnyl') is broadly equivalent in effect to the luteinising hormone, L.H. It is produced by the placenta, the fleshy body which develops in the uterus and which governs the nutrition of the foetus, and is excreted in the urine of pregnant women; this urine is collected from ante-natal clinics and the chorionic hormone extracted from it and prepared in injection form. Chorionic gonadotrophin is used mainly in cryptorchidism (undescended testicle(s)) in adolescent males and is sometimes successful in achieving descent, thus avoiding the need for surgical intervention. The action is explained by the fact that it is the chorionic hormone which is responsible for the descent of the testicles in the male foetus before birth.

It has now been explained that the gonadotrophic hormones of the anterior pituitary lobe, i.e. F.S.H. and L.H., are not available separately, and that two other hormones, which *are* obtainable separately, are used instead of them in certain conditions, i.e. serum gonadotrophin in place of F.S.H., and chorionic gonadotrophin in place of L.H.

It has also been made clear that F.S.H. and L.H. control the production in the ovaries of the female sex hormones, oestradiol and progesterone respectively.

In the male, F.S.H. stimulates the production of the spermatozoa, and L.H. the secretion of testosterone, the male sex hormone; both occurring in the testes.

We can now outline the functions of these sex hormones and the interesting uses to which they, and certain synthetic drugs with equivalent effect, are put in therapy.

### The Oestrogens

The ovarian follicles secrete the oestrogenic hormones, chiefly oestradiol. This hormone is responsible for the development of the organs of generation and the secondary sex characteristics, i.e. the female body shape, the breasts, voice, fine skin, and hair distribution, etc. Oestradiol also controls the condition of the mucus (liquid secretion) in the cervix at the time of ovulation, when it becomes thin and alkaline; this makes it easier for the spermatozoa to pass through the cervical canal in order to fertilise the released ovum in the fallopian tube.

The oestrogenic preparations used are mainly synthetic (but see 'Premarin' later) and are termed the oestrogens, **Stilboestrol** and **Ethinyloestradiol** being conspicuous; they have a special place in the following conditions.

The female menopause occurs in middle age, and is associated with a falling production of oestradiol by the ovaries. Accompanying symptoms may be hot flushes, depression, lethargy, increase in weight, and menstrual disturbance, and these can be helped by replacement therapy, using small doses daily of stilboestrol (e.g. 0·5 mg) or ethinyloestradiol (e.g. 0·05 mg). These drugs are also used for various types of amenorrhea, delayed puberty, dysmenorrhoea (painful menstruation), and other disorders associated with ovarian dysfunction.

A second use of oestrogen therapy is in the inhibition of lactation (production of milk in the breasts) after childbirth. During pregnancy, milk production is suppressed because the secretion of the lactogenic hormone, prolactin (p. 178), is blocked by a high level of oestradiol secretion by the ovaries; the oestradiol level drops sharply at childbirth, lactogenic hormone production then rises as a result, and the breasts fill with milk. This is a source of discomfort when breast-feeding is not being pursued with (or there may have been a miscarriage or stillbirth), and stilboestrol, or ethinyloestradiol, may then be used to "dry-up" the milk, the action being similar to that of the natural oestrogen (oestradiol) during pregnancy, as just referred to. A short intensive course is given, 5 mg of stilboestrol or 0·1 mg ethinyloestradiol two or three times daily for the first few days, tapering off subsequently. **Quinestrol** ('Estrovis') is another synthetic oestrogen, but with such prolonged effect that one tablet of 4 mg given shortly after delivery is normally sufficient.

A point to note is that the use of oestrogens in inhibiting lactation is lessening, due to increasing consideration of the possible effects associated with oestrogen therapy. The use of bromocriptine for this purpose is referred to later.

The third use of oestrogens is in the palliative treatment of certain types of cancer. They may be given occasionally in breast cancer, but are restricted to patients who are several years past the menopause, for oestrogens are held to have carcinogenic (i.e. cancer inducing) effect if taken in high dosage by younger women who may be susceptible. Stilboestrol and ethinyloestradiol have long been in use to treat cancer of the prostrate gland; they arrest or reduce the size of the growth, probably by suppressing production in the testes of testosterone; this hormone is known to be a stimulating factor in the progress of prostatic cancer. High doses of oestrogens are used, and as these drugs are equivalent to the ovarian (i.e. female) sex-hormone they can produce unpleasant side-effects, such as painful swelling of breast tissue. A stilboestrol derivative, **Tetrasodium fosfestrol** ('Honvan'), is comparatively free of this effect, for it is inactive in the body until it is converted to an active form by an enzyme which is present in high concentration in the prostate gland; hence the action is largely localised at the required site. It is thought that the action of this compound, unlike that of the oestrogens generally, is mainly cytotoxic within the cancer cell (p. 203).

Stilboestrol may cause unpleasant side-effects, e.g. nausea and vomiting, and alternatives are **Dienoestrol** and **Hexoestrol**; however, ethinyloestradiol appears to be the favoured drug amongst the synthetic oestrogens.

**'Premarin'** is a preparation of oestrogens obtained from natural sources, and is used similarly to the synthetic oestrogens in conditions already discussed; in high dosage it can inhibit lactation in less than a day, and, being of natural source, it is said to be relatively free of the side-effects associated with the synthetic oestrogens. A further use of 'Premarin' in controlling bleeding is described on page 70.

**Tamoxifen** is a synthetic compound which *antagonises* the activity of the natural oestrogens. Thus, it is employed in appropriate patients *more usually past the menopause* and who have advanced breast cancers which are considered oestrogen dependent and unsuitable for surgery or radiotherapy; the tablets ('Nolvadex') are given twice daily, and the effectiveness of this drug (though also only palliative) is comparable with that of androgens and oestrogens in women of this age group. Advantages of Tamoxifen are that the side-effects of androgen therapy (p. 201) are avoided, and the pattern of life is made more acceptable to the patient.

**Bromocriptine** is a substance derived from ergot (p. 108) and available as tablets ('Parlodel'); it has the effect of suppressing the secretion of prolactin (p. 178) and is thus used to prevent lactation, when one tablet is taken on the day of delivery and then twice daily for the following 14 days. If lactation needs to be suppressed *after* it has commenced, higher doses are given.

The use of bromocriptine as a supportive measure in the treatment of acromegaly is referred to on page 178; it is possible that this important drug will be employed in other conditions, for which it is at present on trial.

### The Progestogens

Progesterone, the hormone produced by the corpus luteum, is the natural progestogen, and, as will be seen, it is essential for the successful initiation and maintenance of pregnancy.

Fertilisation takes place when the ovum (p. 194) unites with a spermatozoon in the fallopian tube, and a vital function of progesterone is to stimulate the growth and condition of the endometrium so that the fertilised ovum can be successfully embedded within the uterus (p. 194). Progesterone continues to be produced as pregnancy proceeds, and its effect is to prevent further ovulation and ensure a full-term delivery.

**Progesterone** is available in synthetic form, and is given by injection. It may be used in habitual abortion, where the patient has repeated miscarriages, treatment being by regular moderate dosage until the end of the eighth month with either progesterone or **Ethisterone,** the latter being an orally effective tablet form. Threatened abortion is an acute phase of the condition and requires hospital admission, when higher doses of progesterone are given until bleeding stops. **Medroxyprogesterone** ('Provera') is a derivative of progesterone with more powerful action; the tablets are used similarly in habitual and threatened abortion, but the high-dose presentation (100 mg) is employed in certain gynaecological cancers which are hormone-dependent, the action being possibly related to suppression of anterior pituitary production of the ovary-stimulating hormones.

Other synthetic derivatives of progesterone are available, and this group of drugs is known collectively as the progestogens. Further indications for their use range from functional uterine bleeding to pre-menstrual tension.

Many commercial combinations of synthetic oestrogens and progestogens are employed in the various types of ovarian and uterine dysfunction that may result from disturbance of the finely balanced hormonal mechanisms involved. The oestrogen, **Mestranol,** and the progestogens, **Norethisterone** and **Norethynodrel,** are examples of those employed in these formulae. An increasingly important use of such combinations forms the subject of the next section.

### The Pill

—is the name commonly given to the combination of oestrogen and progestogen widely used for oral contraception.

A typical such combination is norethisterone or norethynodrel as the progestogen, with a small amount of an oestrogen such as mestranol or ethinyloestradiol, the tablet (i.e. "pill") being usually taken once daily from the fifth to the twenty-fifth day of the menstrual cycle, inclusive. A modified formula contains the progestogen only and may be considered more suitable in certain cases, though it is held to carry a higher risk of failure; an oestrogen content appears to be necessary for maximum effectiveness.

Several factors are considered as contributing to the action of the "pill". Firstly, the presence in the blood of the two synthetic ovarian hormones has a suppressant effect on the production of the anterior pituitary hormones, F.S.H. and L.H. (by the "feed-back" mechanism, p. 175); in consequence, secretion of oestradiol and progesterone in the ovaries is inhibited or greatly reduced. The overall result is that ovulation does not occur, or is less likely, and, in addition, the endometrium fails to be made receptive for implantation of the ovum —this is an important factor. In addition, certain significant and likewise important changes occur in the condition of the mucus of the uterine cervix. This has been mentioned (p. 196) as being normally thin and alkaline at the time of ovulation, so facilitating passage of the spermatozoa through the cervix; during oral contraceptive treatment, however, it becomes acid and viscous (thick), and is thus hostile to movement through it. The progestogen is held to be mainly responsible for these effects, but, as mentioned earlier, the oestrogen component also appears to be a significant factor.

Side-effects of oral contraception are common, e.g. headache, nausea, painful breasts, and weight gain; liver damage and fatal thromboses of various kinds have been reported. The oestrogen content is incriminated as the cause, hence the official recommendation regarding limitation of the oestrogen level in each tablet to a stated maximum (50 micrograms); a lower level still—30 micrograms—is being advised where the higher level is not considered essential.

## The use of hormones in infertility

When the cause of infertility has been assessed as anovulation (inability to ovulate), treatment may be undertaken with injections of F.S.H. and L.H., the gonadotrophic hormones of the anterior pituitary lobe. Although, as stated earlier, these are not obtainable *separately* for use, they can be extracted *in combination* from human menopausal urine, and are available as the preparation 'Pergonal'; this is given as a course of injections and is followed by an injection of chorionic gonadotrophin (p. 195). The effect is to duplicate the functions normal to naturally secreted F.S.H. and L.H., thus stimulating ovulation and encouraging subsequent embedding of the fertilised ovum in the uterus. The treatment is conducted under hospital supervision. It will be appreciated that because, thus far, the delicate process of ovulation cannot be absolutely controlled in the numerical sense, instances of multiple births are possible and very occasionally occur.

## The Androgens

Testosterone is the chief male sex-hormone, or androgen; it is secreted in the testes.

Testosterone is responsible for the development of the organs of generation and the secondary sex characteristics, e.g. the deeper voice, growth of facial and pubic hair, and general masculinity. It is available synthetically as tablets of **Methyltestosterone** and as **Testosterone propionate,** a solution in oil for injection. The tablets are dissolved slowly in the mouth (usually sublingually—p. 2), thus bypassing the stomach where absorption is moderate.

The main use of testosterone is in breast cancer of the inoperable type and when there are bone or lung metastases (secondary growths). High doses are employed, commencing with injections and continuing with a maintenance dose orally; this may be successful in prolonging life for several years. The action is said to be due to suppression of the ovarian production of oestrogens, on the stimulating influence of which the growth of the malignant tissue in the breast may be dependent.

It is interesting to observe the parallel between the treatment of prostatic and mammary cancer. In each case the high blood level of the administered hormone inhibits, by "feed-back" effect (p. 175), the production of the anterior pituitary gonadotrophins (p. 179); lack of these gonadotrophins leads to the required decrease in the secretion of testosterone in the case of prostatic cancer, and of oestrogens in the case of mammary cancer.

Several commercial testosterone preparations are available; some are of the prolonged-effect type (e.g. 'Sustanon'), one injection lasting for several weeks. **Drostanolone** ('Masteril') is a derivative of testosterone with similar androgenic action, but is comparatively free of the virilising effect which is referred to under "Anabolic Drugs" (see below).

## The Anabolic Drugs

Testosterone treatment often stimulates additional protein formation, improved condition of muscle and bone, and an increase in body weight; this is termed the anabolic (building up) effect. This would make testosterone a valuable aid in illness, convalescence, and in geriatrics (treatment of the elderly) but for the fact that in long-term therapy women tend to become masculinised (the virilising effect), the voice deepening and hair growing on the face; also, if given to men with prostatic cancer, it accelerates spread of the disease. However, several synthetic drugs are available, chemically related to testosterone, which have a similar anabolic effect but with less of the masculinising feature; these are used in the circumstances mentioned above, but with prostatic cancer still a contraindication.

Anabolic therapy is also used in osteoporosis, which may follow long-term steroid treatment (p. 191) and which also occurs in old people, protein being essential to the basic foundation of bone structure.

Examples of anabolic drugs are methandienone ('Dianabol') and stanozolol ('Stromba'), both in tablet form, and nandrolone ('Durabolin') which is a long-acting injection.

The building-up effect of the anabolic drugs, or so-called 'steroids' (they, too, have a steroid structure), can be gauged by the allegation that they have been employed in the athletes' preparation for certain events in the Olympic Games entailing great strength.

## Hormone therapy by implantation

Hormone treatment is often long-term, and injections may have to be given regularly and frequently. An alternative in the case of some of the hormones is a long-acting implant; this involves a small incision in the abdomen and the insertion of a sterile, high-dose tablet deep into the tissue. The hormone is released gradually into the circulation, and one implant may last many months. Testosterone may be used in this way in the treatment of breast cancer (p. 200).

## Danazol

—is a synthetic compound which *reduces* the output of F.S.H. and L.H. by the anterior pituitary; it is taken orally as capsules ('Danol') in cases where a reduced output of F.S.H. and L.H. is of benefit. Such conditions include endometriosis (abnormal positioning of endometrial tissue), excessive virginal breast development, gynae-comastia (abnormal quantity of breast tissue in the male) and precocious (unusually premature) development of the secondary sex characteristics. Danazol has some androgenic (male sex-hormonal) activity, hence slight growth of facial hair, voice change, and weight increase may occur as side-effects in certain cases.

# CHAPTER 19

# DRUGS USED IN THE TREATMENT OF MALIGNANT DISEASE—THE CYTOTOXICS

## *With an outline of the immune-response mechanism and related aspects*

Cytotoxic drugs are used in the chemotherapy (see page 127) of malignant disease. They are, in general, synthetic compounds (though certain antibiotics have become prominent in this field), and are employed in the treatment of certain types of cancer which cannot be treated, or treated solely, by surgery, radiotherapy (deep X-Ray), or the use of hormones. This may be due to surgery not being possible because of the site of the growth, or the malignant condition may be too disseminated, or widespread, or it may be one of leukaemia or Hodgkin's disease, where the bone-marrow and the lymph glands are involved. Another aim in cancer chemotherapy may be to prevent, or delay the appearance of metastases (secondary growths). The action of the drugs concerned can be broadly described as either directly injurious to the cancer cells, or interfering with the availability of certain essential substances needed for their further growth. Unfortunately, they have the disadvantage in many cases of affecting the cells of the normal healthy tissue as well, including those of the bone marrow, which is of vital concern in blood cell formation. However, in certain malignant conditions, the revival of the cells of healthy tissue following chemotherapy is far quicker than that of the cancer cells, and in such cases this type of treatment can be a significant factor in prolonging life for several years.

One of the serious side-effects of many members of this group of drugs is that the white cell count may be reduced to a dangerous point during treatment, as a result of bone marrow depression, and in these cases regular laboratory tests are performed on blood samples to ensure that the minimum safety level is maintained. Other side-effects can be extremely distressing, amongst them nausea and vomiting, and the latter may be so acute as to necessitate intravenous fluid therapy to compensate the resultant serious dehydration and electrolyte loss. The value of anti-emetics in these circumstances is referred to on page 17.

It should be made clear that whilst the action of many of the individual members of this group of drugs is broadly of a similar pattern, each has some distinctive feature which makes it especially suitable for certain particular conditions or age groups concerned. Also, the range of dosage employed in cancer chemotherapy is extremely wide, hence these details are not included.

The cytotoxics may be broadly classified into two groups of drugs, the **Antimitotics** and the **Antimetabolites.** The antimitotic drugs can be said to duplicate the effect of deep X-Ray therapy, for they injure the nucleus of the cancer cell in various ways, thus preventing mitosis, i.e. its ability to divide and multiply; they are sometimes called "radiomimetic" because of their action in imitating radiotherapy. The mode of action of the antimetabolites differs in that they do not directly damage the cell structure, but instead interfere with the availability of certain nutritional factors essential to the metabolism of the cell and its normal ability to multiply by division. A further term sometimes used to denote certain of these drugs is *cytostatic*, which implies an action of blocking the functional processes within the cell. It should be emphasised that the above classification is a very broad generalisation, and the differentiation is not always clear cut; also that the aim in the case of all cytotoxic drugs is the same, i.e. the arrest of the progress of the malignant cells, and their ultimate destroyal.

The routes employed in cancer chemotherapy are mainly the oral and intravenous, but other procedures are used which aim to *localise* the action of the drugs in order to enhance the effect and minimise as far as possible the *systemic* damage to healthy tissue already referred to. Thus, a sterile solution of the suitably chosen drug may be allowed to drip (or, more often, be injected from a machine-operated syringe at an extremely slow rate) into an artery leading to the cancer site, examples being the hepatic artery in carcinoma of the liver and the carotid artery in tumours of the head and neck; this is termed "regional perfusion".

The following is a representative selection from this group of drugs.

## ANTIMITOTICS

**Nitrogen Mustard** ('Mustine') was the forerunner in this group; it is available in vials of dry powder, which is dissolved in sterile water or normal saline and given by intravenous injection. This drug is highly vesicant, or blistering, hence the solution must be handled with care and due precaution taken during injection to ensure that it does not leak from the vein. It is used, in dosage varying with the weight of the patient, in a variety of malignant conditions, including certain leukaemias, Hodgkin's disease and carcinoma of the lung, and also as an intra-pleural injection, and in weak dilution for irrigation during certain operations where there is a risk of release of free cancer cells.

**Cyclophosphamide** ('Endoxana') is a similar drug to nitrogen mustard, but is non-vesicant and has far less side-effects; it is given intravenously and intramuscularly, and also orally as tablets. Its mode of action is interesting. Cyclophosphamide is inactive in the form given (and is thus better tolerated by the patient), but is converted in the liver into two substances which appear to enter cancer cells far more easily than into normal healthy cells. They are then converted within these cells into two further substances which have cytotoxic action, one of them being almost identical with nitrogen mustard. Hence the action of the drug is able to concentrate largely in the cancer tissue—where it is needed, and is less likely to damage healthy tissue. A discomforting side-effect of cyclophosphamide is alopecia, fall-out of hair being common during treatment. Special pneumatic head-caps are used, which can be inflated to compress the outer blood vessels in the head and so minimise access of the drug to the scalp; if this is done for several hours after each injection, the alopecia may be resisted.

**Busulphan** ('Myleran') is a cytotoxic drug in tablet form, which is somewhat selective in depressant action on bone marrow, hence its use in appropriate leukaemias. **Chlorambucil** ('Leukeran') is also given orally in the treatment of certain leukaemias; it is related to nitrogen mustard but is effective at dosage levels which are not damaging to the bone marrow. **'Thio-Tepa'** resembles nitrogen mustard in action and effect, but has the advantage of being non-vesicant, and is employed as a suppressant to the spread of the growth in a wide variety of cancer conditions; sometimes, as with other cytotoxic drugs, it is used in conjunction with deep X-Ray therapy or surgery.

**Vinblastine** ('Velbe') is a cytotoxic drug of *natural* origin, being an active principle derived from the common periwinkle plant; the dry powder is dissolved for giving by intravenous injection, and is used largely in Hodgkin's disease. Another active principle from the same plant is **Vincristine** ('Oncovin') which is also given by intravenous injection, mainly in leukaemias in children. Both these drugs are vesicant, and must be handled and given with due care.

**'Bleomycin'** is also of natural source, being an antibiotic; it has an antimitotic effect on malignant tumour cells and is used in the treatment of carcinomas, particularly of the head and neck, and testes. It is given weekly by intramuscular, intravenous or intra-arterial injection, and even into the tumour site itself if suitable; dosage is according to age of patient, except in the case of children, when a nomogram (p. 10) is employed. Bleomycin is non-toxic to the cells of the bone marrow, but side-effects include a dangerous type of pneumonia—hence patients have chest X-Rays taken weekly, this continuing for four weeks after completing the course.

**Doxorubicin** ('Adriamycin') is another antibiotic with antimitotic action, and is used in leukaemias, Hodgkin's disease, and solid tumours—especially of the breast and lungs. Dosage is decided by body surface area (per nomogram, p. 10), and the injection solution is introduced slowly into a fast-running intravenous infusion, e.g. normal saline—this may be once every three weeks (to reduce toxicity to the minimum) or daily for three days. In addition to nausea and vomiting, alopecia (p. 205) may occur during treatment; also, the urine may be coloured red, and patients are warned of this to avoid alarm.

**Daunorubicin,** also known as **Daunomycin** and **Rubidomycin** ('Cerubidin') is closely related to doxorubicin. It is likewise injected into the tubing of a fast-running intravenous infusion, but dosage may be by weight of patient as well as by surface area; alopecia may again be a side-effect.

**Procarbazine** is in capsule form ('Natulan'), and is often used with other cytotoxic drugs in "multiple" therapy (p. 208) in the treatment of Hodgkin's disease and also solid tumours. Commencing with low dosage and then increasing, the course is continued until at least 6 grams has been given; regular blood counts are again necessary to ensure the white cell count has not fallen too low.

**Actinomycin D** ('Cosmegen') is a further cytotoxic antibiotic, and is given by intravenous injection for the palliative treatment of certain malignant conditions, mainly in children; the course is usually short, e.g. one dose daily for five days.

## ANTIMETABOLITES

**Mercaptopurine** ('Puri-nethol') is mainly used in leukaemias in children and is given orally; its action depends on antagonising certain factors essential to cell metabolism.

**Amethopterin** ('Methotrexate') is given orally, and by intramuscular and intravenous injection, and is also frequently the drug chosen for slow intra-arterial perfusion as referred to earlier. The action of antimetabolites is well illustrated by the fact that 'Methotrexate' prevents the conversion of folic acid into folinic acid, the form in which folic acid is utilised in cell metabolism; thus deprived of this essential factor, the cancer cells are unable to function and multiply. A further interesting point is that if a folinic acid preparation ('Leucovorin') is given by injection within a few hours of the administration of 'Methotrexate', the general toxic effect of the antimetabolite on body tissue is reduced, apparently without unduly affecting its anti-tumour activity (tablets of

"Leucovorin", one six-hourly for four doses, may be used in place of the injection); use of this is made in acutely severe cases, and also if overdosage has occurred. Patients who are taking 'Methotrexate' orally may develop pronounced soreness of the mouth and throat; this warning sign is an aid to enabling corrective measures (i.e. stopping the drug and giving 'Leucovorin') to be taken in time before bone-marrow depression occurs.

**Colaspase,** also known as **Asparaginase** and **L-asparaginase** ('Crasnitin'), is an enzyme produced during the growth of certain bacteria. It acts by breaking down an amino compound which is essential to the growth of certain malignant cells, and is used in some types of leukaemia, being given by slow intravenous infusion.

**Cytarabine** ('Cytosar') is powerfully suppressant to the bone marrow and is used in the leukaemias. It is given by intravenous injection daily, commencing usually with a ten-day course and then increasing dosage until toxic effects preclude or satisfactory response is achieved.

**Fluoro-Uracil** is employed in the chemotherapy of carcinomas, e.g. of the breast and intestines; it is given either by intravenous injection or in high dilution as an intravenous infusion, but also by regional perfusion in suitable cases. In addition to the side-effects common to drugs in this section, including reduced white cell count, alopecia may also occur, but this resolves on treatment being discontinued. Fluoro-uracil is also used as a cream ('Efudix') in malignant skin conditions; satisfactory response is indicated by very marked inflammation, and this may take up to two months to heal after ceasing treatment.

**Thioguanine** ('Lanvis') is employed in the leukaemias, usually in "multiple" therapy; again its effect reduces the white cell count, and regular check is made. Thioguanine enhances the effect of several other drugs, e.g. the barbiturates and phenothiazines, hence if also being taken, dosage of these is reduced accordingly.

### Other drugs employed in Malignant Disease

Corticosteroids such as prednisone (p. 189) are also used in high dosage in the treatment of certain leukaemias and generalised cancers, the action, though not completely understood, being probably allied to the inhibiting effect this group of drugs has on tissue activity; they can also be said to enhance the effect of the other cytotoxic drugs used. The use of sex hormones is fully described on pages 197 and 200, the androgenic hormone testosterone and its derivatives in the treatment of mammary cancer, and the ovarian hormone equivalents, ethinyloestradiol and stilboestrol, in the treatment of both mammary cancer and prostatic cancer; the employment of tamoxifen for its inhibiting effect on oestrogenic *activity* in appropriate cases is also explained on page 198.

These drugs are not discussed in this respect in this chapter, because they do not fit neatly into the category of either antimitotic or antimetabolite action. There is, however, one exception, tetra-sodium fosfestrol, which, as will be noted on page 197, appears to have an antimitotic action within the cancer cell in addition to its possible oestrogenic effect.

It will be appreciated that should the white cell count drop significantly, as it may do during intensive treatment with certain cytotoxic drugs, the patient is denuded of his natural defence mechanism, hence, in such cases, nursing in strict isolation is employed in order to minimise any risk of severe infection.

### Multiple therapy

Just as the range of cytotoxic drugs is becoming wider, so too is the pattern of their use changing. Formerly, the agent chosen would be given as a course, with continuation treatment where appropriate; or a cycle of several drugs might be used, a course of each being given consecutively. The advantage to the treatment, and the comfort of the patient, of rest periods in between has also been exploited. More recently, combinations of three or more drugs used concurrently are being employed, but preserving the intermittent-course/rest-period regime.

These combinations vary in composition, and a method used to distinguish them is the use of a short code word made up of the first letters (or syllables) of the names ("trade" or "approved", whichever fits in the better) of the drugs making up the treatment. Thus, for example, the code word COP indicates that the combination comprises cyclophosphamide, "Oncovin" and prednisone; MOPP is made up of 'Mustine', 'Oncovin', procarbazine and prednisone; VAMP refers to vincristine, amethopterin, 'Mercaptopurine' and prednisone; and CON-FU indicates cyclophosphamide, 'Oncovin' (ON) and fluorouracil (FU). Such code words are termed *acronyms*, and their use makes reference to the component drugs concerned easier and less cumbersome. These combination courses are now so concentrated and well devised that patients may only need to be in hospital for as brief a period as a few days.

The potential value of multiple drug therapy in this field is evidenced by the truly significant progress being made in the treatment of acute lymphatic leukaemia in children.

### IMMUNO-THERAPY
Before proceeding to discuss further developments in treatment on

which this Chapter has a bearing, it will be helpful to make a basic point which, if clearly grasped, will enable a readier understanding of what follows. The point is that the vast numbers of cells which make up the organs and systems of a body, all conform, in health, to a particular pattern of behaviour which applies specifically *to that body;* i.e. each body has *its own special code of behaviour,* which all its cells normally observe.

Sometimes a cell may arise which behaves *abnormally,* i.e. deviates from the normal set code of cell behaviour, but in such an event, the body has an inbuilt surveillance (i.e. policing) system which enables it to detect this flaw in the pattern immediately, and the cell concerned is disowned and "shed", to be then destroyed and finally eliminated. This defence system therefore enables the correct pattern of behaviour of all the body cells to be maintained undisturbed; it is termed the **immune-response mechanism.**

Knowledge of this protective mechanism is now being utilised in therapy in two directions; in one the immune-response is stimulated —termed *immuno-stimulation,* and in the other it is suppressed— termed *immuno-suppression.* Both will now be outlined.

### Immuno-stimulation

Under certain conditions, possibly debility, the "running down" of the ageing process, or some other conducive circumstance, it may happen that the body's immune-response mechanism is not sufficiently powerful to cause rejection of the abnormally-behaving cell; this cell may then multiply and result in the formation of a new growth, or neoplasm, which may be benign (non-invasive) or malignant (invasive). In appropriate conditions of invasive type, e.g. certain leukaemias and some solid tumours, one form of treatment that may be employed is the *stimulation* of the immune-response mechanism with the aim of removing these abnormal cells. Such stimulation is done by a combination of *general* and *specific* methods.

Firstly, *general* stimulation. Here, use is made of the fact that vaccines (p. 163), in addition to their own particular immunising effects in the *blood serum,* also have a general "alerting" effect on the *cellular* immune-response mechanism referred to earlier; B.C.G. vaccine (p. 163) is especially active in this respect. Hence, in immuno-stimulation therapy, an injection of B.C.G. is first given in order to condition the body to make maximum use of the specific vaccine—which is then given immediately or soon after.

The *specific* vaccine is a further injection which contains a large number (several millions) of malignant cells *of the same kind as those in the condition being treated,* e.g. leukaemic cells in leukaemia. The cells themselves may have been obtained from the patient concerned (i.e. be autogenous—p. 164) or from another patient, and they will have been killed and made safe by irradiation. The aim of this specific vaccine is to stimulate an immune-response *specific to the actual malignant cells causing the condition*, and so lead to their rejection and destruction.

This form of therapy is employed only in certain designated centres, but, as of significant interest, merits reference in this Chapter.

**Immuno-suppression**

Appreciation of what has been said regarding the special code of behaviour to which the body cells normally conform will make it clear why the transplantation of an organ, e.g. a kidney, may not be successful. In short, the organ is "rejected" because the significantly different pattern of behaviour of its cells is immediately detected by the body, and the immune-response mechanism then ensures that no "take" is achieved; as an eminent medical authority has put it "the body detects self from non-self".

Now it so happens that cytotoxic drugs, in addition to their inhibiting effect on cell growth and survival, also suppress, in varying degrees, the immune-response mechanism of the body.

Particularly powerful in this respect are actinomycin-D, cyclophosphamide, mercaptopurine and methotrexate, and various combinations of these and other cytotoxics, together with azathioprine ("Imuran") and a corticosteroid such as prednisolone in very high dosage, are employed before, and following the transplant process; the immune-response is thereby suppressed, leading to greater probability of the organ being accepted. Azathioprine, a drug with cytotoxic action, has an extremely specific immuno-suppressive effect and is a standard drug in these procedures; the steroid, by its restrictive effect on tissue activity, is likewise an essential factor in preventing immune-response and rejection of the organ transplant. Cytotoxic/steroid therapy also has a suppressant effect on the patient's ability to resist infection, and in such cases special care is taken to maintain conditions in the unit as near sterile as possible, thereby reducing the risk of infection.

It is interesting to note that if azathioprine therapy is stopped for some reason (it is normally continued after the transplantation) it is possible for the organ concerned to be rejected, even after it has been accepted successfully for quite a long period.

An additional point is that whilst immuno-suppression by drug therapy is of great value in organ transplant surgery, the unfortunate possibility exists that should a cell of abnormal behaviour appear in another part of the body during the same period, the suppression of the immune-response may allow this cell to proliferate (i.e. multiply) and a malignant condition result. However, such happenings are rare, and are mentioned here merely to complete an understanding of the background to immuno-therapy.

# CHAPTER 20

# DRUGS USED BY LOCAL APPLICATION

## —the sites involved
## —the types and forms of drugs employed

This chapter resumes where Chapter 1 left off. In that chapter were described the major routes by which drugs are administered, together with the forms in which they are given; the effects concerned were mainly *systemic,* the drugs discussed being absorbed or introduced into the circulation. This chapter proceeds to deal with the several sites in the body to which drugs are applied *for local effect.* It outlines the forms and ways in which the drugs are used and gives a few prominent examples in each case.

### Drugs used—in the EYE

These are discussed at some length, for they are of particular importance, their proper use having been the subject of much interest in recent years. Drugs applied to the eyes are mainly in the form of drops (in Latin "guttae"); they cover a wide range of effect.

### Mydriatics

—dilate the pupil of the eye, and are employed in the treatment of inflammation of the iris and also to facilitate examination of the interior of the eye. The best known is **Atropine** (obtained from the belladonna plant, p. 14), which is commonly used as drops of 0·5% or 1%; a disadvantage is its prolonged action, hence blurring of vision and an inability to read and withstand strong light can be discomforting to the patient. **Homatropine,** a derivative of atropine, is both quicker and shorter acting and is thus preferred for use prior to examination; the usual strength employed is 2%. **Hyoscine** (p. 93) is another mydriatic of quicker and shorter action than atropine; drops are used at strengths of from 0·25% to 1%. Synthetic mydriatics are also available, e.g. **cyclopentolate** ('Mydrilate') which is used as drops of 0·5% and 1%.

## Miotics

—have the opposite effect to mydriatics and thus contract the pupil of the eye; this results in freer drainage of fluid from within, accompanied by a lowering of intra-ocular pressure, and this is a valuable effect in the treatment of the painful swelling and hardening of the eye-ball known as glaucoma, which is a primary cause of blindness throughout the world. Two examples, also obtained from plant sources, are **Eserine** (also known as physostigmine) and **Pilocarpine,** average strengths used being 0·5% and 2% respectively, though up to 8% is sometimes met in the case of pilocarpine. Eserine solutions tend to become pink during use; this should be watched for and a fresh supply obtained at first sign. A synthetic miotic is **Neostigmine** ('Prostigmin'), which is related chemically to eserine and is available as 3% drops. Miotics may also be used at the completion of eye examinations in order to reverse the disturbance of vision caused by the mydriatic (e.g. atropine) which has been employed.

**Ecothiopate** ('Phospholine') is a powerful miotic with very prolonged action, which ensures that the effect of the drops instilled at bedtime continues through the night; this is a marked advantage in certain cases of glaucoma.

## Antiseptic and anti-inflammatory preparations

Antiseptic drops are used in infections of the eye and include many antibiotics, e.g. chloramphenicol, framycetin and neomycin; in the case of resistant infections, the appropriate antibiotic is used, e.g. gentamicin in infections due to pseudomonas (p. 126). Antibiotics are sometimes given by subconjunctival injection, i.e. into the inner lining of the lower eyelid. The use of the sulphonamide, sulphacetamide, in eye infections is mentioned on page 130.

Idoxuridine (also known as I.D.U.) is a chemical compound which is active against the virus which causes *herpes* infections. Such an infection may occur in the cornea, the outer lining of the eye-ball, when the condition is known as keratitis, and in such cases idoxuridine is used as drops of 0·1% or as an eye ointment of 0·5%. The use of idoxuridine in shingles, the herpetic condition of the skin, is referred to on page 221.

Inflammation of the eye may be caused by infection or by a "foreign body", and preparations of various steroid drugs are used for their anti-inflammatory effect, examples being hydrocortisone, prednisolone ('Predsol') and betamethasone ('Betnesol'); reference has been made (p. 192) to the value of incorporating an antibiotic, e.g. neomycin in 'Predsol-N' and 'Betnesol-N', to ensure that spread of infection (if present) is prevented. Drops of castor oil are occasionally used for their soothing effect in conditions such as burns.

## Fluorescein

—is a dye which is used as 2% drops during eye examination in order to locate minute foreign bodies, these are then indicated by a surrounding green ring; corneal ulcers are also made distinguishable by being stained green. It is most essential that fluorescein solutions be sterile, due to their being mainly used in *damaged* eyes, and in order to avoid risk of infection via contaminated drops either "one-use" disposable units or impregnated paper strips can be employed in place; the latter are applied dry to the eye and the tears extract the stain from the paper, or the strip is premoistened in sterile water or saline.

## Anaesthetic drops

Anaesthesia of the eye is also a requirement during certain examinations and surgical procedures, and, as mentioned on pp. 123–4, cocaine and amethocaine are used as eye drops at the strengths indicated. Oxybuprocaine ('Benoxinate') is used as Minims (p. 215) of 0·4% in many procedures, e.g. the fitting of contact lenses, and has the advantage of not causing subsequent irritation as can occur with amethocaine. Lignocaine (p. 124) is employed as eye drops of 4% to aid removal of foreign bodies, etc.

## Adrenaline

—is used as eye drops at strengths of from 1 in 1 000 to 1 in 10 000 to reduce bleeding during surgery by its constricting effect on the vessels. The commercial preparation 'Eppy', a stable 1% solution of adrenaline, is employed to reduce intra-ocular pressure, or tension, by this same effect. 'Eppy' is frequently used with a miotic (e.g. pilocarpine) in the treatment of certain types of glaucoma. 'Simplene' drops are almost identical with 'Eppy', but are viscous (thickened) and thus more comfortable in use; they are packed in a convenient plastic dropper bottle.

## The administration of eye drops

Protection of the eye from infection is of extreme importance, and the following points should be closely studied.

Out-patients are usually issued with eye drops in the customary bottle with screw cap and dropper insert. They should be as recently prepared as is practicable, and be dated to enable this to be checked; the bottle should always be issued with contents sterile and cap sealed, again to ensure freedom from contamination. Eye drops in this form usually contain a preservative, which prevents the growth of any organism that may be introduced into the solution during use, but, even so, the out-patient should be advised to use a "clean" routine during the drop procedure and reclosure of bottle, etc.; likewise that cool conditions are best for storage, and that the eye drops should not be used for longer than one month after opening.

In the hospital ward, should similar eye-drop bottles with dropper insert be in use, the patient should have his own individual bottle (and separate ones for each eye if both are being treated), and this should be replaced with a fresh supply as frequently as possible, official direction being not less than once fortnightly, though once weekly is often customary and good routine. Stock bottles of eye drops with dropper insert should *not* be kept in the ward, for the use of the same dropper from patient to patient may result in contamination and cross-infection; this applies also to Out-Patient Clinics and Casualty Departments. Far preferable is a bottle with a plain cap (i.e. without dropper insert), together with dropper pipettes separately packed and pre-sterilised; a fresh dropper is then used for each patient (and each treatment) and subsequently collected for cleansing and re-sterilisation or discarded as a "disposable". Regular and frequent replacement of such stock bottles is likewise essential, the ideal being a fresh bottle for each Out-Patient Clinic. When drops are used in eye surgery, or where there is eye damage (as may be the case in the Casualty Department), a fresh unopened container is essential *for each separate occasion.*

The increasing accent laid on the danger of infection has led to the availability of a wide range of eye-drops in *single-use* presentation, and this is the ideal routine for all eye drops used in hospitals; 'Minims' are a prominent example; 'Opulets' are also in use.

### Irrigation Solutions

When irrigation of the eye is required, sterility of the solution used, e.g. normal saline, is equally essential, therefore, should a bottle be opened and partly used for one treatment, any remaining solution should be discarded; a sterile glass or stainless-steel undine is used for the irrigation procedure. Strips of plastic sachets (p. 173), each containing 25 ml of sterile normal saline ('Normasol'), are available and make for both safety and convenience.

### Eye ointments and lamellae

Two other forms of drugs used in eye treatment are the eye ointment (in Latin, oculentum) and the lamella; both are applied to the lower conjunctiva, the inner lining of the lower eyelid. Recognised eye drugs such as atropine and eserine are used in oculentum form in small tubes with elongated nozzles for ease of application; so also are corticosteroids and antibiotics, e.g. betamethasone ('Betnesol') and chloramphenicol ('Chloromycetin'). Several eye ointments, e.g. atropine and chloramphenicol, are available in the 'Opulet' range of small one-use gelatine capsules; these are cut with sterile scissors and the ointment squeezed out. Sterile glass or plastic eye-rods with smooth rounded ends are sometimes used to apply eye-ointments.

A lamella is a tiny thin disc of gelatine which contains an eye drug such as homatropine, and which is picked up with the moistened end of a small, clean camel-hair brush and applied to the lower conjunctiva; it then melts at the body temperature and releases the drug contained. Lamellae (plural) are now but rarely employed.

### Carbonic-anhydrase inhibitors

Although they are not drugs which are applied locally, it may be of interest here to note the use of acetazolamide ('Diamox') and dichlorphenamide ('Daranide') in the treatment of glaucoma; both are taken in tablet form and are absorbed into the circulation. The secretion of aqueous humour (fluid) in the outer chamber of the eye is influenced by the high level of bicarbonate usually present; acetazolamide (p. 30) and dichlorphenamide are carbonicanhydrase inhibitors, hence, as explained on page 95, they reduce the level of bicarbonate and therefore also the secretion of aqueous humor. The desired lowering of intra-ocular tension (or pressure) then results.

### —in the EAR

The drugs used in conditions of the outer ear are usually in the form of drops or ointments; powders for insufflation (puffing in) are just occasionally used. Steroids and antibiotics are employed when inflammation and infection are present, e.g. hydrocortisone with neomycin, but the laboratory report on a swab taken from the ear may indicate the need for a specific antiseptic, e.g. fungal infections will respond only to an appropriately chosen drug.

In conditions of wax accumulation, drops of warm glycerin, liquid paraffin or arachis oil are instilled for their softening effect, before syringing out with warm normal saline. Commercial preparations are also available for softening and "dissolving" wax, an example being 'Cerumol'.

### —in the NOSE

Drops or sprays are the forms mainly used. Ephedrine is employed as a 0·5% solution to treat the inflammation and "running nose" of rhinitis, as in hay-fever; the effect is to constrict, or "shrink", the nasal mucosa and so clear the airway, and also to block the further secretion of fluid. Commercial preparations are available as drops or convenient squeezer-pack sprays (nebulisers), and are based on phenylephrine (e.g. 'Fenox') and other compounds, e.g. xylometazoline ('Otrivine'), which have a similar decongestant action to ephedrine; some also contain an antihistamine for its anti-allergic effect, e.g. 'Otrivine-Antistin'. A disadvantage of many of these preparations is that whilst they provide quick relief, it is often followed in a few hours by a "rebound" swelling of the mucosa, which again makes breathing through the nose difficult; this can lead to an unhealthy condition of dependence.

The use of sodium cromoglycate in the prevention of allergic asthma (p. 86) has been extended to include the allergic, inflammatory condition of the nasal mucosa commonly known as hay-fever. The drug is again in cartridge form ('Rynacrom'), one of which is placed inside the insufflator supplied; the powdered drug contained is then puffed into each nostril in turn, following the directions provided, the nasal mucosa being thus protected against the inflammatory effect of the allergen concerned with the hay-fever, e.g. pollen. A solution is also available as nasal spray or drops.

Infection can be a factor in these nasal conditions, and some commercial decongestant sprays incorporate antibiotics (e.g. 'Soframycin'), and occasionally a steroid as well for its anti-inflammatory effect.

Nasal douches, or washes, are used to clear the naso-pharyngeal passage by "sniffing" the liquid from the cupped hand and expelling from the mouth. They are usually solutions of simple formula, e.g. sodium bicarbonate and borax, which liquefy tenacious mucus, with a little phenol for its antiseptic effect.

Menthol is used as an effective method of clearing the nasal and upper respiratory passages; a few crystals, or a teaspoonful of a solution in spirit (the B.N.F. Menthol Inhalation), are added to hot (not boiling) water, and the steam containing the menthol vapour inhaled.

A nasal condition which may be serious is the persistent presence of a staphylococcal infection (p. 126). This is detected by laboratory investigation of a swab, which is usually taken in cases of significant frequency of "staph." infections in a ward; the "carrier" can be a danger if present at operations or dressing procedures. The regular application to the nostrils of an ointment containing chlorhexidine and neomycin ('Naseptin') is used to clear the condition.

## —in the MOUTH

Mouthwashes are often used as routine in the hospital ward, and generally contain an antiseptic such as phenol or thymol; a time-honoured preparation of the latter is Compound Glycerine of Thymol ('Glyco-thymoline'), which is diluted with warm water for use. Hydrogen peroxide in "2½ volume" strength (p. 171) is also an excellent cleansing solution. The use of the antibiotics nystatin, amphotericin and natamycin in "thrush", and similar yeast-type infections which may accompany "broad-spectrum" antibiotic treatment, has been described on page 143–4.

In conditions of mouth ulcer, tablets containing an anti-inflammatory drug are used; the patient retains the tablet at the site whilst it dissolves. One preparation ('Corlan') employs the steroid hydrocortisone; another ('Bioral') contains carbenoxolone, which is referred to on page 15.

### —in the THROAT

Lozenges or pastilles are mainly used, and contain a variety of antiseptics and sometimes mild surface anaesthetics such as benzo-caine; they are slowly sucked for prolonged effect, and may be of some value in the common "sore throat". Menthol in pastille form is used to clear the air passages and in "loss of voice". Gargles, e.g. of Compound Glycerine of Thymol, are also used in "sore throat", and aspirin in the form of a thick mucilage is sipped for its analgesic effect following tonsillectomy (removal of tonsils). A preparation of iodine still occasionally prescribed is the compound paint, also known as Mandl's paint; this has a thick glycerine base, and is applied to the throat with a long brush in tonsillitis and other septic conditions of the pharynx.

### —in the RESPIRATORY TRACT

The use of menthol by inhalation in clearing the respiratory passages has been referred to (p. 217). Eucalyptus oil may also be combined in this inhalation (as the B.N.F. Inhalation of Menthol and Eucalyptus), which is added to steaming water in the customary china Nelson Inhaler. Compound Tincture of Benzoin is used in the same manner as a soothing agent in bronchitis and laryngitis.

The mucolytic drugs used by inhalation or instillation to liquefy sticky bronchial mucus are described on page 84.

Appropriate antibiotics, e.g. neomycin, are used by inhalation as a fine mist for local effect in the lungs when these are involved in the condition of cystic fibrosis (p. 18), and anti-fungal antibiotics, e.g. amphotericin and natamycin, are used similarly in yeast and fungal infections.

### —in the ANUS and RECTUM

A common cause of anal and rectal irritation and pain is the condition of haemorrhoids or "piles", and the preparations used in suppository and ointment form contain drugs with astringent, or shrinking, action, e.g. hamamelis (witchhazel), tannic acid, and compounds of bismuth and zinc, together with local surface anaesthetics such as benzocaine, lignocaine and cinchocaine (p. 124); a steroid is also included in certain preparations to enhance the anti-inflammatory action. Examples of commercial preparations are 'Anusol' and 'Proctosedyl'. A solution of phenol 5% in almond oil is occasionally used by direct injection into the haemorrhoid, the effect being to harden and shrink the swollen vein concerned so that it becomes occluded, i.e. sealed off; this is termed a *sclerosant* effect. Counter-irritants and antipruritics (p. 223) are used to relieve the itching in pruritus ani.

*Sclerosants* are also used by injection in the treatment of varicose veins (commonly in the **leg**); examples are ethanolamine oleate and sodium tetradecyl sulphate ('S.T.D.'), the latter being supplemented by maintaining firm pressure for a period of several weeks, employing crêpe bandages over pads of rubber.

## —in the URETHRA and BLADDER

Antiseptic solutions are used for irrigation in infections involving the bladder; this is referred to on page 146.

Lubricant jellies containing the local anaesthetic lignocaine ('Xylocaine') are often inserted into the urethra beforehand in order to relieve the pain which may be associated with the introduction of a catheter or cystoscope (particularly); a sterile introducing nozzle is attached to the tube of jelly before use, and it is a common and safe, aseptic routine for a fresh tube to be used on each occasion.

## —in the VAGINA

Infections and irritation comprise the main indications for local treatment of this organ. In yeast-type infections, due to the candida (or monilia) organism (p. 127), the antibiotics nystatin, natamycin and amphotericin (pp. 143–4) are used as pessaries or ointment; pessaries are similar to suppositories, but are larger in size, and melt within the vagina after insertion, so releasing the drug contained.

A chemical compound which has wide use in candida infections of the vagina is miconazole ('Gyno-daktarin', 'Monistat') which is supplied as a cream with applicator, and as pessaries.

In trichomonas infections (p. 146), certain compounds of arsenic (acetarsol, 'S.V.C.') or mercury (hydrargaphen, 'Penotrane') have specific effect and are used as vaginal tablets or pessaries. Creams are also used; some are packed in collapsible tubes together with disposable applicators for ease of deep placement. The oral use of metronidazole in this condition is referred to on page 146.

Trichomonas and candida infections of the vagina are also treated with clotrimazole ('Canesten'), the tablets being used by insertion;

the cream is employed if inflammation is present (vaginitis) and also applied appropriately if a sexual partner is involved, this to avoid cross-infection and persistence of the condition.

A common condition affecting the vagina is pruritus vulvae, which is associated with inflammation and causes intense irritation; this often occurs during the menopause and later in life, possibly as a result of progressive deficiency of oestrogen production (p. 196). Thus, oestrogenic compounds, e.g. dienoestrol and oestrone, are used as pessaries or creams for local effect, together with oestrogen therapy by mouth (p. 196), the aim being to improve the tone of the vaginal tissue concerned and render it less prone to infection, which is often the cause of irritation. The other approach to vulval irritation is the use of antipruritic preparations (p. 223).

## —on the SKIN

Drugs are used in several forms for application to the skin. Ointments, which are semi-solid preparations, are the most common. Pastes are thicker and more solid forms of ointment, and thus remain at the site of application longer. Creams are softer and thus more soothing; they are often non-fatty, hence many commercial preparations are available in both ointment and cream form for the prescriber to choose from. The use of tulle-gras dressings continues to increase in various forms. Thus, the plain type (the old "vaseline gauze") is still a routine application in many conditions, and those incorporating antibiotics are firmly established in treatment.

Liquid applications are also used. Lotions may contain an insoluble ingredient, e.g. calamine, and, in any case, should always be shaken; liniments are normally intended to be massaged into the part affected; and paints are usually applied with a brush and allowed to dry on the skin. Antibiotic and steroid, etc., preparations are now much used together in pressurized container form (aerosols); this greatly increases the ease of application, but caution is necessary in the disposal of empty containers, as referred to on page 145.

Dusting powders may contain starch, zinc oxide and talc, and are used in the hospital ward for their soothing and toning effect on backs, etc.; certain "puffer" preparations (e.g. 'Cicatrin') contain a spreading powder plus antibiotics for application to the affected part.

### Steroid and antiseptic preparations

Anti-inflammatory and anti-infective agents again play a major part in the treatment of skin conditions. A wide range of steroid preparations is available (p. 190), often incorporating antibiotics such as neomycin and antiseptic compounds such as clioquinol

('Vioform'), the overall effect being one of reduction of inflammation and treatment or prevention of infection. Concerning the application of such steroid preparations, as creams, etc., it is worth repeating that a thin layer only should be used, for reasons of both cost and risk of excessive absorption (p. 190).

Following the introduction of the antibiotics and corticosteroids, the use of the drug ingredients formerly contained in ointments and lotions, etc., is diminishing; examples of those still employed are coal-tar and salicylic acid, which have antiseptic effect, and zinc oxide and calamine (also a zinc compound), which are astringent in action.

## Drugs used for specific effect

Certain drugs continue to be used for their effect in specific conditions, e.g. dithranol, which is a standard ingredient of ointments employed in the treatment of psoriasis.

Chlorphenesin ('Mycil') and tolnaflate ('Tinaderm') are further examples; they are used as ointments, creams and powders in fungal infections of the skin, and, in particular, "athlete's foot". The B.N.F. Compound Ointment of Benzoic Acid, which also contains salicylic acid, is still prescribed for fungal infections; it has long been known as Whitfield's ointment. Miconazole (p. 219), too, is employed as a cream ('Dermonistat', 'Daktarin') in fungal conditions of the nail and skin.

Cases of severe burns may be treated with 'Flamazine', a cream containing a compound of silver and sulphadiazine (p. 128); it is used in hospitals only and gives specific protection against the organisms likely to complicate such conditions; it also promotes the healing process.

The painful condition of shingles (herpes zoster) is treated effectively with idoxuridine (I.D.U., p. 213). The commercial preparation 'Herpid' contains 5% I.D.U. in a special penetrating solvent which enables the drug to reach the deeper layer of tissue where the virus is active. The solution is applied for four days, and a side-effect possible is the experiencing of an unusual taste.

## Preparations with protective and soothing effect

Ointments and creams of mild action are much used for their soothing effect on the skin, a popular example being zinc and castor oil ointment. Creams containing dimethicone (silicone) are an aid in preventing the breakdown of skin and tissue, e.g. in cases of colostomy and ileostomy, where leakage of intestinal fluid may have a damaging effect around the opening. Dimethicone acts by preventing fluid settling on the skin, and so protects the area concerned, hence its further use on the buttocks of babies to prevent napkin rash, and on long-term incontinent patients. The customary use of surgical spirit to protect "pressure areas" is referred to on page 241.

## Poultices

—are still occasionally employed for application to septic wounds, the one chiefly used being kaolin poultice. This is warmed to a comfortable heat, spread on lint and covered with a layer of gauze, and then applied to the affected part. Kaolin poultice contains thymol for its antiseptic value, glycerin to draw fluid from the wound, and kaolin for its absorbent effect.

## Anti-parasite preparations

Head lice are effectively treated with commercial preparations containing benzene hexachloride ('Lorexane', 'Derbac Soap'), carbaryl ('Suleo', 'Derbac Shampoo'), or malathion ('Prioderm', 'Derbac Liquid'). Benzyl Benzoate Application B.N.F. is a standard treatment for scabies.

## Warts

Preparations containing a high percentage of salicylic acid are used to remove warts, either in ointment form or as a solution in collodion for applying as a paint; collodion being a thick clear liquid which dries rapidly to leave a protective film over the area concerned (the solvents in collodion are inflammable—n.b.). Podophyllin is a powdered resin obtained from a plant source and is effective in the treatment of warts, particularly in the ano-genital area; it is used in the form of an ointment or, mixed with liquid paraffin, as a paint, and removes the wart by its destructive effect on tissue growth.

Other applications employed are silver nitrate, in the form of the "caustic pencil" which is moistened before using, and strong acids such as trichloracetic acid, which are applied neat on a cotton wool applicator after smearing a little vaseline around to confine the corrosive action to the wart. Warts which resist such treatment may involve attendance at a clinic, where they may be removed surgically; or one of three methods may be employed, each involving the use of a gas. Carbon dioxide is normally a gas, but when compressed in a special unit it becomes a solid "snow"; this is applied to the wart and acts as an effective caustic. Likewise, the gases oxygen and nitrogen each become liquid when compressed, and when applied on a cotton wool applicator remove the warts by similar caustic action.

## Counter-irritants, Antipruritics and Rubefacients

—are terms which refer to certain preparations applied to the skin, generally for their sedative effect in the relief of irritation or pain.

Counter-irritants are used in conditions of extreme irritation, as in pruritus vulvae (p. 220) and pruritus ani (p. 219). They may produce an initial stinging effect, or a sensation of warming or cooling, but this is then followed by a period of relief from the original irritation; examples are menthol, which may be incorporated in creams or lotions, and preparations containing crotamiton (e.g. 'Eurax').

As already mentioned, counter-irritants may be used to treat pruritus and are thus themselves antipruritic. Other drugs also have antipruritic effect, but may act in a different way. Thus, oestrogens are used by application in pruritus vulvae, and their probable mode of action is described on page 220. The antihistamines (p. 101) are applied externally (though with caution, p. 102) as creams and lotions, and are also given orally for their general sedative effect. Corticosteroid preparations are applied for their anti-inflammatory effect (p. 190) and local anaesthetics (e.g. lignocaine) may be incorporated in creams and lotions when the irritation is pronounced, as in haemorrhoids and pruritus vulvae and ani.

"Rubefacient" means "reddening", and rubefacients do this to the skin by causing the blood vessels to dilate locally, hence improving the blood supply; in addition, they induce a feeling of warmth and stimulation, and often relieve pain. Examples are menthol, camphor (as the time-honoured camphorated oil, which is used as a chest rub in bronchitis), certain derivatives of nicotinic acid (through their local vasodilating action (p. 58), and the local analgesic, methyl salicylate (p. 116).

## The use of Zinc in wound healing

The metal zinc is present as a trace element in the body tissues, and it has been found that the administration of its compound, zinc sulphate, may reduce the time taken for wounds to heal by almost half. Thus, capsules of 220 mg are taken three times daily for this purpose, and also to accelerate the so-often slow healing of varicose ulcers, etc.

# CHAPTER 21

# DRUGS USED IN DIAGNOSIS
## —general—urine examination—radiological

## GENERAL

In addition to their use in the treatment of disease, the actions of certain drugs and other substances are utilised in diagnosis. This frequently occurs in the hospital ward, and it will be of both interest and value for the student nurse to have an acquaintance with the technique employed and the interpretation of the results.

**A.C.T.H.** is used to test the function of the cortex of the adrenal glands. A.C.T.H. (either the natural or synthetic substance) is given by intramuscular injection, and this is normally followed by stimulation of the output of the steroid hormones from the adrenal cortex (see page 178). This output can be measured by estimation of the plasma cortisol (hydrocortisone). If the hormones are absent, this indicates lack of response to A.C.T.H. due to complete inactivity of the adrenal cortex, as in Addison's disease.

**Alcohol** stimulates gastric secretion, and may still be used in testing for the presence of acid in the gastric juice. It is given as 100 ml of a 7% solution, and samples of the stomach contents are taken at intervals; assessment of high acid levels (hyperchlorhydria), if present, may assist in the diagnosis of gastric or duodenal ulcer. However, pentagastrin (p. 226) is now generally the gastric stimulant of choice.

**Ascorbic Acid** is vitamin C (p. 79). It is used as a test when deficiency of the vitamin is suspected. A large dose is given, and the urine produced about 6 hours later is examined for ascorbic acid content. This is repeated daily until a certain definite level of ascorbic acid is obtained in the urine. This will take merely a day or two if the patient has been receiving adequate amounts of vitamin C in his diet. In extreme deficiency, however, it may take up to one or two weeks of daily tests before the body is "saturated" sufficiently to excrete the required level in the urine.

**Carmine** may be used as a "spotting" device in the investigation of faeces. It is a dye in powder form (colour as name) which passes through the gastro-intestinal tract unchanged, and if given in a capsule with any particular food, the faeces which correspond to that food are easily recognised by the colour. This test has also been used to confirm suspected leakage of fluid from the intestine, e.g. through a fistula.

**Edrophonium** ('Tensilon') is used in the diagnosis of myasthenia gravis (p. 108), a condition in which there is pronounced muscle weakness. It is given by intravenous injection and its potent anticholinesterase action (see also p. 107) releases acetylcholine activity, which, in turn, strengthens muscle tone. If the muscle response is powerful and very quick (within 5 minutes), this indicates the probability of a positive diagnosis (i.e. that the disease is present).

**Glucose** is used in the glucose tolerance test. A blood glucose estimation is performed after fasting, and the patient is then given 50 grams of glucose dissolved in water. Further blood glucose estimations are done at several half-hourly intervals. If the patient is producing normal levels of insulin, the blood glucose level will rise after absorption of the glucose and will then fall steadily back to normal. If, however, the blood glucose rises to an unusually high level, and remains at this level for some time before tailing-off very gradually, then this will indicate that the patient has diabetes mellitus and has not been producing sufficient insulin to deal with the intake of the glucose.

In this test, glucose estimations are also performed on the urine as additional evidence; firstly on a fasting specimen (when none of the sugar should be found), then on specimens taken 1 hour and 2 hours after the glucose has been taken. If the second and third specimens contain glucose, this is an indication that the patient may be diabetic. However, this is not to be absolutely relied upon, for the patient may not be a diabetic but merely happen to pass the sugar into the urine more readily than is normal.

**Gonadorelin** ('H.R.F.', 'Relefact LH—RH') is a synthetic compound equivalent to the hypothalamus factor (p. 176) which stimulates the release of F.S.H. and L.H. (p. 179) by the anterior pituitary; it is administered by injection to test pituitary function, a sample of blood being taken before and after, and the levels of F.S.H. and L.H. measured in each case. If there is little or no increase, this indicates *lack* of pituitary function, which may then be diagnosed as the cause in a number of conditions in either sex, e.g. poor development of the sex glands, in both male and female; amenorrhoea and anorexia nervosa (persistent lack of appetite) in the female; and cryptorchidism (undescended testicles) and Frohlich's syndrome (a feminising condition) in the male.

**Histamine** increases the secretions of the stomach glands, and may be used when a sample of gastric juice is required for testing in the diagnosis of certain conditions. 1 ml of the injection is usually given subcutaneously, and successive samples of gastric fluid are then withdrawn through a stomach tube for laboratory investigation. Absence of hydrochloric acid (normally present in gastric juice) is known as achlorhydria and is significant of pernicious anaemia or gastric cancer.

Occasionally, larger amounts of histamine may be given, even up to 3 or 4 ml, and at such high dosage the unpleasant side-effects associated with histamine (p. 102) are likely, and an injection of one of the antihistamines is given beforehand as a preventive measure. An interesting point is that the action of the antihistamine is confined to the unpleasant side-effects of the histamine injection, and does not interfere with the required secretion of gastric juice.

**Insulin** indirectly stimulates the passage of impulses along the vagus nerve which increase the secretion of acid in the stomach. Thus it is used to confirm whether the operation for resection of this nerve has been successfully performed (this is sometimes the surgical treatment for duodenal ulcer). Insulin is given intravenously to the fasted patient, and the gastric fluid removed at intervals and examined for acid content; if the operation has been successful, there will be no increase in acid secretion. A validity check of the test itself is also made by taking a sample of blood during the procedure and measuring the glucose content; due to the effect of the insulin, this will be expected to have reached a low level.

**Pentagastrin** ('Peptavlon') is a synthetic equivalent to the natural body substance which stimulates gastric secretion. It is given by subcutaneous injection in order to induce an increased secretion when this is needed for examination, and thus may be used in place of histamine for this purpose (see earlier). The advantage of pentagastrin is the absence of side-effects, especially in patients who have allergic conditions such as asthma, which may be precipitated by histamine; as indicated earlier, it is increasingly the gastric stimulant of choice.

**Phenolsulphonphthalein** (Phenol Red) is a dye which is used to test kidney function. It is given by intravenous injection, and the urine (which is coloured red) is collected twice at hourly intervals afterwards and tested for the percentage of the dye it contains. If the kidneys are functioning normally, at least 50% of the amount injected should be contained in the first collection, and be made up to 75% in the second, otherwise some impairment is indicated.

**Phentolamine** ('Rogitine') is used in the diagnosis of phaeochromocytoma, a condition of tumour in the medulla of the suprarenal (adrenal) gland. It is given by intravenous or intramuscular injection, and if the blood pressure falls decidedly this is an indication that such a tumour is present. The test is explained by the fact that phentolamine is anti-adrenergic in action (p. 56), i.e. it blocks the effect of adrenaline and noradrenaline. These hormones are produced by the medulla of the suprarenal gland, and if a tumour is present excessive secretion will have been stimulated, and the blood pressure will be abnormally high in consequence. Success of phentolamine in blocking the action of these two hormones is indicated by a dramatic fall in blood pressure; this is a pointer to a positive diagnosis.

**Saccharin** (gluside) is used to test the circulation time in patients with heart disease. It is given by injection (2.5 grams in 4 ml) into the appropriate vein in the arm, and a stop-watch is used to record the time it takes to reach the mouth, the patient signifying as soon as the sweet taste of the saccharin is apparent. An average time in health is between 10 and 15 seconds, but much longer is taken in the slower blood circulation of failing heart.

**Sulphobromophthalein** ('Bromsulphalein') is a dye used for testing liver function. It is given intravenously into an arm following a fat-free breakfast, and, after 5 minutes, a sample of blood is taken from the other arm; this is done to confirm that an adequate level of the dye has been reached in the blood. After a further 40 minutes, a 10 ml sample of blood is taken and the amount of dye in the serum estimated. Sulphobromophthalein is normally taken up by the liver and excreted via the bile, hence if serum levels are found to be above a specified percentage, this will indicate that the dye has not been taken up to the normal extent and that impaired liver function is probable.

**Thyrotrophic Hormone** (thyrotrophin, 'Thytropar') p. 178—is used to distinguish between a basic inability of the thyroid gland itself to secrete thyroxine (as in myxoedema—p. 179) and a non-production of thyroxine due to lack of the thyrotrophic hormone (which is normally secreted by the anterior pituitary in order to stimulate activity of the thyroid). Thyrotrophic hormone is given by injection, together with a dose of radioiodine (a special form of iodine which may be traced, or "tracked", during its stay in the body), and the take-up of the iodine by the thyroid is later measured by a "scanning" device. If the thyroid *is* active, it will have collected the iodine (which it utilises to manufacture thyroxine) and the condition will appear to be one of lack of thyrotrophin production by the anterior pituitary; if, however, the iodine is *not* taken up, this will indicate that the thyroid has ceased to function adequately and there is therefore a probability of myxoedema.

**TRH** (or 'TRH-ROCHE') is a synthetic equivalent to the thyro-trophin-releasing factor produced by the hypothalamus (p. 176); when administered orally, as tablets, or by intravenous injection, it normally stimulates an increase in the secretion of thyrotrophin (TSH) by the anterior pituitary, and this, in turn, stimulates the thyroid to produce extra thyroxine (p. 179). Thus, whilst thyrotrophin is the agent normally employed in the investigation of thyroid disease (see prev. para.), the use of TRH gives a finer degree of assessment, should this be required, and in addition provides a check regarding the degree of activity of the anterior pituitary and the hypothalamus. Blood samples for examination are taken at appropriate intervals after administration.

**Tolbutamide** ('Rastinon') is used for the diagnosis of moderate diabetes mellitus, i.e. where the islets (see page 181) may be partially active but would appear to be producing insufficient insulin. The patient's blood glucose is taken in the morning, fasting, and one gram of tolbutamide is given intravenously; the blood glucose levels are further estimated at intervals afterwards. There is a rapid and pronounced fall in blood glucose level if the insulin-producing islets are functioning normally. A slow fall will indicate that part of the islet tissue is inactive and the patient is not secreting sufficient insulin. The explanation of this test is that the action of tolbutamide is to stimulate the functioning beta cells of the islets to produce more insulin; thus, if the islet tissue is functioning normally, there will be a rapid fall in blood glucose levels due to greatly increased insulin output, whereas if only *part* of the tissue is active the extra insulin produced will be appreciably less and the fall in blood glucose levels will be equivalently slower in consequence.

**Vasopressin** ('Pitressin'), the anti-diuretic hormone secreted by the posterior pituitary (p. 177), is used for its effect not only in the treatment of diabetes insipidus (p. 37) but also in the diagnosis of the disease. In this condition there is a high output of urine, and if an injection of vasopressin is followed by a marked decrease in urinary flow, this is an indication that the patient is not producing sufficient, if any, vasopressin himself and is thus confirmed as likely to be suffering from diabetes insipidus.

**Xylose** is a sugar which, unlike other sugars (e.g. dextrose), is not metabolised (i.e. broken down) in the body; hence it is excreted unchanged in the urine. It is used to test certain conditions of malabsorption, in which carbohydrates and fats are not being ingested from the intestine. Five grams, dissolved in a glass of water, are given to the patient (fasted and with an empty bladder), and all the urine produced during the first two hours is collected, and also that produced during the next three hours, each lot being examined for xylose content. Absence, or a low result, will indicate an impairment of the absorption mechanism in the intestine. An interesting point is that the first sample (hours 0–2) provides an indication of the degree of function of the *upper* part of the small intestine, and the second sample (hours 2–5) that of the *lower* part; this may provide a useful lead to the location of the disease.

In the case of children under 30 kg, the test may be done on blood, a single specimen being taken one hour after the xylose is given.

## REAGENTS USED IN THE EXAMINATION OF URINE

The testing of urine has, in the past, involved the use by the nursing staff of a variety of reagents, e.g. Fehling's solution, Benedict's solution and sodium nitroprusside, etc. In the case of many of these reagents the success of the examination may be dependent on a degree of care in the technique of measuring, heating and timing, etc.; this can be frequently a problem under busy ward conditions. These former reagents have now been largely superseded by commercial tablets and "strips", which are dropped or dipped, respectively, into the urine (or in some cases a drop of urine is placed on the tablet); the resultant colour change is compared with the chart supplied and may indicate a positive reaction, i.e. confirmation of the presence of what is being looked for, e.g. glucose in diabetes mellitus. The examples given are from a much used range.

The following notes will help the student nurse to appreciate the background to each investigation. The directions regarding use are omitted, for these are clearly explained with each container.

'**Clinitest**' tablets are the most commonly employed of these commercial reagents. Diabetics use them daily, for they indicate not only the presence of sugar in the urine, but also the approximate amount, and this is a most helpful aid to the necessary adjustment of their carbohydrate intake (p. 186). If sugar is newly found in the urine, this may indicate the possibility of diabetes mellitus and will invite further investigation to confirm (see also 'Acetest'). An interesting point is that other substances can give a positive reaction to 'Clinitest', e.g. salicylates in the urine following the taking of aspirin, and confirmation that it is *glucose* (p. 181) that is present can be obtained with the aid of 'Clinistix' (see following), which reacts only to this particular sugar.

'**Clinistix**' strips indicate the presence of glucose (and also provide a rough guide to the amount, if this is small). They are specific for this sugar and are thus more sensitive than 'Clinitest' tablets, and more reliable in detecting small amounts of glucose in the urine. A point to note is that if the patient is being given ascorbic acid (vitamin C), the presence of this in the urine may interfere with the 'Clinistix' colour change.

'**Diastix**' strips provide a test for the presence of glucose in the urine which is so sensitive that they may give a positive result, i.e. that glucose is present, when tests with 'Clinitest' have been negative; they also give an approximation of the *amount* present.

Diastix are particularly intended for the type of diabetic whose condition is controllable by diet alone or, at most, by oral hypoglycaemic drugs (p. 185) or low dosage of insulin, the sensitivity of the test giving timely warning of significant presence of urine glucose.

'Acetest' tablets are used to detect the presence of acetone and other ketone bodies, which result from the metabolism (i.e. breakdown) of fat. This occurs in people who are starved of food, and also in diabetics, who, although they may have adequate glucose in the blood, cannot utilise it (due to insufficiency of insulin). In both cases the body falls back on breaking down fat for energy. If glucose is newly found in the urine as well as ketones, this is a strong pointer towards the condition being one of diabetes mellitus.

'Ketostix' strips provide a rapid test for the presence of ketones (see under "Acetest").

'Keto-Diastix' strips cover urine glucose as do Diastix, but also supply similar sensitive information regarding presence of ketones.

'Albustix' strips detect the presence of protein. If a trace is found, further investigation in the laboratory will be indicated, for this can be a pointer to several serious conditions, including cardiac failure, anaemia, nephritis (inflammation of the kidneys), and urinary infections.

'Hemastix' strips detect the presence of blood in the urine, and also give a rough guide to the concentration. This may be due to several causes, including damage to the kidneys following crystalluria during treatment with systemic sulphonamides (p. 128). As with 'Clinistix' (see earlier), the presence of ascorbic acid in the urine may interfere with the 'Hemastix' colour change.

'Ictotest' tablets provide a colour test for the presence of bilirubin, a pigment (i.e. colouring matter) contained in bile. A positive reaction denotes the possibility of liver disease or an obstruction of the biliary duct.

'Urobilistix' strips are used to test for the presence of another bile pigment, urobilinogen. A strongly positive result is indicative of liver disease or haemolytic disease, but in bile-duct obstruction the colour change is not significant.

'Urobilistix' are frequently used in combination with 'Ictotest'. In liver disease, results with both reagents are strongly positive; in bileflow obstruction, 'Ictotest' give a positive result and 'Urobilistix' an almost negative one; and in haemolytic disease, 'Ictotest' give a negative result and 'Urobilistix' a strongly positive one. If these facts are matched up with the results obtained on testing the urine with both reagents, this is often a useful guide to the diagnosis of which one of the three conditions mentioned is probably present.

'**Phenistix**' strips are used to test for the presence of phenylpyruvic acid; this substance is excreted in the urine of children suffering from phenylketonuria, a rare condition in which there is a failure to metabolise the amino-acid, phenylalanine, and there is consequent brain damage and mental deficiency. If P.A.S. or another salicylate (e.g. aspirin) has been taken beforehand, this may also give a positive reaction with 'Phenistix', hence it is usual to examine the *blood level* of phenylalanine for confirmation that the condition is one of phenylketonuria.

The following "compound strips" provide a means of performing several tests in one operation; a colour change occurs on the appropriate part of the strip for each substance detected.

'**Uristix**' detect the presence of protein and glucose.
'**Hema-Combistix**' detect the presence of protein, blood and glucose.
'**Labstix**' detect the presence of protein, blood, glucose and ketones.
'**Bili-Labstix**' provide the same information as 'Labstix', plus the detection of bilirubin.
'**Multistix**' provide the same cover as 'Bili-Labstix', but with the additional detection of urobilinogen, thus completing the provision of information regarding pancreatic, kidney and liver function.
*N.B.* 'Hema-Combistix', 'Labstix', 'Bili-Labstix' and 'Multistix' also give an indication of the "pH" of the urine, by which is meant its level of alkalinity or acidity. A pH of 7 is neutral. Lower numbers are progressively acid, and higher numbers are increasingly alkaline. The use of litmus (see later) merely decides whether the urine is acid or alkaline, whereas 'Hema-Combistix', 'Labstix', 'Bili-Labstix' and 'Multistix' also show *how* acid or alkaline it is, it being possible to recognise pH levels of 5, 5·5, 6, 6·5, and so on up to 9.

The prefix '**N-**' in the case of further reagents, e.g. '**N-Multistix**', indicates that the presence of nitrites in the urine may also be read; the value of this coverage is explained under 'Microstix' below.

'**Microstix**' strips are distinct in this section because they not only supply information about the presence of *nitrites* in the urine, but, in addition, indicate if a urinary tract infection (if Gram-*negative*) is actually present or has been successfully treated. The nitrite substances will have been formed by the action of such bacteria on the *nitrate* substances commonly present in urine, and this is an immediate indication that infection is, or has recently been present; the urine should be the early morning specimen, or have been in the bladder for at least 4–6 hours, for the organisms concerned will have then had time to convert sufficient nitrates to *nitrites* to give a significant reading. The test for actual presence of bacteria then takes from 12 to 18 hours before results can be assessed; the strip is placed in a transparent pouch (provided) and this is incubated at body temperature for at least 12 hours, when coloured areas (usually pink) indicate presence of bacterial colonies. Microstix is also useful in confirming that treatment of urinary infections *has been successful,* the test being made at least 48 hours after ceasing therapy; presence of bacteria then indicates that treatment has not been complete.

### Litmus

Litmus is a dye which is in frequent use in the examination of urine; it indicates by a colour change whether it is acid or alkaline. It is commonly used in the form of books of paper strips ("litmus papers") which are either blue or red. The blue paper will turn red if dipped into urine which is acid; conversely, the red paper will turn blue if the urine is alkaline. Urine is normally slightly acid, and any change in this respect is sometimes a guide in diagnosis; thus, in some infections, e.g. those caused by the proteus organism, it becomes alkaline. Similarly, it is useful to be able to confirm, for example, that the urine of a patient taking Potassium Citrate Mixture (p. 29) has become alkaline (as it should), or that the desired acidity has been achieved if ammonium chloride (p. 30) has been given for this purpose.

## CONTRAST MEDIA
### —Drugs used in Radiography (X-Ray examination)

These preparations differ widely in form, in the method and route of administration, and in the organ or part of the body concerned in the examination; they are based on either **Barium** or **Iodine,** and all are X-Ray opaque, i.e. X-Rays do not pass through them. They are administered to the patient so as to fill the organ or part to be examined at the appropriate time, and the X-Ray film is positioned behind the patient at the site concerned and then exposed to X-Rays, which are directed through the body from the other side. The contrast medium blocks the passage of the X-Rays, and the shape of the organ or vessel concerned is thus clearly outlined on the film. Or the Radiologist may himself watch the passage of the contrast medium by a technique known as screening, as in the case of a barium meal given for examination of the oesophagus or stomach. The X-Ray report, together with the film, is a valuable diagnostic aid.

In the case of some of the contrast media, appropriate preparation of the patient is required beforehand, and this is mentioned where it is of significance and may concern the ward nurse.

## Barium Contrast Media

—are used in the X-Ray examination of the alimentary tract, i.e. the oesophagus, stomach, and small and large intestines. The compound used is barium sulphate, a heavy white powder which is insoluble and not absorbed, and is thus safe in use. It is administered as a suspension, either by mouth (the "barium meal") for examination of the oesophagus, stomach or small intestine, or per rectum (the "barium enema") if the colon is concerned. A thick paste may be used if the lower pharynx and oesophagus are to be filmed, because of its slower movement along these organs. 'Baritop 100' is a suspension of barium sulphate which contains also carbon dioxide, this is liberated in the gastro-intestinal tract and the effect provides an improved picture with better definition.

For preparation, the patient does not eat or drink anything for at least six hours before the examination if the stomach or small intestine is to be filmed, for it is essential that they be empty. In examination of the colon, further measures have to be taken to completely empty the channel of faecal, liquid and air residue. A typical routine is to give two tablets of bisacodyl (p. 22) by mouth, together with a suppository of bisacodyl per rectum the night before the examination, followed by a further suppository in the morning; or 'X-Prep' (p. 21) may be used for its similar highly effective action.

## Iodine-containing Contrast Media

These are compounds of complex chemical composition, and are used in the examination of many remotely different sites in the body. The iodine they contain is held in close combination and is not released as the free substance during their stay in the body, hence their safety in use in this respect. Nevertheless, a small test dose is sometimes given well beforehand to ensure that the patient is not allergic, i.e. sensitive to the preparation.

In order to clarify the use of the contrast media in this group it will be helpful to separate them according to the X-Ray process in which they are used; it will be noted that some are employed in several of these processes.

**Urography** is the radiography of the urinary system, and **Pyelography** refers specifically to that of the kidneys. Examples of contrast drugs used are—

Sodium Diatrizoate         —'Hypaque', 'Urografin'
Iothalamate compounds—'Conray'
Metrizoate        „        —'Triosil'

These are issued in ampoules (e.g. 20 ml) and given by intravenous injection. They are quickly excreted via the kidneys, and several pictures are taken at short intervals following the injection.

For preparation, the patient is kept free of fluid for at least six hours before the examination; the object is to reduce the urinary output to the minimum and so concentrate the contrast drug and obtain a clearer picture.

The above routine is termed "intravenous" or "excretion" pyelography. "Retrograde" pyelography is also used, whereby the same drugs are introduced towards the kidneys from the opposite direction, i.e. through ureteric catheters inserted into the ureters via the urethra and bladder.

The retrograde routine may also be used to X-Ray the bladder; this is termed **Cystography,** and involves the use of a comparatively large volume of the contrast medium, e.g. 250 ml, which is run in through a catheter.

The retrograde route is naturally further indicated for examination of the male urethra, this is termed an urethrograph; 40 ml of the medium, 'Umbradil Viscous', is introduced with a syringe via the penile orifice, and its thick consistency effectively ensures the required coating of the urethral wall.

The number which follows the name in the case of many contrast media indicates the concentration of iodine contained in terms of mg per ml, e.g. 'Conray 420', 'Urografin 310'.

**Cholangiography** is the radiography of the bile ducts, and **Cholecystography** that of the gall bladder; **Cholecystangiography** covers both systems. Contrast media used are—

Iopanoic Acid          —'Telepaque'    —oral—tablets
Sodium Ipodate         —'Biloptin'     —  „ —capsules
Calcium   „             —'Solu-Biloptin'—  „ —powder
Meglumine Ioglycamate—'Biligram'      —i.v injection &
                                           infusion

The oral preparations are given well beforehand, i.e. up to 15 hours prior to the examination, this allows for absorption and full concentration in the gall bladder. Food rich in fat, such as a glass of milk or about 30 ml. of the fat emulsion 'Prosparol', is given during the examination, and this causes the gall bladder to contract and expel its contents (including the contrast medium) into the bile ducts, which are then more clearly pictured.

For preparation, the patient is sometimes purged (e.g. with mag. sulph.—see page 20) the morning of the day before the examination, and fats are withheld from the light meals allowed. Note the subsequent giving of fat during the examination, for the reason mentioned.

The intravenous route is employed when the use of oral contrast media is unsatisfactory, as in impaired function of the gall bladder, or when this has been removed and the ducts need to be radiographed. The injection is given shortly before the examination, and quickly reaches the liver via the circulation and thence proceeds to the bile ducts and gall bladder (if present). The giving of a laxative is the only preparation required for this examination.

**Bronchography** is the radiography of the bronchial tree. Contrast media used are—

    Iodised oil    —'Lipiodol Viscous'
    Propyliodone—'Dionosil'        —in either oily or aqueous
                                              (watery) base.

Introduction into the bronchi (one or both) is effected through a catheter fed through the mouth or nose and downward via the trachea. A spray, or a few drips, of a local anaesthetic are first used to enable the patient to tolerate the examination and to prevent coughing. Alternatively, the contrast medium can be injected directly into the trachea with a syringe, using a large needle which has been inserted through the crico-thyroid membrane following infiltration with a local anaesthetic. Propyliodone may be preferred as there is less tendency to clog the alveoli (air sacs); it is also more quickly absorbed and eliminated.

For preparation, the patient does not eat for several hours before or after the examination. A sedative (e.g. a barbiturate) is sometimes given beforehand, and also an injection of atropine to prevent secretion of bronchial mucus.

**Myelography** is the radiography of the spinal canal.
    The contrast media used are—

    Iophendylate        —'Myodil'
    Meglumine Iocarmate—'Dimer X'
    Metrizamide        —'Amipaque'

Iophendylate is given by means of a lumbar puncture; being an oil, it does not mix with the cerebrospinal fluid (C.S.F.). It is injected into the lower part of the spinal canal, and because the oil is heavier than the C.S.F. the patient is tilted so that it flows slowly towards the site, when the picture is then taken; an interruption of flow of the medium indicates the level of obstruction. For preparation, patients are sometimes fasted for a few hours.

Meglumine iocarmate differs from iophendylate in being non-oily, and therefore miscible with water and, in turn, the cerebrospinal fluid. Again a tilting table is employed following the injection, and it is required that the patient be taken back to the ward either on a chair or by helped walking; for the next eight hours he should sit upright, and for a further six hours lie on a sloping bed if needing to rest, but not horizontal. Meglumine iocarmate is also used for examination of the cavities of the brain, following which the patient should, again, be nursed with the head and upper parts of the body suitably raised and kept so for twelve hours. A further use is in examination of the knee joint, and here, before and after its introduction, an injection of air is given so as to improve the contrast effect.

Metrizamide is an aqueous solution again employed in conjunction with tilting of the patient; likewise, the patient remains in bed for 24 hours afterwards with the head of the bed elevated for the first 6 hours. Features of metrizamide are that it must be freshly prepared for use, i.e. just prior to injection, and that drugs of the phenothiazine type, e.g. chlorpromazine, are contra-indicated both before and after the examination due to possibility of untoward reaction.

**Angiography** is the radiography of the vessels of the circulation. If the heart and immediate arteries are concerned, it is called **Angio-cardiography;** if the aorta alone is to be filmed, **Aortography;** if the arteries generally, **Arteriography;** and if the veins, **Phlebography.**

In these examinations, the intravenous contrast media used are the diatrizoate, iothalamate and metrizoate compounds already described under urography. Some of the procedures involve only an injection directly into the artery or vein concerned, the patient being conscious. Other examinations (e.g. of the heart or aorta) are more intricate and may entail general anaesthesia and the introduction of long catheters, even into the chambers of the heart itself.

**Hysterosalpingography** is the combined radiography of the uterus (by itself called **Hysterography)** and the fallopian tubes (**Salpingography**). The contrast medium employed is sodium acetrizoate ('Diaginol Viscous'); as the name indicates, this is a thick solution, about 10 ml of which is slowly injected via the cervix with sufficient pressure to fill the uterus and fallopian tubes.

# CHAPTER 22

# "WATER" AND "SPIRIT"
## —the various forms explained

## WATER

—is a combination of two atoms of hydrogen and one of oxygen ($H_2O$), and is often thought of as merely either tap water or distilled water; the need for it to be sterile for certain procedures is also generally known. However, a fuller knowledge of the several types of water used, and the reservations attached to each, will be of interest and practical value to the student nurse.

### Tap Water

—is broadly of two kinds, hard or soft, depending on the source from which it is collected. Hard water contains a variable amount of calcium, and often also magnesium and iron, in the form of soluble compounds. When it is boiled, the dissolved compounds become insoluble and deposit (the calcium as chalk), resulting in the common "scaling" or "furring" of the containers; also, soap does not lather readily in hard water, and a scum or deposit is formed. In contrast, soft water contains but a minute amount of the compounds mentioned, hence the smooth feel and ease with which soap lathers, and the absence of deposit after boiling.

Tap water is normally used in the ward for general drinking purposes and for diluting medicines if ordered to be taken "in water"; it may also be employed in the preparation of dilutions of antiseptics and disinfectants, unless there is a risk of deterioration due to formation of sediment, e.g. in the case of the antiseptic chlorhexidine, which deposits when mixed with hard water.

### Distilled Water

—is prepared by boiling tap water in a "still", and leading the steam through a cooling tube where it condenses to form distilled water. The calcium and other compounds which may be present do not "come off" with the steam, and thus the distilled water collected is pure $H_2O$.

Another method of obtaining water free from dissolved substances is by deionisation (sometimes termed demineralisation). Tap water is passed through a unit containing commercially prepared resins which absorb, and so remove, the calcium, magnesium, iron, bicarbonate, chloride and sulphate, etc., constituents present in the water (these are called "ions"), and the end product is thus pure $H_2O$, or **"deionised water"**. The resins in these units have a limited life of effectiveness, and when exhausted it is necessary for them to be replaced by a fresh re-charged batch obtained from the supplier on an exchange basis.

In hard-water districts, a supply of distilled or deionised water is particularly valuable if instruments or surgical equipment have to be sterilised by boiling (as may be the case in hospitals where newer methods of sterilisation have not been installed), for the deposit from hard water can be extremely detrimental to such items.

### "Sterile Water not for Injection"

Sterile water is widely used in hospital theatres and maternity units, and also in the wards, e.g. in such procedures as rinsing sterile instruments, irrigation of body cavities, and douching, etc. Water that has been boiled and cooled has some merit, but can rarely, if ever, be termed sterile, because of the exposure and contamination which occur during the cooling process; likewise boiling itself cannot be fully relied upon as a sterilising process. Some hospital theatres have employed urn units, in which water is boiled and drawn from via a tap, the air that replaces the water (as it is drawn) usually having to pass through a special filter and being thus freed from bacteria. This method is an improvement in that the water is protected whilst cooling, but the tap outlet is still constantly open to risk of contamination from the air, and the sterility of the water when drawn cannot be guaranteed. Hence, hospitals are now generally organised to provide a service of "Sterile Water Not For Injection" in sealed 1 litre bottles; this has been sterilised by a special high-temperature process. The bottles are etched clearly with the wording **"Non-injectable Water"**, in order to avoid any risk of use in error for intravenous injection. Distilled or deionised water is preferably employed, except in districts where the water supply is extremely soft and deposit on the bottles during sterilisation therefore insignificant. An additional necessity in this bottled-water service is a warming cabinet, in which the water is kept at a convenient temperature ready for use.

### "Water for Injections"

So far, the presence of bacteria and other organisms in water has not been referred to. Tap water contains a varying "count" of living organisms, which is duly kept under observation and control by the Water Authority, and this is of little or no concern in the uses to which tap water is normally put. Thus, the common organisms normally met in drinking water are generally of little significance, except occasionally during travel abroad, when troublesome organisms are not infrequently encountered. Likewise, the bacteria, etc., contained in the water used to prepare "Sterile Water Not For Injection" are killed during the sterilising process and present no risk, even though possibly present in some number. In contrast, however, it is of the utmost importance that **"Water for Injections"**, i.e. water used for preparing injections, contains the very minimum trace possible of dead micro-organisms and associated waste matter. Thus, the student nurse should be fully aware of what is meant by water "fit for injection".

Firstly, it will be helpful to know that bacteria multiply by division, i.e. one divides into two, the two become four, and the four become eight, and so on; and that if this division process occurs every hour, one such organism can increase to over sixteen millions in 24 hours! It can be added that many bacteria split up at a faster rate than once every hour, providing the temperature and the medium they are growing in are suitable.

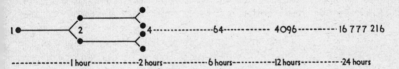

Fig. 9. Illustrating how one organism may increase to over 16 millions in 24 hours by hourly division.

Now "Water for Injections" must be distilled, sterile and *apyrogenic*. Apyrogenic means *non*-pyrogenic, or free from "pyrogens", which are substances that, if present in injections, may cause pyrexia (rise in temperature). The pyrogens concerned with here are dead organisms, e.g. bacteria, together with the waste products which have been excreted by them, and it will be appreciated from the description (and diagram) of the speed with which bacteria multiply how *essential* it is that water used for injection must be freshly distilled *and sterilised as soon as possible afterwards* (remember that one bacterium entering freshly distilled water can become over sixteen millions in 24 hours). Hence, all injection solutions received ready for use in the ward or department, whether made up commercially or in the hospital Pharmacy, have been prepared with freshly distilled water, followed by *immediate* sterilisation in the sealed container, thus ensuring maximum freedom from possibility of pyrogen source. This applies whether in glass ampoules, rubber-capped bottles of the various sizes, or the large "infusion" containers of $\frac{1}{2}$ litre or 1 litre. Likewise the ampoules of "Water for Injections" so frequently used by the nurse for preparing injections herself are of the same unvarying high quality.

The presence of pyrogens in intravenous infusions (which are so often given in large volumes) is particularly dangerous and has been the cause of several fatalities. Hence the advice on page 46 merits repeating—that, before use, each bottle (or plastic bag) *must* be examined against strong light for the slightest sign of cloudiness, which may indicate contamination after sterilisation, via a crack or flaw in the container or an imperfect seal, and subsequent over-growth of organisms which have entered. It is worth repeating also that *all* injections should be used, or put into use, *as soon as possible* after the container has been opened, for the longer it is kept after breaking the seal the greater is the possibility of bacterial contamination from the air and consequent risk of infection or pyrexia.

Sterile water for injection may still be occasionally encountered in rubber-capped bottles of 25, 50 or 100 ml, from which the amount required on each occasion (e.g. to dissolve penicillin for injection) is withdrawn by inserting the needle through the bung. Such "multi-dose" bottles of water (and also of ready prepared injections) usually contain a preservative, e.g. chlorocresol (this is always stated on the label), and this prevents the development and growth of any organism which may obtain access via the needle. Even so, it is unwise to keep multi-dose bottles of water or ready prepared injections over-long, once use has commenced.

If a bottle of "Water for Injections" gives no indication on the label that a preservative has been included, then it should be discarded immediately after its first use, even though this may appear wasteful. Likewise, when using a fresh bottle it should be examined to ensure that the seal has not been previously opened.

## SPIRIT

As in the case of water, there are several types of spirit in use in the Hospital Theatre, Wards and Departments.

### Alcohol

—is another word for spirit. It usually refers to ethyl alcohol, the form of alcohol or spirit which is used in the manufacture of ingredients of liquid medicines (e.g. tinctures), and is also contained in "alcoholic" beverages. Ethyl alcohol is occasionally used in the ward in the form of brandy for its resuscitating value, and also as a 7% alcohol "test meal", which is referred to on page 224. It is also included (as "ethanol", another term for alcohol) in intravenous solutions of protein and sugar, and provides a source of extra calories in this type of post-operative nutrition (see page 46).

## Methylated Spirit

Methyl alcohol is closely related to ethyl alcohol but, in contrast, is highly toxic even in small quantities. When it is added to ethyl alcohol the latter is said to be "methylated", hence methylated spirit is *ethyl* alcohol which has been methylated by the addition of 5% of *methyl* alcohol. Methylated spirit (also known as industrial spirit) is a clear colourless liquid which is employed to make preparations for external use, e.g. solutions of iodine and dilutions of chlorhexidine and other antiseptics, and is valued in the hospital theatre, wards and departments for its cleaning properties wherever oil, fat or grease is involved. It has some antiseptic value, and this is highest at a 70% dilution with water (see page 172), hence the popular use of "70% spirit" as a swab or pressurised spray for cleansing the skin pre-operatively and before giving an injection, and also for spraying or wiping trolley tops prior to dressing procedures; chlorhexidine is often incorporated to increase the antiseptic value. Methylated spirit is also used for burning in the spirit lamps occasionally used during urine examination; it should be pure and undiluted for this purpose.

## Methylated Spirit—as obtainable in retail trade

—is "mineralised" methylated spirit, and consists of industrial methylated spirit to which have been added ingredients which make it highly distasteful to drink, non-miscible with water, and distinguishable by its violet-pink colour. It is intended for use by the public for burning in lamps and various cleansing purposes.

## Surgical Spirit

—is sometimes assumed to be industrial methylated spirit, but this is not so. Surgical spirit is industrial methylated spirit to which have been added castor oil, methyl salicylate, and a bitter tasting ingredient; it is used for regular massaging of backs, buttocks and heels, i.e. the "pressure areas", in order to keep the skin in firm condition and prevent it breaking down when patients are long-stay in bed. The castor oil helps to keep the skin supple, and the methyl salicylate provides analgesic effect (see page 116).

# CHAPTER 23

# WARD MEDICINE ROUTINE

*—requisitioning—storage—administration—*
*patient counselling*

A full understanding of the procedures involved in the ordering, storage and administration of drugs is essential to the proper completion of a nurse's training; firstly because of the important position drugs occupy in the treatment of patients, and secondly because of the dangers associated with wrong handling of them.

## Requisitioning

In most hospitals the custom is (or has been) for ward requirements to be obtained each week-day morning from the Pharmacy (Dispensary), using the appropriate receptacle for transport. This will hold the various empty containers (medicine, lotion and tablet bottles, etc.), together with prescription charts where appropriate, plus the requisition book in which each item will have been written and duly signed for, thus keeping the necessary record. A separate requisition book for Scheduled Poisons (as distinct from Controlled Drugs) may be the custom, and this is an excellent routine, as making queries easier to settle. When the receptacle is returned to the ward it should be checked against the requisition book(s) immediately, so that the Pharmacy staff can be contacted in good time if there is any discrepancy.

It is sensible policy to look ahead and provide for the needs of the day or weekend by requisitioning in good time, but it is bad practice to empty any remaining tablets, etc., into a spoon or measure to enable the sending of an empty container to the Pharmacy; any such balance must be sent in its labelled container, thus avoiding the possibility of mixing stocks when putting back from the spoon or measure on return. Night doses have sometimes been seen in the past put out in separate spoons ready for the check before administration, and this again is to be deplored as allowing possibility of wrong medication. The dose should always be checked *from the container at the time of giving.*

## Storage

It has been said that all nurses are "magpies", from their apparently ingrained tendency to hoard their drugs! The intention is understandable, i.e. to ensure that everything possible that may be required is on hand, but this can be carried to excess, and a commonsense approach is far preferable—and indeed essential; freshness of stock is an important consideration, and unnecessary hoarding of expensive and/or "dated" drugs can be a significant drain on the hospital's economy. Thus, drugs not officially kept as stock items should be returned to the Pharmacy when discontinued, and a further aspect of good stock-keeping is the using up of a "started" bottle before commencing a new one. The need for neatness and cleanliness covers such simple points as always pouring *away from* the label side and wiping the neck and shoulders of bottles after use; also the replacing of lids, caps and stoppers on containers. Due notice should be taken of the requirement to store certain items in the refrigerator, e.g. penicillin solutions and insulin.

An important precaution against wrong use is that drugs for *internal* use should be kept in separate cupboards from those intended for *external* use, i.e. lotions, etc. The latter are normally dispensed in bottles distinguishable by colour, e.g. brown, green or blue, and also by touch, i.e. they have ribbed sides, which is an additional warning to the person handling. Bottles of white glass are sometimes used to contain substances for external use, e.g. methylated spirit, but these are usually ribbed and appropriately labelled. However, a new factor may now have to be taken into consideration, it is that amber-coloured bottles are gaining some favour for containing oral liquid medicines; this is because they protect any maybe sensitive drugs from the effect of light. The need for vigilance in handling *all* containers of drugs is further stressed in view of this possible trend in policy.

Labels should always be read carefully, and particular note taken of such wording as "Not to be taken" or "For external use only"; the need for care in handling bottles labelled "Inflammable", e.g. those containing cleaning ether (p. 122), is especially stressed.

In the next Chapter, when discussing the Regulations concerning Poisons, particular emphasis will be laid on the need to keep these drugs in locked cupboards, but it should be clearly understood that *all* medicines, whether for internal or external use, should be kept under safe lock and key, even if they do not contain a Poison and are thus not controlled by the legal requirements.

The reason for this is, of course, that there must be no possibility of unauthorised handling, for misuse of *any* drug is fraught with danger.

It may not always be practicable (though best if possible) to keep in locked cupboards those lotions and antiseptics, and methylated spirit, etc., which are in frequent use, but, even so, a place constantly under supervision is essential for their storage.

## Administration

With the exception of certain simple items, e.g. a dose of peppermint water for flatulence, the ideal and safe routine is that all drugs should be administered only on a doctor's prescription, and the prescription sheet referred to *before and after the administration of each dose*. In the past, a popular custom has been for a member of the nursing staff to re-write on the "medicine list" all the drugs to be administered during the medicine round; this practice carries with it the risk of error during transcribing, and is now forbidden.

Many of the drugs administered may be from containers dispensed individually for the patients concerned, and labelled with the directions; this is the theoretical ideal. However, it is rarely practicable to have all the items dispensed in this way, due to the numbers involved or because several patients are on the same drug regularly; in such cases administration has to be from ward-stock containers, and it will be left to the nursing staff to interpret the prescription. The writing may not always be clear (although block lettering is increasingly favoured in Medical Schools), and it cannot be emphasised too strongly that if there is any doubt on the part of the nurse administering or checking as to the drug intended, or the amount or frequency of dosage, confirmation should be obtained from the prescriber or a member of the Pharmacy staff.

As to checking, it is advisable that at all times possible a second person should be present on the medicine round to confirm that both drug and dose coincide with the prescription; at least one of the two persons should be as senior as the ward staff situation allows. It is also an obviously cardinal rule that the correct patient is given the medicine, and that he is seen to have taken the dose.

When measuring liquid doses, the measure should be held at eye level. If a clear liquid, there will appear to be two "levels", due to the fact that the surface "curls" upwards where it meets the glass around the measure, thus making it saucer-shaped; this is called the meniscus, and when measuring, the correct level of the liquid is "the bottom of the meniscus", i.e. the lower of the two levels. Finally, a good nurse is always observant of the effect of the drug on the patient, for this can be not only instructive to her but often helpful to the doctor, e.g. in the case of a patient on digitalis therapy who feels a sense of nausea—which can be a warning of impending symptoms of overdosage and consequent need for counter-measures.

## The Medicine Trolley
—is a fairly modern innovation. Until its introduction, the ward medicine round entailed laying out an ordinary trolley with all the drugs needed, after searching for them in the stock cupboards, then returning them to their places in the cupboards after completing the round; this being repeated several times daily. The idea of a mobile drug arrangement was conceived by Miss Joan Hobbs, then Matron of Warwick Hospital, who, with the author, devised the original medicine trolley; this, together with modified versions, is now established as a conventional unit in the hospital ward. These trolleys hold all the drugs, including Scheduled Poisons (but not Controlled Drugs), needed for the current patients on a ward, *but nothing else;* when a drug is not further needed on the ward (e.g. due to discontinuation), the bottle is returned to the stock cupboard, or to the Pharmacy if it has been individually dispensed for the patient. Such restriction *to drugs in use only* is itself a helpful factor in avoiding error in administration. An important point is that when not in use all the compartments are kept locked, and in addition the trolley itself is kept padlocked to a fixture in the ward. The medicine trolley is a real advance in reducing the time and labour involved in the administration of medicines.

The routine outlined for the ordering, storage and administration of drugs in the ward has been the one basically employed for many years in the majority of hospitals, but efforts have been concentrated in recent years on improving, in particular, accuracy in administration. Investigation in several hospital centres had revealed the startling fact that as many as 15% of errors in administration could occur on a single ward medicine round; these involved such factors as loose writing of the prescription by the doctor, wrong interpretation of the prescription by the nurse administering, mistaken reading of the label on a container, omitting to administer, interruption during the medicine round, shortage of staff, and lack of check, etc. Delay of as long as an hour or more in administering a dose (although less serious) was also taken into account in estimating the percentage of error. Thus, several new systems have been devised which alter the basic routine already described in one way or another. The system in use in the Aberdeen Group of Hospitals (the "Aberdeen System") employs a separate administration sheet, on which the giving and checking of each dose of each drug is recorded. The London Hospital system is another which provides for the recording of each dose administered, and may be preferable in one important respect—prescribing and recording are on the one sheet. Other hospital centres have produced systems, all with the same aim, i.e. the reduction of errors in drug administration to the absolute minimum possible. This is the position that obtains at the time of writing, and it is possible, and would seem logical, that a *standard* prescribing and administration record system may eventually apply to the hospitals within the National Health Service, incorporating all the best features of the excellent systems already in use, with the added advantage that nursing staff moving from one hospital to another would then not have to re-adapt themselves to new routines.

Another relevant trend which is becoming established is the regular attendance on the ward of a member of the Pharmacy staff; this service has become an important feature of hospital routine, though it may vary in its scope, depending on such factors as the size and type of institution concerned. Thus, the Ward Pharmacist (official title) may visit the wards once or twice daily at regular times and scan the prescription sheets, checking for clarity and accuracy of dosage and directions, etc., and, if needed, conveying advice or explanation to the nursing staff—and medical staff on occasion. He may also take copies of the prescriptions, and prepare the labels relevant to them, so that they can be dispensed in the Pharmacy without the drug sheets having to leave the ward. In the latter connection, also, systems are in use whereby the drug sheet can be placed on a relaying unit in the ward, to be seen at once on a screen in the Pharmacy and dispensed accordingly from it.

The supply picture, from Pharmacy to ward, is also changing in many hospitals; pre-packed drugs are, in most cases, replacing the usual re-filling of tablet containers, etc., and routine topping-up of intravenous solutions and disinfectants, etc., is being instituted in place of the normal requisitioning, and may even spread to certain drug stocks.

Whilst these new ideas (and others surely still to come) are signs of real progress from the point of view of both avoidance of error and the smooth running of ward medicine routine, accuracy in drug administration must always depend in the final event on the personal vigilance of the nurses themselves, and utmost care in reading prescription and label will always remain the absolute essential.

### Abbreviations used in prescribing

The layout of the new types of drug prescription/administration sheets mentioned earlier implies the use of *figures* for indicating the number and timing of doses to be taken daily; this replaces the former custom of prescribing directions in abbreviated Latin. However, the use of the latter may still occasionally persist, and a familiarity with those which were commonly employed is still useful to the hospital nurse in case she may be required to administer drugs from ward stock containers according to her interpretation of such forms of direction on the patient's drug sheet.

The following list includes the abbreviations most likely to be met:—

| | | | |
|---|---|---|---|
| o.d. | —every day | a.c. | —before food |
| b.d. | | p.c. | —after food |
| or b.i.d. | } —twice a day | | |
| or b.d.s. | | p.r.n. | —when required |
| t.d. | | s.o.s. | —if necessary |
| or t.i.d. | } —three times a day | | |
| or t.d.s. | | o.m. | —every morning |
| q.d. | | o.n. | —every night |
| or q.i.d. | } —four times a day | | |
| or q.d.s. | | h.s. | —at bedtime |
| q.h. | } —every four hours | stat. | —immediately |
| or q.q.h. | | | |

Some confusion has occasionally arisen as to the interpretation of the difference between "p.r.n." and "s.o.s.". A useful distinction made in some hospitals is that "p.r.n." should mean that a dose may be repeated "when required", e.g. in the case of a simple cough linctus; whereas if "s.o.s." the dose should be given only the one time, i.e. "if necessary", subsequent doses being re-prescribed each time if intended to be given "s.o.s.".

## PATIENT COUNSELLING

Patients returning home following a stay in the ward are commonly given medicines "to take out", and a little explaining as to how or when they are best taken, or applied, or stored, etc., can often be helpful, and even essential. The Ward Sister or her deputy, or perhaps the Ward Pharmacist, will usually see to it that the patient is fully conversant with any special points, but the personal interest of the Nurse-in-Training is also of value in this connection, though always observing the deference due to the senior staff and the need to have advice given checked as correct. Examples of points to ensure are—

(1) that the patient (or relative) clearly understands the directions on the label.

(2) that any *special* directions are emphasised, e.g.—
—to "shake the bottle",
—to "keep in a cool place", e.g. eye drops,
—"to be dissolved under the tongue", e.g. certain tablets.

(3) that the medicines *are* taken and at the proper time(s). Haphazard taking of medicines, or, worse still, omitting to take, is an increasingly recognised problem in domiciliary drug medication, and discussion with the patient on how to ensure that each item is duly and properly taken is a valuable exercise. Thus, even if only one tablet is to be taken daily (e.g. digoxin), a safe and easily ensured routine is for 7 tablets to be transferred to an empty vial each Sunday, to be drawn from daily, commencing Monday. Other suitable systems can be worked out if needing to cope with the several items often prescribed, e.g. each day's quota can be laid out on a strip of paper ready marked by the nurse with drug names and times—the latter, again, always with the confirmation of Sister or her deputy.

(4) that certain medicines directed to be taken once daily are best taken in the morning, and *not* at night, e.g. frusemide taken at night can lead to disturbed sleep due to diuresis calls.

(5) that the expected effect of certain drugs is fully appreciated, e.g. the increased output of urine in the case of a diuretic.

(6) that the patient is conversant with significant side-effects associated with a drug, and, if possible, how they may be lessened or prevented—as in the case of hypotensive treatment (p. 56).

(7) that *all* medicines (and particularly if potent or attractive, e.g. iron preparations) are kept locked up or in a safe place away from the reach of children.

(8) that medicines left over are best disposed of via the toilet. Incidentally, if capsules (often potent), these should be first slid apart and the contents emptied out, because capsules contain some air and may float for some time.

(9) that there is special need for aseptic care in handling and administering certain items, e.g. injections of insulin, and eye drops.

(10) that the patient knows how to cope with any special packaging, e.g. strip-packs and the child-resistant containers now becoming popular.

With regard to Out-Patient Clinics, the doctor and the Pharmacy staff normally emphasise special instructions where indicated, but, even so, a supporting word from the Sister or Nurse in attendance can do much to ensure that treatment is given every chance to achieve success.

Likewise, the points made are equally important in the case

of the District Nurse who may have the responsibility of the regular supervision of the patient at home, for so often such patients are needing all the help they can get, as well as being on heavy and perhaps potent medication.

# CHAPTER 24

# POISONS REGULATIONS
## —as they apply to the Hospital Ward

The laws which govern the manufacturing, sale and handling of medicinal substances are many and complex, but fortunately those parts of the Regulations which deal with the use of medicines within the hospital sphere are clear and straightforward.

Two classes of poisons are concerned, the "Scheduled Poisons", and those further governed by the Controlled Drugs section of the Misuse of Drugs Act, 1973.

### Scheduled Poisons

These are drugs contained in certain Lists or Schedules attached to the Poisons Rules and drawn up by the authorities; they comprise a very large number, and common examples are the barbiturate hypnotics, tranquillizer drugs such as chlorpromazine, the analgesic pentazocine, the sulphonamides, and atropine and hyoscine, etc. It would be impossible for the nurse to know every one of the drugs and preparations which are "Scheduled", and it is the onus of the Pharmacy staff to label each container concerned with a clear indication that it is a Scheduled Poison.

The following regulations apply—

1. Scheduled Poisons can be obtained from the Pharmacy only on a requisition duly signed by a Doctor, or, as is more usual, the Sister or Nurse in charge of the ward. Thus, if a stock bottle of phenobarbitone tablets needs refilling, it will be sent to the Pharmacy with the appropriate entry duly signed for in the normal requisition book; better still, as mentioned earlier (p. 242), if a separate requisition book is kept for Scheduled Poisons. Although not legally necessary, many hospitals require the recording, on a special sheet, of the administration of each dose of certain selected Scheduled drugs which are particularly liable to abuse, e.g. the hypnotics and tranquillizers, and before the stock bottle is filled or replaced the Pharmacy staff will need to satisfy themselves that the previous issue has been properly accounted for in detail.

If a patient is prescribed a Scheduled drug which is not kept as stock in the ward, the Pharmacy staff will supply on the prescription itself, and usually record the issue thereon, but, even so, it is wise to order in the requisition book as well, in order to ensure a record of the supply.

2. Scheduled Poisons should be taken to the Ward or Department by a responsible person, either an official messenger or a nurse, and in some hospitals a receipt form is returned duly signed. It is now an official directive that if drugs liable to abuse (e.g. the barbiturates and other hypnotics, and tranquillizers and anti-depressants such as chlordiazepoxide and amitriptylene) are included in the ward's requirements from the Pharmacy, a locked container must be used as the means of transport. As these drugs are frequently in use in most wards, this will doubtless have become a *routine* method of conveyance.

3. Scheduled Poisons must be kept in the appropriate cupboard assigned to them, and the key should be kept on the person of the Sister or Nurse in charge.

4. Scheduled Poisons may only be administered on a written order duly signed by the Doctor, although, in emergency, a dose may be given on verbal instructions, with the proviso that it is written up as soon as possible and within 24 hours.

5. Each dose of a Scheduled Poison must be checked at the time of giving, with due scrutiny of label, dose and prescription sheet, *and* identification of patient.

### Controlled Drugs

The former Dangerous Drugs Act, which covered the established drugs of addiction, e.g. morphine, heroin, pethidine, cocaine, etc., has been entirely replaced by a section of the Misuse of Drugs Act, 1973. This section still deals specifically with the major addictive drugs, i.e. all the former "D.D.A." drugs, *but with the addition of others now decided as also needing the same stringent control,* prominent examples being the amphetamines, dihydrocodeine (in *injection* form only), and methaqualone (e.g. in 'Mandrax'). All these are now designated as **Controlled Drugs,** and this title now replaces the term "Dangerous Drugs"; likewise, the abbreviation **"CD"** replaces the former "D.D.A.", or "D.D.", which is now obsolete.

As in the case of Scheduled Poisons, containers holding Controlled Drugs must be clearly labelled so by the Pharmacy staff.

The procedures governing the ordering, storage and administration of Controlled Drugs (CD) in hospitals remain essentially the same as applied formerly to the "D.D.A.'s"; they are as follows:—

1. CD drugs can be obtained from the Pharmacy only on a

written, fully-signed order from the Sister or Acting Sister in charge of the ward, and the Requisition book is a special one used only for this purpose. The order is written in duplicate, and one copy remains in the Pharmacy for record purposes and is retained for two years.

2. It is customary for CD drugs to be taken to the ward by a responsible person such as a State Registered Nurse or other nurse of experience and standing, or by a member of the Pharmacy or messenger staff duly authorised by the Pharmacist. Acceptance for delivery is signed for, as is also the final receipt at the ward end.

3. CD drugs must be kept under lock and key in the special cupboard allotted to them (which must contain nothing else, not even "Scheduled Poisons"), and it is usual for *this* locked cupboard to be sited within a further locked cupboard (customarily the Scheduled Poisons cupboard), thus storing the drugs under double lock and key. The CD cupboard keys must be kept on the person of the Sister, or Acting Sister or Nurse in charge of the ward, who alone may open the cupboard; thus, if a Doctor requires a CD drug for use, the Sister, or Acting Sister or Nurse concerned, will unlock the cupboard door and remain present.

4. CD drugs can be administered only on a prescription signed in full by a Doctor, but, as in the case of "Scheduled Poisons" mentioned earlier, a dose may be given on verbal instructions in emergency, with the proviso that it is written up for as soon as possible afterwards and within 24 hours.

5. The administration of each dose must be checked by a nurse of appropriate rank (this is discussed later), and such check includes the prescription sheet, the label of the container, the dose, the administration itself *and* identification of the patient.

6. Although not now legally required under the CD Regulations, it is still an excellent and safe routine to enter the administration of each dose in the Administration Record book—as was customary in the former "D.D.A." routine; this contains details of the date, patient's name, time given, dose, prescriber, names of nurses (or doctors) administering and checking, *together with balance left.* An important point is that the custom of merely deducting from the previous balance (e.g. $9-1 = 8$), and entering this, is quite wrong, the balance should be *counted* each time before entering; any shortage is then discovered promptly, and investigation (possibly a dose may not have been recorded) is made very much easier.

7. The CD cupboard (and also the "Scheduled Poisons" cupboards) is inspected by a Pharmacist, or a duly appointed

person, at regular intervals; this is usually once every three months. It is customary for the balances of the Controlled Drugs in stock to be checked at each visit against the balances recorded in the Administration Record book.

Occasionally a patient will be prescribed a special CD preparation which is not kept as stock, e.g. a mixture containing morphine and cocaine, and whilst the Pharmacist will dispense these from the prescription sheet, providing it is properly signed, etc., it is good routine to treat such medicines in the same way as CD *stocks,* i.e. for the Sister or Nurse in charge to order and record, in the CD Requisition and Administration Record books, respectively, in the usual way. This ensures complete control of the use of these potent medicines.

Should there be no Pharmacist or appropriately authorised Dispenser on the staff, as in the case of some small hospitals, the Nursing Officer may then be in charge of the stock of Controlled Drugs and Poisons, and of the issues to the wards, though fresh requirements may only be purchased on a Doctor's signed order.

District Midwives (certified and practising) are allowed to administer pethidine (and 'Pethilorfan') on their own responsibility, but can only obtain supplies of the drug on the signature of the appropriate Medical Officer. It is required that a record be kept of supplies received and of each dose administered.

As a timely and necessary point relative to Poisons and CD Regulations, it is often not clearly understood what is meant by the "Nurse in charge" or "Acting Sister in charge", and, in consequence, confusion arises as to whether, for example, a State Enrolled Nurse (S.E.N.) can administer or check a dose. The regulations themselves, and, likewise, the report of the Aitken Committee in 1958, do not lay down specifically what the terms "Nurse in charge" or "Acting Sister in charge" mean, and it must be accepted that the S.R.N. or S.E.N. qualification is not legally enforceable. Thus, a logical interpretation of the position is that whilst the theoretical ideal may be for CD drugs to be administered by a State Registered Nurse and checked by a State Registered Nurse, the need for a student/pupil nurse to be one of the team of two, as part of her training, must be borne in mind; and that, accordingly, it should suffice that either administration or checking be performed by a State Registered Nurse. Then, failing the availability of a State Registered Nurse, State Enrolled Nurses should administer and/or check. Circumstances should rarely be so extreme as to require a CD drug to be given without the presence of a person holding a nursing qualification. In many hospitals it is the excellent custom, in the absence of qualified nursing personnel, for such cover to be supplied from adjoining wards when necessary, e.g. when Controlled Drugs are concerned.

Similar problems of interpretation arise concerning the custody of the keys. Ideally, again, these should be kept on the person of a State Registered Nurse, or a State Enrolled Nurse if the latter is in charge of the ward, but this does not rule out the possibility that a duly appointed person who may not necessarily hold any qualification *can* hold the Scheduled Poisons and CD keys if she is left "in charge of the ward", always providing the Nursing Officer is satisfied she is a fit and proper person for such responsibility. In short, commonsense must prevail and reliance placed on the best possible use being made of the qualifications and personal levels of responsibility which are available on the ward, for the work of the hospital must go on.

As a final word on the position, it is emphasised that the ordering, safe custody, and correct use of Controlled Drugs and Scheduled Poisons are the personal responsibility of the Sister, or her official deputy, in charge of the Ward; the highest standard of control in these respects must never be relaxed.

# CHAPTER 25

# CALCULATIONS

The calculations which need to be performed by the nursing staff are often of a simple arithmetic order, e.g. if a dose of 500 mg is ordered and 250 mg tablets are in stock, *two* tablets are given; if 750 mg., then *three* are needed. Again, if a 2% aqueous lotion is in stock and a 1% strength is needed for use, it is obvious that the 2% strength will need to be diluted with an equal part of water. Calculations of this type can usually be done mentally, but if any doubt exists, it is always wise to perform the arithmetic on paper.

In hospitals which have a Pharmacy, the lotion dilutions, etc., are usually ready prepared or so organised as to be easy for the nursing staff to perform, but, even so, the student nurse should have a practical knowledge of calculations, not only for Examination Question purposes, but also to enable the standard of accuracy which is necessary in ward routine to be maintained at all times.

In the small hospital without a Pharmacist or Dispenser, an adequate knowledge of how to perform calculations is even more important, for the nursing staff will be more greatly self-dependent in this respect.

### Percentage

Percentage refers to the *strength* of a preparation, i.e. the proportion of the ingredient contained in it. "Per cent" means "per hundred" and is usually abbreviated to "%"; thus 1% means 1 in 100, i.e. one part in every hundred; 2% means 2 in 100; $\frac{1}{2}$% (0·5%) means $\frac{1}{2}$ in 100 (or 1 in 200). Now one millilitre of water weighs one gram, and 100 ml weighs 100 g, and if this is duly noted the following examples of percentage solutions will be grasped quite easily:—

A 5% dextrose solution contains 5 grams of dextrose in every 100 ml.

A 50% dextrose solution contains 50 grams of dextrose in every 100 ml.

"Normal Saline" (0·9%) contains 0·9 gram (i.e. 900 mg) of sodium chloride in 100 ml.

"Double-strength Saline" (1·8%) contains 1·8 grams of sodium chloride in 100 ml.

"Half-strength Saline" (0·45%) contains 0·45 gram (450 mg) of sodium chloride in 100 ml.

**Further examples:—**
Hibitane 1 in 200 contains 1 gram of Hibitane ín 200 ml

i.e. 0·5 g (500 mg) in 100 ml, or 0·5%.

and, conversely, Hibitane 0·5% = 0·5 g (500 mg) in 100 ml = 1 g in 200 ml = 1 in 200.

Hibitane 1 in 2 000 contains 1 g Hibitane in 2 000 ml

i.e. 0·1 g (100 mg) in 200 ml, or 0·05 g (50 mg) in 100 ml = 0·05%.

and, conversely, Hibitane 0·05% = 0·05 g (50 mg) in 100 ml = 0·1 g (100 mg) in 200 ml = 1·0 g in 2 000 ml = 1 in 2 000.

Note that if the active ingredient is a liquid, making it "liquid dissolved in liquid", then 1% means that 100 ml contains 1 ml of the active ingredient.

Thus:—
Savlon 1% contains 1 ml of Savlon in 100 ml.
Milton 5% contains 5 ml of Milton in 100 ml.
N.B. Milton "1 in 20" also contains 5 ml of Milton in 100 ml, because 1 in 20 = 5 in 100 = 5%.

**Examples of calculations:—**
Q.    How much dextrose in $\frac{1}{2}$ litre of 5% solution?

100 ml contains 5 g

$\frac{1}{2}$ litre, i.e. 500 ml, contains $5 \times \dfrac{500}{100} = 25$ g dextrose.

Q.    How much dextrose and sodium chloride in 1 000 ml of dextrose 4·3% with sodium chloride 0·18%?

100 ml contains 4·3 g dextrose

1 000 ml contains $4·3 \times \dfrac{1\,000}{100} = 43$ g

100 ml contains 0·18 g (180 mg) sodium chloride

1 000 ml contains $0·18 \times \dfrac{1\,000}{100} = 1·8$ g.

It will be noted that in the calculation examples so far, amounts of less than 1 gram have been expressed as decimal fractions of a gram, followed in brackets by the equivalent in milligrams, e.g.

"0·5 g (500 mg)", whereas the official preference (see page 9) is for such amounts to be in milligrams only. The decimal fraction has been deliberately included here to simplify understanding of the calculations.

## Percentage in Small Volumes

Referred to here are small ampoules, e.g. from 1 ml to 20 ml, with contents expressed in percentage, from which it may seem difficult to calculate dosage; however, it is helpful to note that:—

1% is 10 milligrams in 1 millilitre—explained as follows:—

1%, as we know, is 1 g in 100 ml
$$= 1\ 000 \text{ mg in } 100 \text{ ml}$$
$$100 \text{ mg in }\quad 10 \text{ ml}$$
and $\quad 10 \text{ mg in }\quad 1 \text{ ml.}$

**Examples:—**

Q.   How much Largactil is there in 2 ml of a 2·5% solution?

1% is 10 mg in 1 ml

$$2\cdot5\% \text{ is } 10 \times \frac{2\cdot5}{1} = 25 \text{ mg in 1 ml}$$

$$\text{or } 50 \text{ mg in 2 ml}$$

or, worked out the alternative way:—

2·5% is 2·5 g in 100 ml
$$= 2\ 500 \text{ mg in } 100 \text{ ml}$$
$$250 \text{ mg in }\quad 10 \text{ ml}$$
$$25 \text{ mg in }\quad 1 \text{ ml}$$
or $\quad 50 \text{ mg in }\quad 2 \text{ ml.}$

Q.   How much potassium chloride in 10 ml of a 15% solution?

1% is 10 mg in 1 ml
15% is 150 mg in 1 ml
$$= 1\ 500 \text{ mg in } 10 \text{ ml}$$
or 1·5 grams potassium chloride.

or, alternatively:—

15% is 15 g in 100 ml
or 1·5 g in 10 ml.

## How to dilute solutions from one strength to another

If using solutions labelled in terms of percentage, the volume of stock solution needed may be calculated as follows:—

$$\frac{\text{required \%age}}{\text{stock \%age}} \times \text{volume required}$$

**Examples:—**

Q.  How would you prepare 500 ml of 1% cetrimide from a 5% stock solution?

$$\frac{1}{5} \times 500 = 100 \text{ ml of 5\% solution;}$$

add    400 ml of water (i.e. make up to 500 ml),
= 500 ml of 1% solution.

Q.  How would you prepare 1 litre of Hibitane 0·1% in spirit from a 5% stock solution?

$$\frac{0·1}{5} \times 1\,000 = \frac{1}{50} \times 1\,000 = 20 \text{ ml of 5\% solution;}$$

add 980 ml spirit (i.e. make
up to 1 litre),
= 1 000 ml of 0·1% solution.

If using solutions with strengths expressed in terms of "parts" (e.g. 1 in 20), the amount to be taken of the stock solution is calculated

by using the formula $\dfrac{S}{R} \times N$,

where $\underline{S} = \underline{S}$tock strength (i.e. what "1" is in)

$\underline{R} = \underline{R}$equired strength (i.e. what "1" is in)

and    $\underline{N} = \underline{N}$umber of millilitres required.

Thus, to make 1 litre (1 000 ml) of Milton 1 in 80 from a 1 in 20 solution—

$$\frac{S}{R} \times N = \frac{20}{80} \times 1\,000 = \frac{1}{4} \times 1\,000 = 250$$

i.e. measure 250 ml of stock solution 1 in 20,
and make up to 1 000 ml with water.

### To prepare Solutions from "neat" or pure substances

This is simply a matter of measuring the calculated amount of the ingredient, and dissolving (or mixing, if a liquid) and making up to volume.  Thus, if 2 litres of Stericol 1 in 200 are required—

For 200 ml one needs 1 ml Stericol

for 2 000 ml one needs  $1 \times \dfrac{2\,000}{200} = 10$ ml or, to put the question another way—how would you make 2 litres of Stericol 0·5%?

In a 0·5% solution, 100 ml contains 0·5 ml Stericol,
and 2 000 ml contains 20 × 0·5 = 10 ml.

If a powder (e.g. dextrose) is concerned, the same routine applies, except that the calculated amount will be in terms of weight, not volume. Thus, to make 500 ml of dextrose 10%—

100 ml contains 10 g dextrose
500 ml contains 50 g dextrose.

## Injection Calculations

—or how to calculate a smaller (or larger) dose than is contained in an ampoule.
This is again simple arithmetic.

Q. How would you give 6 mg of morphine from an ampoule containing 10 mg in 1 ml?

10 mg in 1 ml

6 mg in $1 \times \dfrac{6}{10} = \dfrac{3}{5}$ ml (or 0·6 ml).

Q. How would you give 75 mg pethidine from an ampoule containing 100 mg in 2 ml?

100 mg in 2 ml

75 mg in $2 \times \dfrac{75}{100} = \dfrac{150}{100} = 1\frac{1}{2}$ ml (or 1·5 ml).

Q. How would you give 0·6 mg (600 micrograms) atropine, using ampoules containing 0·4 mg (400 micrograms) in 1 ml?

400 micrograms in 1 ml

600 micrograms in $1 \times \dfrac{600}{400} = 1\cdot5$ ml (i.e. using two ampoules).

Q. How would you give 15 mg of papaveretum from an ampoule containing 20 mg in 1 ml?

If there are 20 mg in 1 ml

there are 15 mg in $1 \times \dfrac{15}{20} = \frac{3}{4}$ ml (or 0·75 ml).

## Temperature

As already mentioned (p. xv) the term Celsius has now replaced Centigrade, but as the degree and the symbol (C) remain the same, this change presents no problems. Thermometers marked in the old Fahrenheit scale may just still be met on occasion, however, and the following is a useful conversion table to have on hand.

### Fahrenheit to Celsius

| | |
|---|---|
| 70°F = 21°C | 99°F = 37°C |
| 75°F = 24°C | 100°F = 38°C |
| 80°F = 27°C | 102°F = 39°C |
| 85°F = 29°C | 104°F = 40°C |
| 90°F = 32°C | 105°F = 40·5°C (accepted bath |
| 91°F = 33°C | 106°F = 41°C        temperature) |
| 93°F = 34°C | 107°F = 41·5°C |
| 95°F = 35°C | 108°F = 42°C |
| 97°F = 36°C | 109°F = 43°C |
| 98·4°F = 36·9°C (normal | 110°F = 43·3°C |
| body temperature) | |

# FACTORS WHICH MAY INFLUENCE DOSAGE

Despite the general employment of tablets and capsules, etc., in standard strengths, dosage still needs judgement, and the following are factors which may be taken into consideration by the prescriber.

*Age* is an important factor, especially in paediatrics. Several formulae have been devised to estimate how much of the normal adult dose of a drug is suitable for the various age levels, and one still quoted is Young's Rule, which is—

$$\text{Adult dose} \times \frac{\text{age of child}}{\text{age} + 12.}$$

For example, adult dose 100 mg and age of child 3 years. Then—

$$100 \times \frac{3}{15} \ (3+12) \quad = 100 \times \frac{1}{5} \quad = 20 \text{ mg}$$

Such dosage calculations obviously serve for guidance initially, and other factors, referred to later, may also need to be considered. However, awareness itself of the wide differentials between infant and adult doses can help to prevent serious errors—such as have occurred in the case of digoxin, for example.

Age considerations also apply at the other end of the scale, i.e. *in the case of the elderly*, when, for example, deteriorating kidney function may lead to raised blood levels of drugs which possess severe side-effects, as with certain antibiotics where ototoxicity (p. 138) is a problem; dosage is then carefully assessed.

*Weight* can be a factor in two directions. Thus, if the patient is grossly overweight, dosage may need to be higher than normal. Secondly, dosage of certain potent drugs is actually based on the weight of the patient, e.g. that of gentamicin is 2 mg per kg bodyweight for children up to 12 years.

*Surface Area* is the deciding factor in the dosage of certain potent drugs, e.g. the cytotoxic, doxorubicin. Here, the height and weight of the patient are ascertained, and the body surface area of the patient estimated in terms of square metres by means of a nomogram—as described on page 10; dosage of the drug being based on a specified amount "per square metre".

*Severity of the patient's condition* is obviously an important factor, and common examples are the variation in dosage from patient to patient of insulin, and warfarin, in diabetes mellitus and long-term anticoagulant therapy, respectively.

*Route of administration* may frequently govern the amount of a drug to be given. Thus, if by injection, the more certain absorption may normally indicate a smaller dose than if given by mouth; and if per rectum, where full absorption is less certain, the dose is normally higher than if by the oral route. Again, the implantation route (p. 201) normally implies a large dose, for the tablet concerned may need to continue effective by slow-release over many months.

*Tolerance* to the effect of a drug indicates the possibility of increased dosage need. Thus, children tolerate belladonna and atropine better, and hence accept higher doses, weight for weight, than do adults; this is an example of *natural* tolerance. Tolerance may be *acquired* as in the case of drug addicts and in terminal disease, where ever-increasing doses of narcotic drugs may be needed.

*Intolerance* to the effect of a drug may also be termed *sensitivity*, and the need for caution in dosage of the narcotic drugs (morphine, etc.) in the case of children, who are very sensitive to them, is a typical example. An extreme level of sensitivity may be described as an *idiosyncrasy*, where an unusually severe reaction may contra-indicate any further use of the drug concerned; penicillin sensitivity (p. 137) is a case in point.

*Toxicity* indicates caution re dosage levels, thus certain antibiotics, e.g. gentamicin and streptomycin, can cause ototoxicity (p. 138) if given too freely.

*Cumulative effect* indicates that a drug may not be "used up" at the same rate as it is being given. Thus, accumulation of digoxin may lead to the typical side-effects (p. 51), and possibility of overdosage is kept routinely in mind by both doctor and observant nurse. Poor or reduced kidney function may also induce cumulative effect, as mentioned earlier.

*Absorption or non-absorption*—most drugs taken by mouth are absorbed from the gastro-intestinal tract and thus act *systemically*, others are not absorbed and are intentionally prescribed for their effect within the bowel. Thus, average dosage of the systemic sulphonamide, sulphadimidine (p. 128), is a total of 4 grams daily, whereas the bowel sulphonamide, succinylsulphathiazole, is not absorbed and 12–15 grams may be given daily. Obviously, the safety factor of non-absorption allows of a far higher dosage regime.

*Speed of absorption* may also affect dosage levels. For example, the traditional sublingual tablets of trinitrin (p. 52) contain 0·5 mg and give immediate but brief effect in angina, whereas the commercial tablet "Sustac" (p. 52) contains up to 6·4 mg, the drug being slowly released along the intestinal tract over a period of several hours.

*Combination treatment* may indicate reduction of dosage of one or more of the drugs employed; this has been referred to in the case of the anticonvulsants (p. 96) and the hypotensives (p. 58).

These, then, are general factors which may have a bearing on drug dosage levels, and appreciation of the points made will not be unrewarding to the nurse concerned with drug administration.

# AN OUTLINE OF THE PRINCIPLES OF THE EMERGENCY TREATMENT OF POISONING

The initial measures taken when a case of poisoning is discovered may be life-saving. The following are situations that may present themselves, together with the relevant guide-lines and broadly in order of priority—this may, of necessity, be modified by circumstances prevailing.

## Respiration

The automatic first reaction should be to ascertain that respiration is proceeding satisfactorily, and that there is a clear airway. Breathing may be weak and critically shallow (e.g. if a barbiturate has been taken), or may even be imperceptible, and its prompt restoration to adequate strength is vital; this can be achieved by the mouth-to-mouth technique or artificial respiration.

## Identifying the poison: summoning help

The label on the container (or gas may be the involvement) should enable quick identification, and this information should be included in the message got through speedily to the appropriate or handiest authority, as, for example, doctor, hospital, or ambulance depot as the case may be.

## Presence of Poison in Stomach

In the case of poisons such as aspirin (which stays in the stomach for several hours), it may be decided to attempt emptying the stomach and so avoid danger of further absorption; similarly in the case of iron tablets or berries, when frightened children may sound the alarm in time. Hence, depending on degree of alertness of patient,

(a) a finger may be used to tickle the back of the throat; or
(b) an emetic may be given, e.g. salt, a tablespoonful dissolved in a glass of warm water, or mustard, the same amount, first made into a cream with a little water before filling the glass.

One of these two is normally to hand in the home, though it

should be borne in mind that *too lavish* a use of salt as an emetic solution can promote the absorption of toxic levels of sodium; serious results have occurred following highly excessive administration.

*Note* that in the case of patients in stupor or hysterical, an emetic carries the danger of vomit being aspirated into the lungs; this is particularly serious if petrol or paraffin has been swallowed. Secondly, that if the poison taken is a strong acid (e.g. spirits of salts), a strong alkali (e.g. strong ammonia solution), or other corrosive substance (e.g. Lysol), emetics should *not* be used except under medical decision, for an already damaged stomach may well perforate under strain of vomiting.

If unconscious, the patient is best in a semi-prone position (on side), so that saliva or vomit will then run out of the mouth and not be aspirated back into the lungs.

Keep all vomit, etc., for later examination.

## Shock

This is typified by pallor, cold skin, weak rapid pulse, shallow breathing and "pinched" features, and is due to insufficient force of circulating blood flow. Helpful measures are—

(a) Lay the patient flat, with head lower than trunk, and limbs well raised to an upward slope.

(b) Maintain normal body temperature—using blankets if necessary.

*Note* that in the case of gas poisoning, removal of patient to fresh air is important.

It is again stressed that the foregoing are broad initial principles only and that specific treatment may also be necessary, as determined by individual circumstances.

It is useful to know that Poisons Centres exist (e.g. at Guy's Hospital) which can be telephoned for specific advice (24 hour service) if an uncommon substance has been swallowed—as may be met in the case of admissions to Casualty Departments. The telephone number of the appropriate Centre is invariably and prominently available in such Departments.

# INDEX

N.B. Where two or more page numbers are given as references, and one is in **bold type**, this is intended to be the principal reference.